W9-CZY-977

The Missing Pieces
of the Fibromyalgia Puzzle

Exposing The Fallacy of Pain From Nowhere
Revealing The Failure of The Fibromyalgia Diagnosis
Elucidating The True Cause of Fibromyalgia Pain
Real Treatment for What's Really Going On

by

Jeff Sarkozi, M.D.

F.R.C.P.C., F.A.C.R.

Copyright © 2009 Jeff Sarkozi

No part of this publication may be reproduced, stored in a retrieval system, or transmitted in any form or by any means, electronic, mechanical, photocopying, recording or otherwise, without the prior permission of the publisher. Permissions may be sought directly through the publisher as noted below.

Permissions and Licensing:

Sagecoast Publishing
801 North Tustin Avenue
Suite 503
Santa Ana, California 92705

Phone: (714) 973-0106
Fax: (714) 973-0129
Email: permissions@missingpiecesfibromyalgia.com

Designed by Teresa Trujillo
Book Workshop, Inc., Fullerton, CA

This publication is designed to provide complete, accurate, and authoritative information with respect to the material presented. The author has taken great care to confirm the accuracy of the information presented and to describe generally accepted, evidence based practices. However, the author assumes no liability and is not responsible for errors, omissions, loss, damage, or any consequences from the information or application of the information presented in this book and makes no warranty, express or implied, with respect to the contents of this publication. Furthermore, the author is not engaged in rendering professional advice or services to the reader.

The author has exerted every effort to ensure that product recognition, drug identification, treatment routines, or drug dosages set forth in this book are in accordance with current treatment recommendations and practice at the time of publication. Medicine, however, is an ever changing science and in view of evolving new information related to treatment modalities including drug therapy, ongoing research, as well as changes in government regulations, the reader is urged to consult with a treating physician regarding the introduction and maintenance of treatment modalities including medications. The reader is advised to check the most current product information provided by the manufacturer of each drug under consideration for use to verify the recommended dose, method and duration of use, warnings, precautions, and contraindications.

The concepts, procedures, treatment suggestions, and medication suggestions described in this book are not intended as a substitute for the medical advice of physicians. The reader is advised to regularly consult a physician in health related matters and particularly in regard to symptoms that may require investigation, diagnosis, treatment, or other medical attention.

All product brand names mentioned in this book are registered trademarks of their respective owners.

Acknowledgements

I am honored and privileged by the many influences in my life that have allowed this book to take form and evolve. I want to thank my parents, George and Etel Sarkozi for instilling in me, through their example of survival against all odds, the immense power of courage combined with determination. I want to thank my wife, Marla, for the love and happiness that inspires me to reach higher, dig deeper, and grow further. I want to thank my children, Tara, Jason, Aaron, and Ashley, for always asking questions, for having the wisdom to listen to the answers, and most importantly, for then asking better questions. To my mentor, Hugh Smythe, thank you for your insights. Finally, I wish to thank all my patients for allowing me the confidence and trust to share in their lives, and for giving me the gift of allowing me to help them to heal.

Contents

Chapter 8—Step 2: Why Biomechanics and Posture Affect Pain and How to Optimize Them 169

Chapter 9—Step 3: The Real Facts About Weight Management, Pain, and What To Do 211

Chapter 10— Step 4: Ergonomics: Understanding How Pain Interacts With The World At Large and What To Do About It 239

Chapter 11—Step 5: How Sleep Disturbances Adversely Affect Pain and Effectively Managing Them to Reduce the Hurt 255

Chapter 13—Step 7: Sex Reduces Pain: Approaches to Bring Pleasure Back Into Your Life 339

Part One

The Dead End That Is Fibromyalgia

Chapter 1

Pain From Nowhere: Fibromyalgia is A Failure of Medical Science

"Be careful what you wish for." —Anon

Pain from nowhere. This is what doctors expect individuals with fibromyalgia and many other forms of chronic widespread pain to believe. Why? Because doctors and other healthcare providers believe it as well. As bizarre as it sounds, the health care system in 2008 actually accepts as reasonable the notion that over six million Americans diagnosed with fibromyalgia have pain that apparently nobody knows the cause of or how it even develops. This, despite the fact that the concept of fibromyalgia consisting of muscular rheumatism and tender points has been noted as far back as 1816. This, despite the fact that fibromyalgia is one of the most prevalent rheumatic diseases encountered. This, despite the fact that research into fibromyalgia over the past two hundred years has identified many physiologic abnormalities in fibromyalgia, yet not one has been shown to cause fibromyalgia or even occur consistently in all patients.

We Know Much Less About Fibromyalgia Than We Think We Do

Chronic Widespread Pain and Fibromyalgia Are Common

Chronic generalized or widespread musculoskeletal pain is common in the general population. It has been noted to be present in about 10-20% of the population in developed countries and in up to 36.2% in developing countries. Studies using the definition of widespread pain as described in the 1990 American College of Rheumatology (ACR) criteria for the classification of fibromyalgia identify the presence chronic widespread pain in about 10-11% of the population. When the subjects with chronic widespread pain were further examined for tender fibromyalgia points, about 1 out of 5 individuals had 11 or more tender points consistent with fibromyalgia. Significantly, the tenderness had little relationship to the pain itself and was better correlated with depression, fatigue, and poor sleep. So, where did the pain come from and what did it correlate with? This has never yet been answered.

By using the ACR criteria of widespread musculoskeletal pain and painful tenderness in at least 11/18 fibromyalgia points to diagnose the presence of fibromyalgia, the overall prevalence of fibromyalgia in the United States is estimated to be about 2% and ranging from 0.7% - 7.3% in the Western world at large. Clearly, widespread pain and tenderness are common musculoskeletal complaints. Indeed, fibromyalgia is considered to be one of the top three most common diagnoses amongst rheumatology patients. It is identified in even higher prevalence amongst hospitalized patients.

The mean patient age at the time of diagnosis is in the forties to fifties range and the predominant age at the time of diagnosis is in the fifties. The prevalence of fibromyalgia notably increases with age reaching nearly 8% by 70-80 years of age. The clinical features of fibromyalgia have been reported to occur in children as well.

Fibromyalgia occurs much more commonly in females with a female to male ratio of about 8-9:1.

While fibromyalgia is identified as a condition unto itself, many other disease states, predominantly rheumatologic conditions, have been associated with the presence of fibromyalgia. Fibromyalgia has been reported to occur in about 18-44% of patients with other rheumatologic conditions. It has been reported to occur in patients with rheumatoid arthritis, Sjogren's syndrome, and systemic lupus erythematosus. It has also been reported to occur in association with hypermobility syndromes, localized osteoarthritis, neck and back pain, hepatitis C infection, Lyme disease, parvovirus B19 infection, and HIV infection. Nobody has yet explained how the exact same symptoms and findings of fibromyalgia could occur independently and in concert with a wide variety of diverse known diseases.

The Cause, Mechanism, and Relationship of Fibromyalgia Symptoms Are Unknown

The core and cardinal symptom of fibromyalgia is the subjective reporting of chronic, widespread pain. Patients generally report widespread, generalized pain in the soft tissues, especially in muscle areas. They often report that they have "pain all over". Often, not all sites of pain have the same degree of pain and frequently there are one or several pre-eminent regions with more severe symptoms. The pain can be variable in intensity and the severity can shift amongst different regions. Pain can vary over the course of a day as well as over days and weeks. Patients report factors that modulate their symptoms to include physical exertion, infection, injuries, sleep disruption, weather changes, and psychological stressors. The pain quality is subjectively reported by patients to vary from soreness or aching to burning, gnawing, radiating, and even "screaming". The intensity of subjectively reported pain is greater than reported in rheumatoid arthritis. However, despite its pre-eminence, no study to date has identified the nature, source, or cause of the pain in patients with fibromyalgia.

Stiffness is subjectively reported along with the pain frequently. The stiffness is usually worse in the morning, especially on wakening, and improves in the middle of the day. It may worsen later in the day. The nature or cause of stiffness in fibromyalgia also remains unknown.

Another prominent manifestation of fibromyalgia is fatigue. It is noted especially in the morning and can persist throughout the day. Physical exertion, mental exertion, and psychological factors aggravate the fatigue. The cause of the fatigue has not been identified to date, however, multiple factors adversely affecting fatigue have been identified. These include disrupted sleep, deconditioning, depression, psychological distress, and neuroendocrine dysfunction with abnormalities of the hypothalamic-pituitary-adrenal axis and reduced growth hormone. As a seeming contradiction, both activity and inactivity promote the fatigue in fibromyalgia. As with pain and stiffness, it is important to take note that fatigue is also a subjective symptom with no hard objective correlate.

Sleep disruption is a significantly prominent and frequent feature of fibromyalgia. The characteristic feature of this sleep disruption is the feeling of being unrefreshed on wakening in the morning with feeling tired on wakening. This may be noted even if the individual reports sleeping through the night. Patients often report feeling as if they do not sleep well and they report having a poor quality sleep. Patients describe light sleep and being easily aroused from sleep by pain, noises, or thoughts. Wakening from sleep may occur multiple times nightly. The presence of a poor quality sleep is noted to cause worsening of the fibromyalgia symptoms. It is also associated with cognitive impairment, fatigue, and negative mood. Polysomnography, a procedure that studies brain wave electrical activity when sleeping, shows that many, but not all, patients have electroencephalogram (EEG) brain wave patterns showing a wakening alpha wave pattern intrusion on the stage 3 and 4 Non-Rapid Eye Movement (NREM) deep sleep delta wave pattern. This finding, however, is neither diagnostic of fibromyalgia, as it is not seen in all patients with fibromyalgia, nor is it specific to fibromyalgia, being seen in other conditions as well. However, it is of significant note that the experimental disruption of slow wave, stage 3 and 4 NREM sleep in healthy, normal individuals produces muscle aching, stiffness, and increased tenderness. The cause and significance of the sleep disturbances in fibromyalgia is unknown.

Cognitive impairment is also subjectively reported by many fibromyalgia patients. Patients describe difficulty with short term memory, concentration, and logical thinking. Deficits have been noted in working memory, episodic memory, and verbal fluency. The problems with impaired memory and impaired concentration have been related to the severity of the pain, mental fatigue, and psychological distress. However, it is not known how or why cognitive deficits occur.

Psychological distress is another common and significant feature of fibromyalgia. Clearly, there is a higher prevalence of psychological symptoms in those with fibromyalgia compared to controls. Patients with fibromyalgia have a greater number of lifetime psychiatric diagnoses compared to controls, especially mood disorders such as depression and anxiety disorders. The psychiatric symptoms correlate with health-care seeking behavior, the perceived severity of the symptoms of pain and fatigue, and perceptions of environmental stress. Fibromyalgia patients are reported to have major depression in 20-30% and anxiety disorder in 10-20% at the time of assessment. A prior diagnosis of psychiatric disorder is identified in 90% of patients diagnosed with fibromyalgia. A lifetime diagnosis of major depression is noted in 68%-86% of fibromyalgia patients. Furthermore, psychiatric disorders including depression, anxiety, stress disorders like posttraumatic stress disorder, and sexual and physical abuse are identified in 75% of dysfunctional fibromyalgia patients. Somatization, the expression of physical complaints not fully explained by a medical or psychiatric disorder or the direct effects of a substance is noted in 14-23% of patients with fibromyalgia. In chronic musculoskeletal disease, psychological status is a major determinant of health status along with physical functioning and the pain itself. It is clear that anxiety, stress, and depression significantly affect the appreciation of pain and its presentation in fibromyalgia, but does not cause pain in and of itself.

It should be noted that the diagnostic criteria for major depressive episode as well as generalized anxiety disorder includes features of sleep disruption, fatigue, and psychomotor changes as seen in Chapter 12, Tables 12.1 and 12.2. Thus, depression and anxiety from any cause independent of fibromyalgia can independently produce a significant overlap in the clinical features of fibromyalgia. Importantly, the presence of a diagnosis of fibromyalgia does not exclude depression and anxiety as independent conditions even when fibromyalgia directly contributes to the depression and anxiety. This has not been explored in fibromyalgia.

Other symptoms reported by individuals with fibromyalgia include headaches; restless legs syndrome; irritable bowel syndrome; irritable bladder or female urethral syndrome; cold sensitivity along with cold hands and feet; sensitivity to chemicals, weather, medications, loud noises, and bright lights; dry eyes and mouth; dizziness; paresthesias and dysesthesias (needles, pins, numbness, tingling or unusual skin sensations) without obvious neurologic abnormality; skin photosensitivity; skin rashes; and mouth ulcers. How these develop and relate to other fibromyalgia symptoms such as widespread pain is unknown.

Despite Widespread Pain, the Only Physical Examination Finding Identified is Widespread Soft Tissue Tenderness

In patients with fibromyalgia, the physical examination is reported to be virtually unremarkable with no significant findings on general examination as well as on specific neurological and musculoskeletal examination with regard to the fibromyalgia itself. The only finding specific to fibromyalgia is widespread soft tissue tenderness. This tenderness has been qualified and quantified by the ACR criteria for the classification for fibromyalgia to include the 9 paired fibromyalgia tender points as noted in Chapter 3, Table 3.1 and Figure 3.1. The painful tender points are clinically identified by applying pressure with the thumb or first 2 or 3 fingers to produce a pressure of approximately 4 kilograms or less. The subjective patient response to the pressure is noted. The presence of at least 11/18 painfully tender fibromyalgia points fulfills the second ACR classification criterion for fibromyalgia. Clearly, the examination for soft tissue tenderness identifies increased sensitivity to a painful stimulus compared to normal individuals. This is known as hyperalgesia. In some patients, even a light touch, which would not be considered a painful stimulus by normal individuals, may be perceived as painful by patients with fibromyalgia. This phenomenon is known as allodynia. There has been no correlation identified between the severity of the subjective complaints of widespread pain and the degree of tenderness elicited.

There may also be findings of occasional deep muscle nodules or knots known as myofascial trigger points as seen in myofascial pain syndromes. Trigger points are regional in location and are not widespread and generalized. They are not the same as fibromyalgia tender points. Skin and soft tissue sensitivity with skin roll tenderness of the upper back and reactive hyperemia or dermatographism producing exaggerated redness with rolling the skin between the thumb and other fingers is often noted.

The bulk of the physical examination and remainder of the history is devoted to assessing for the presence of diseases associated with fibromyalgia including rheumatologic diseases such as rheumatoid arthritis, systemic lupus erythematosus, Sjogren's syndrome, and infectious diseases such as hepatitis C, parvovirus B19, HIV, Lyme disease as well as fibromyalgia-like diseases that are not fibromyalgia. Fibromyalgia-like diseases that are not fibromyalgia include rheumatologic diseases such as rheumatoid arthritis, systemic lupus erythematosus, Sjogren's syndrome, ankylosing spondylitis, polymyalgia rheumatica, polymyositis; neurologic diseases; chronic active infectious diseases; hormonal disorders such as hypothyroidism or disorders of bone metabolism; metabolic disorders such as diabetes mellitus; malignancies; vascular diseases; and psychiatric abnormalities such as malingering, hypochondriasis, or conversion disorder.

Pain and Tender Points Are Two Different Things

A common feature of fibromyalgia is the presence of painful tender fibromyalgia points. However, they do not correlate well with widespread pain and can be found in patients independent of the presence of widespread pain. More significantly, the presence of tender points correlates strongly with psychological and generalized distress independent of the pain status of the individual as well as sleep difficulties, fatigue, and depression. Clearly pain and tenderness are two different things. Doctors simply ignore this.

Laboratory Investigations Tell Us Nothing About Fibromyalgia

Laboratory investigations are unrevealing with regard to fibromyalgia itself. There are no identified laboratory abnormalities that help diagnose, treat, or define prognosis in fibromyalgia. The same holds true for other studies including radiological studies, neurodiagnostic studies, sleep studies, or biopsies in the clinical setting. The role of laboratory investigation in fibromyalgia is to assess for the presence of other conditions that co-exist with fibromyalgia or conditions producing fibromyalgia-like syndromes as above.

It makes no plausible biological sense that a chronic, painful disease process does not cause a single lab test abnormality that links all the patients together. Yet, doctors readily accept the notion that the pain comes from nowhere. Therefore, it is acceptable that there be no objective measures of the pain.

The Trigger for Fibromyalgia Is Unknown

Fibromyalgia is characterized as a medically unexplained disease. The cause of the pain and other symptoms is not known. Many patients cannot identify any particular event that precipitated the onset symptoms. Of the patients that do identify a factor associated with the onset of the fibromyalgia symptoms, the commonest are: flu-like viral type illnesses; onset after successful treatment of active Lyme disease; associated with viral infections related to parvovirus B19, infectious mononucleosis, and hepatitis C; physical trauma and surgery; emotional stress; and medication related. However, these are retrospective, subjective associations. The recall of, or actual occurrence of, events preceding the onset of fibromyalgia symptoms does not mean that there is a causal relationship by the preceding events and the development of fibromyalgia. There is no evidence in the medical literature that identifies any common link between the highly disparate processes that have been reported with the onset of fibromyalgia symptoms. There is no biologically plausible explanation as to how these factors could possibly contribute to the cause of fibromyalgia pain and symptoms, especially given the cause of fibromyalgia is unknown.

The Mechanism of How Fibromyalgia Develops Is Unknown

A genetic predisposition to the pain and tenderness of fibromyalgia has been reported in familial studies. Amongst individuals with pain, the family history correlates with increased pain complaints. Family studies in patients diagnosed with fibromyalgia show that first-degree female relatives of patients with fibromyalgia have findings consistent with fibromyalgia with evidence of increased tenderness and lower pain thresholds. Sex differences in pain sensitivity are also reported with evidence showing that women have more tenderness and lower pain thresholds compared to men with fibromyalgia. While a genetic predisposition to the tenderness of fibromyalgia appears to exist, it does not explain the cause or mechanism of disease of fibromyalgia.

Given the widespread nature of the soft tissue pain and tenderness noted in patients with fibromyalgia, much work has gone into identifying a muscle abnormality to explain these. The bulk of the evidence supports the conclusion that the abnormalities of muscle found in patients with fibromyalgia are the result of inactivity and pain, and are not primarily due to an intrinsic problem related to the muscles themselves.

Multiple neuroendocrine abnormalities have been documented in patients with fibromyalgia. There is no evidence that these findings cause fibromyalgia.

Women with fibromyalgia have been shown to have increased heart rate variability compared to normal, healthy females. Abnormal heart rate responses to being upright for prolonged periods have been documented. There is no evidence that these changes cause fibromyalgia.

The Diagnosis of Fibromyalgia Has Become Superficial, Expedient, and Filled With Complacency

The diagnosis of fibromyalgia, ideally, has always been a clinical diagnosis based upon the constellation of features derived from the patient history and physical examination looking for clinical features identified to be associated with fibromyalgia as well as disease processes producing a fibromyalgia-like syndrome in concert with laboratory testing limited to looking for other disease processes producing a fibromyalgia-like syndrome. The current concept of fibromyalgia is one of a subjective disease based on purely subjective characteristics of unexplained pain and tenderness. It is important to recognize that tenderness itself is subjective as it is a subjective response to pain stimulated by someone else looking for a pain response. Neither widespread pain of origin undefined and unknown nor tender points are, in and of themselves, diagnostic of fibromyalgia and are seen in many patients who do not have fibromyalgia. Adding to the problematic nature of fibromyalgia, as we currently know it, is that no clear characteristic risk factors to developing fibromyalgia have been identified. Further, the natural history of fibromyalgia is a highly variable and inconsistent process, although over long periods of time almost all patients do not enjoy improvement and many worsen. Finally, there is no specific or consistent response to treatment interventions.

Due to the highly variable and inconsistent clinical picture of presented by patients diagnosed with fibromyalgia, the ACR undertook a multicenter study to "provide a consensus definition of fibromyalgia" and to "establish new criteria for the classification of fibromyalgia" (Wolfe et al., 1990). The results of this watershed study were published in 1990 and became the basis of the ACR Classification Criteria for Fibromyalgia as described in Chapter 3, Table 3.1. It must be noted that it was not the intention of the study to develop diagnostic criteria. The ACR criteria were never intended to be diagnostic criteria. They were simply classification criteria for the purpose of research studies to hopefully stratify patients with a common set of symptoms and findings. Over time, however, the ACR criteria have been erroneously converted and misused as diagnostic criteria for fibromyalgia.

This has led to the over-simplistic reduction of the assessment of a patient with complaints of widespread musculoskeletal pain. In essence, no matter the character, distribution, duration, and factors influencing the pain, all pain symptoms are lumped into the category of widespread pain. Once the physical examination identifies widespread tenderness and normal joint ranges, all pain findings are attributed to the tenderness regardless of their nature and distribution. Once the combination of widespread pain and tenderness are found, the ACR criteria are blindly invoked to make a diagnosis of fibromyalgia. Once a diagnosis of fibromyalgia is made, all other and subsequent complaints and findings that cannot be otherwise explained are attributed to fibromyalgia. Forever.

However, in reality, there are no such things as diagnostic criteria for fibromyalgia including the ACR criteria. While widespread pain and tenderness are cardinal features of fibromyalgia, they fail to diagnose, explain, or even identify whatever fibromyalgia truly is. Indeed, it defies logic and common sense that a two criterion classification composed of one nonspecific, common symptom characterized by the presence of widespread pain the origin of which is unknown and one non-specific finding of least 11/18 painful tender points could possibly define a uniform and homogeneous rheumatologic disease. To put this in context, well described rheumatologic conditions such as rheumatoid arthritis and systemic lupus erythematosus also have classification criteria that are used for purposes of research. The criteria for the classification of rheumatoid arthritis comprises 7 criterion elements of which at least 4 have to be satisfied. The criteria for the classification of systemic lupus erythematosus are even more complex comprising 11 criterion elements many of which have subelements and at least 4 criterion elements must be satisfied to be so classified. Despite their detail and complexity, the classification criteria for rheumatoid arthritis and systemic lupus erythematosus are also not diagnostic criteria. They, too, were developed for purposes of research studies to attempt to stratify patients with a common set of symptoms and findings. Even these more complex criteria are not validated to make a diagnosis of their respective diseases when relied upon solely to make that diagnosis.

Unfortunately, the realities of modern health care severely constrict the duration of office visits. In particular, patients with chronic medical problems, especially those that are insufficiently or inadequately treated, and specifically patients with diseases in which the cause of the symptoms is unknown such as individuals with a diagnosis of fibromyalgia, do not get the type of quality assessment their symptoms warrant and deserve. To the contrary, doctors and other healthcare providers make every effort to limit and control the duration of office visits to one or a few issues and never get to review or understand the true nature of the many and complex complaints of individuals with fibromyalgia. This is further promoted by the fact that absent a known cause for the symptoms, absent any specific or effective treatment based on an identified cause, absent organ or life threatening complications, and absent a significant impact on disease outcome or healthcare utilization, treatment is nonspecific and patients are advised to develop "acceptance" and to "learn to live with it". In essence, why not give patients a quick and easy diagnosis, rather than spending a great deal of time explaining nothing much is known about what they have, especially if it doesn't make much difference? Unfortunately, whether patients get better, worse, remain unchanged, indeed, no matter what happens, once patients are labeled with the diagnosis of fibromyalgia, everything that happens in their lives that can't be explained otherwise is attributed to fibromyalgia. Thus, patients accumulate an ever growing list of symptoms that can't be explained and are attributed to a single diagnosis that itself can't be explained or satisfactorily treated.

Fibromyalgia is Controversial

There exists significant controversy in the medical community as to whether fibromyalgia is indeed a discrete and distinct entity. There are those who feel: fibromyalgia is nothing more than an accumulation of common symptoms; and/or the complaints are magnified by psychological problems; and/or fibromyalgia is a garbage bin diagnosis to collect symptoms that have no explanation. Others feel there is value in the fibromyalgia diagnosis to establish validation to patients that their symptoms are real, to provide reassurance that they are not alone, and that treatment directed at getting them to "learn to live with it" is available. Neither view is appropriate. There is no doubt that the symptoms and tenderness in fibromyalgia are real. The real unanswered issues are what causes them and how do they occur.

The Diagnosis of Fibromyalgia Is Not a Means To An End, It Is The End

Invariably, patients who have been diagnosed as having fibromyalgia are initially grateful to receive the diagnosis. Rather than being told that their symptoms are all in their head, they are thrilled and relieved that there is a diagnostic label for their condition. In time, however, such gratitude wanes as the hope and promise of the diagnosis fails to materialize in substantial improvement. Frustration follows at the lack of significant improvement, or worse, ongoing progressive symptoms. Eventually, such frustration leads to resignation about the inability to impact the disease process. In some, such resignation leads to hopelessness and fear. In all, the initial optimism is shattered by an insidious and creeping pessimism regarding the utility of the diagnosis of fibromyalgia. While there are many things in medicine that are worse to have than fibromyalgia, it is clear that there is nothing gratifying or relieving in receiving such a diagnosis. Indeed, who would want a disease or a diagnosis of a disease that has been described for almost two hundred years, that correlates with widespread pain and causes widespread tenderness, is associated with a significantly disrupted sleep pattern, has no identified known cause, has no known treatment, is chronic, and will persist for the rest of one's life? The diagnosis of fibromyalgia is not a means to an end. In the current state of affairs, sadly, it is the end.

Fibromyalgia: The Need for Substance Over Style

Fibromyalgia is not a fatal disease or syndrome. It does not shorten one's life. Yet, it just feels that way to many patients. The current lack of knowledge or understanding as to the cause, mechanism, or treatment of fibromyalgia has a significant impact on the fibromyalgia patient's quality of life. The increased demand over life devoted to dealing with this essentially unknown syndrome takes more time from life's normal activities than it should simply because so little is known about the cause, mechanism and treatment of fibromyalgia. Thus, there is a clear and overwhelming need for a breakthrough in the understanding of just what fibromyalgia really is and how to effectively treat it. Patients and doctors are in dire need of something new, different and more effective than the current thinking and treatment related to fibromyalgia.

Chapter 2

Three Things We Know About Fibromyalgia

"The good news is you have fibromyalgia. The bad news is that you have fibromyalgia."—Jeff Sarkozi, M.D.

Fibromyalgia stands alone amongst disease entities in the vacuum of knowledge that surrounds it. When AIDS was first reported in the early 1980s, it was only several years later that its cause was identified. Similarly, within several years of its first reporting, the cause of Lyme disease was identified and effective treatment protocols were developed. Yet, despite being the second most prevalent rheumatologic disease, there has been relatively little research undertaken to understand fibromyalgia. Furthermore, the research that has been done has failed to elucidate a direction, let alone an answer, as to how and where fibromyalgia pain arises. While the work into fibromyalgia has raised many more questions than answers, three things have become very clear.

First, Fibromyalgia is Associated With Disordered Pain Processing

Patients With Fibromyalgia Process Pain Sensations Differently

Patients with fibromyalgia have widespread, and even generalized, tenderness in response to pressure stimulation of soft tissues such as when examining for tender points. The evidence in the medical literature is strongly supportive of abnormal processing of pain information in the central nervous system to physically induced pain such as pressure, heat, cold, or electrical stimulation resulting from generalized lowered pain thresholds in fibromyalgia. Importantly, these studies have all used an extrinsic stimulus to trigger or provoke a pain response. However, there has been no convincing or consistent evidence of an intrinsic repetitive or ongoing painful stimulus occurring in fibromyalgia and no intrinsic trigger that produces pain in fibromyalgia has yet been identified.

Neurotransmitter abnormalities have been identified in patients with fibromyalgia. These include low serum levels of serotonin, low central nervous system levels of a serotonin metabolite, and elevated central nervous system levels of the neurotransmitter substance P. These findings are consistent with abnormalities in the processing of pain information, but do not identify where such pain arises.

Enhanced response to evoked pain by laser stimulation of the skin has been reported in fibromyalgia patients as demonstrated by measuring brain electrical activity through somatosensory evoked potentials.

In response to painful electrical stimulation or painful injection of hypertonic saline into a non-painful muscle of patients with fibromyalgia, patients were noted to have lower pain thresholds to the external stimulation of pain and it was further noted that the induced pain was sensed to extend beyond the stimulated area in a process known as referred pain. The induced pain was noted to persist longer after the stimulation stopped compared to normal individuals. The referred pain and prolonged persistence of pain following a painful stimulus relates to a process of pain amplification.

Functional abnormalities or differences have been identified on brain imaging studies in patients with fibromyalgia compared to normal individuals as identified by single photon emission computed tomography (SPECT) studies. Such findings, however are not specific to fibromyalgia and are seen in other painful conditions such as neuropathic pain, metastatic cancer pain, and spinal cord injury. In these non-fibromyalgia pain situations, such changes are related to the presence of an identified source or cause of pain, contrary to fibromyalgia in which no source or cause of pain has been identified. When exposed to a painful stimulus, patients with fibromyalgia show abnormalities or changes in SPECT scanning studies and functional MRI studies but normal controls also show similar responses if the stimulation was severe enough to produce pain. The fibromyalgia patients, however, demonstrated changes at a lower intensity of stimulation than did normal individuals indicating increased sensitivity to that stimulation.

Patients with fibromyalgia also demonstrate temporal summation of pain. In response to repeated thermal stimulation or pressure in fibromyalgia patients, the pain intensity to any one stimulation is greater than the response to the preceding stimulus. In other words, the second painful stimulus hurts more than the first one, the third painful stimulus hurts more than the second one, and so on. This process is also known as wind-up.

In addition, fibromyalgia patients display impairment in diffuse noxious inhibitory control, a central nervous system pathway that normally suppresses the severity of a painful stimulus through the application of of a painful or non-painful stimulus locally or to another site. This is the mechanism through which pain is reduced in situations such as when you stub your toe and then grab it and squeeze it to make it feel better, when you hit your thumb with a hammer and squeeze it, when you bite your lip or dig your nails into your skin in the face of pain, or when you feel better after counter-irritation treatments like massage, cupping, and acupuncture.

Patients With Fibromyalgia Feel Pain More Readily and With Greater Sensitivity

Clearly, the evidence is strongly supportive of an abnormality in the central nervous system pain processing known as central nervous system sensitization or central sensitization for short. Basically, patients with fibromyalgia or fibromyalgia-like syndromes feel a painful stimulus more readily and with a much higher sensitivity to the threshold of pain than individuals who do not have fibromyalgia. In other words, they have a lower pain threshold and are more tender to a painful stimulus. Figure 2.1 depicts a low level painful stimulus, identified by the circle, that is below the pain threshold of individuals classified as having fibromyalgia and normal individuals classified as not having fibromyalgia. In this circumstance, despite the low level pain stimulus, it does not exceed the pain threshold of individuals classified as having fibromyalgia nor the pain threshold of normal individuals and pain is not sensed as painful by either group.

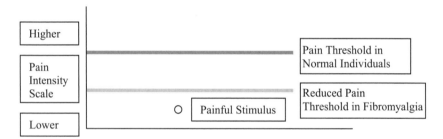

Figure 2.1: Pain stimulus below threshold of fibromyalgia and normal individuals. No pain sensed in fibromyalgia or normal individuals.

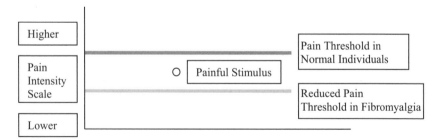

Figure 2.2: Pain stimulus above threshold of fibromyalgia but below threshold of normal individuals. Pain sensed in fibromyalgia but not normal individuals.

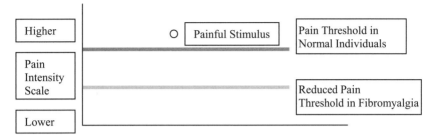

Figure 2.3: *Pain stimulus above threshold of fibromyalgia and normal individuals. Pain sensed in fibromyalgia and normal individuals.*

Figure 2.2 depicts a more intense painful stimulus, identified by the circle, that is above the pain threshold of individuals classified as having fibromyalgia to which these individuals would be aware of having pain but below the pain threshold of normal individuals classified as not having fibromyalgia, with no awareness of pain in this group of normal individuals. It is this circumstance that distinguishes individuals with fibromyalgia and fibromyalgia-like syndromes from non-fibromyalgia individuals. Figure 2.3 depicts an even more painful stimulus, identified by the circle, that is above the pain threshold of the individuals classified as having fibromyalgia as well is the normal individuals classified as not having fibromyalgia with awareness of pain in both groups of individuals. Thus, the presence of a lowered pain threshold leading to increased tenderness and an increased painful response to tenderness is a relatively characteristic feature in patients with fibromyalgia and fibromyalgia-like syndromes.

However, in no instance has a study identified the source or cause of the seemingly spontaneous pain reported in fibromyalgia. Indeed, to this day, the cause of the pain in fibromyalgia remains a mystery and is unknown. The painful stimulus as shown in Figures 2.1-2.3 remains the great question. No study has identified what it is fibromyalgia patients are tender to, absent the external induction of pain such as when looking for tenderness when examining for tender points or when examining for pain thresholds as noted in the research studies and as depicted in Figures 2.1-2.3 as above.

Think of a surround sound system tuner tuned into a radio station. When the volume is turned up, the sound gets louder and louder, and eventually becomes painful. This is what happens in fibromyalgia. The body is tuned into pain and then turns the volume up. But, what if the sound system was not tuned to a station signal? Then turning the volume up wouldn't matter as there would be no sound to get louder. Thus it is with fibromyalgia. Pain thresholds are like the volume control and determine the intensity of the pain. The pain itself is like the radio station signal, waiting to be received and interpreted. In fibromyalgia, however, the origin of the signal is unknown and there is no understanding of how to change the station or turn the signal off.

All this data is consistent with the presence of abnormal pain processing in patients with fibromyalgia in the central nervous system referred to as central nervous system sensitization. There is clear evidence for increased sensitivity to external painful stimuli in patients with fibromyalgia with processes of referred pain and pain amplification. However, and most critically, there is no intrinsic source of pain or cause of pain identified in fibromyalgia to which this sensitivity develops. Central nervous system sensitization explains in part how patients with fibromyalgia are sensitized to pain but in no way explains where the pain arises from.

Second, The Treatment of Fibromyalgia is Profoundly Disappointing

Patient education forms the foundation for all treatment programs in fibromyalgia management protocols. The role of such patient education is to validate the reality of the symptoms; to emphasize the chronic nature of fibromyalgia; to emphasize it is not life threatening; to emphasize that there is no specific treatment; and that symptomatic treatment used may improve, but does not necessarily eliminate, symptoms. Studies in patients with fibromyalgia have supported the value of such education, especially in the context of broader treatment programs. However, beyond validation and providing some semblance of hope, it defies common sense that such education, in the current state of affairs, can be of any therapeutic value as inherently patients are being told they have a chronic painful disease that may impair their ability to function with no known cause, cure, or highly effective treatment and that they must learn to live with it.

Medications Do Not Seem To Help Much

Nonsteroidal anti-inflammatory drugs (NSAIDs) are frequently pre-scribed to manage the symptoms of fibromyalgia. This is done despite the evidence indicating that NSAIDs are no better than placebo as a single modality of treatment. Indeed, while NSAIDs may be recommended as a potential initial therapy, they are not promoted as first line treatment.

Prednisone has not been shown be of benefit in treating fibromyalgia.

Analgesics are also frequently used in managing fibromyalgia symp-toms despite little data regarding their effectiveness. Acetaminophen is frequently used by patients and the majority of users report lesser subjec-tive benefit than NSAIDs. Tramadol (Ultram) is a weak opioid medication with additional properties of inhibiting the reuptake of serotonin and nore-pinephrine in the spinal cord pain message processing areas. It has been shown to be of some benefit in helping manage symptoms of fibromyalgia alone or in combination with acetaminophen. Other narcotic class opioid medications such as morphine are used frequently to manage chronic pain conditions such as temporomandibular joint disease and chronic low back pain. A survey of academic medical centers found that this class of drug is used in 20% of fibromyalgia patients. However, a study of intravenous morphine was found to demonstrate no beneficial effect in treating fibromyalgia. Indeed, the use of narcotic class analgesics is shunned by the medical community out of concern, primarily, regarding addiction.

Thus, it is a seeming twist of irony that one of the pre-eminent and characteristic features of fibromyalgia, the pain component, does not ap-pear to respond well to the use of NSAIDs and analgesics. This has led to the reverse logic argument that because the pain of fibromyalgia is not very responsive to analgesics that there is no source of pain itself. This fallacy has led to the strong de-emphasis of NSAIDs and analgesics in treating fibromyalgia. However, this is contrary to the intuition of many patients and some clinicians who continue to use analgesics to treat the unexplained pain of fibromyalgia.

Antidepressant and other psychoactive medications are used fre-quently to manage the symptoms of fibromyalgia. The most frequently studied medications in the management of fibromyalgia are the tricyclic antidepressant amitriptyline (Elavil) and the muscle relaxant cyclobenzaprine (Flexeril). Placebo controlled studies of amitriptyline, in low doses ranging from 10-50 mg daily have shown improved pain, sleep, and global well-being. In addition, the use of amitriptyline has been associated with improved pain thresholds and reduced tender point counts. Not all studies confirm the benefit of amitriptyline, however. Further, the long term benefit of amitriptyline in fibromyalgia to six weeks or beyond is unclear. Notably, the beneficial effect is not related necessarily to the antidepressant features of amitriptyline.

Cyclobenzaprine, although classified as a muscle relaxant, shares similar structural and pharmacological properties with the tricyclic antidepressant group of medications with the additional benefit of muscle relaxing properties. In doses ranging from 10-40 mg daily, placebo controlled studies have reported improvement in pain, sleep, global well-being, and fatigue. Not all studies confirm an improvement in pain, however. Like amitriptyline, the long term benefit of cyclobenzaprine is unclear.

Selective serotonin reuptake inhibitors (SSRIs) are a class of drugs that have been highly successful in treating psychiatric conditions such as depression, anxiety, and phobias. Their primary mode of action is to selectively inhibit the reuptake of serotonin in the central nervous system producing increased levels of serotonin. Fluoxetine (Prozac), citalopram (Celexa), and sertraline (Zoloft) have all been studied in patients with fibromyalgia in placebo controlled trials. Controlled studies with fluoxetine consistently show improvement in sleep and depression but are not consistent in showing improvement in pain. Amitriptyline combined with fluoxetine was more effective in reducing pain and symptoms than either drug alone. Two controlled studies of citalopram revealed no significant improvement in pain, fatigue, or sleep but one of the two studies demonstrated improved mood. A controlled trial of sertraline showed no benefit over placebo on pain and mood but revealed improvement in pain thresholds. Three meta-analyses (a meta-analysis is a study that groups the results of multiple prior studies) have been performed looking at randomized placebo controlled trials of tricyclic antidepressants, SSRIs, and s-adnosyl-methionine in fibromyalgia. It was estimated that about one in four patients experienced improvement in sleep, fatigue, pain, and global well-being in that order.

Venlafaxine (Effexor) is dual reuptake inhibitor similar to some tricyclic antidepressants in that it also inhibits the reuptake of serotonin and norepinephrine. Results of studies in treating fibromyalgia with venlafaxine have been mixed and inconsistent. Duloxetine (Cymbalta) also inhibits the reuptake of serotonin and norepinephrine. A controlled trial in fibromyalgia has shown improvement in some but not all pain measures, reduction in tender point counts, and some improved quality of life measures in women with fibromyalgia but not in men. Another controlled trial of duloxetine in fibromyalgia demonstrated some significant improvement in some patients in pain severity independent of the effect on depression. Milnacipran (Savella, Ixel, Midalcipran) is another dual reuptake inhibitor that has shown improvement in pain, fatigue, physical function, and global well-being in a randomized, placebo-controlled study of fibromyalgia patients.

S-adenosyl-L-methionine (SAMe) is a compound that has antidepressant, anti-inflammatory, and analgesic properties. Again, the results of controlled studies are inconsistent. One trial showed improved mood and tender points; another showed improvement in mood, pain, overall disease activity, and fatigue; and a third study showed no benefit.

Moclobemide (Manerix, Aurorix) is a reversible monoamine oxidase inhibitor. In a controlled trial comparing it to amitriptyline and placebo, no benefit was noted in fibromyalgia patients.

The antiepileptic medication, pregabalin (Lyrica), is a gamma-aminobutyric acid (GABA) analogue similar to gabapentin (Neurontin). A randomized controlled trial in fibromyalgia demonstrated improvements in pain, sleep, fatigue, and global symptom severity in higher doses. A second larger randomized placebo controlled trial to assess the benefit of pregabalin in patients with fibromyalgia showed that 63% of patients achieved significant reduction of pain initially, and after 26 weeks of treatment, 32% of those patients lost the therapeutic response achieved at onset but significantly more patients sustained a defined improvement compared to placebo treatment. Based on these data, pregabalin has become the first drug approved by the United States Food and Drug Administration with a specific indication for treatment of fibromyalgia. However, further studies are required to distinguish the mechanisms of symptom improvement in fibromyalgia as the high doses of pregabalin at which benefit is identified may also be associated with sedative effects.

The expectorant guaifenesin has been used to treat fibromyalgia on the assumed, but unproved, theory that there is an excess accumulation of phosphate in the muscles and that this can be excreted by the action of guaifenesin. A one year double blind controlled trial failed to demonstrate any improvement in global functioning or tender point counts.

The use of medications to successfully treat the symptoms and findings of fibromyalgia has been dismally inconsistent. Given the population prevalence of fibromyalgia at about 2% or more, the number of well designed study trials is exceedingly small. The situation is further complicated by the fact that there are very few long term studies of efficacy and of those available, the results are not promising. The treatment trial data clearly tell us that fibromyalgia is not a homogeneous disease or process and that we have no clue as to what to target our medications against. This situation is made all the worse by the fact that the treatments employed carry significant potential toxicities that require scrupulous monitoring to ensure safety and tolerability. If we are to ever find an effective medication or medication program, then we surely need a better understanding of what fibromyalgia is. This being said, the medication trial data do show that amitriptyline and cyclobenzaprine appear to be the most helpful drugs in managing fibromyalgia for reasons to be yet determined.

Aerobic Exercise May Help Some Patients, But Worsens Others

Aerobic cardiovascular fitness training exercise programs have been evaluated in multiple controlled studies involving fibromyalgia patients. The programs studied provided exercise about 1 to 3 times weekly for a range of about 6 weeks to 6 months and involved either walking, bicycling, dancing, or swimming with or without accompanying education. Several studies noted improved cardiovascular fitness with benefit persisting up to 2 years after treatment. The studies expectedly suffered from high dropout rates and problems with compliance and adherence to the exercise programs. Common problems limiting participation included lack of time and too intense exercise with worsening of symptoms. In the remainder group that did not drop out for these reasons, improvement in pain, pain threshold, tender point counts, fatigue, quality of life, and psychological distress is reported. However, improvement is not uniformly noted. Further, maximal exercise has been shown to increase pain sensitivity in patients with fibromyalgia. Also, the degree of improvement, when it occurs, is not dramatic. Tender point pain threshold improves by 28% and pain is reduced by 11%. Once again, the data tell us that fibromyalgia is not a homogeneous disease or process and we have no clue as to what it is we are targeting these exercise programs to. We do know, however, that some patients receive nominal benefit from aerobic cardiovascular fitness training while others cannot tolerate such programs.

Cognitive Behavioral Therapy Helps Some Patients, But Not Many

Cognitive behavioral therapy (CBT) is based on the premise that beliefs and the attendant subsequent behavioral responses to them are affected by an individual's cognitive and perceptual interpretation of symptoms as reinforced by environmental and societal influences. The programs are generally multidisciplinary involving integration of mind and body to restructure maladaptive and counterproductive coping strategies. The fundamental components of CBT programs include education, coping skills training, cognitive and behavioral retraining, and relapse prevention. Skills that are addressed include education in what is known regarding symptoms of fibromyalgia, pacing activities in terms of time and intensity, incorporation of scheduled activities that are pleasurable, developing problem solving skills specific to fibromyalgia issues, improving communication skills regarding fibromyalgia issues, and improving sleep hygiene and sleep related behavior. Additional components may include relaxation training, stress management, biofeedback, meditation, exercise, physical therapy, or occupational therapy.

Studies showing benefit from CBT have identified improvement in pain, tender point counts, stiffness, stress when stress management is incorporated, distress, functional ability, sleep, mood including depression and anxiety, and general health assessment. Improvements in pain or function have been reported to be sustained up to 30 months following completion of the program. However, meaningful outcomes occur in the minority of patients undergoing CBT. Unfortunately, it is very difficult to compare outcomes between studies as the treatment protocols are too different to permit such analysis. Clearly, some patients have clinically meaningful improvements with various CBT interventions, but many do not and many of the reported benefits, while statistically relevant, have little or no clinical impact on major symptoms.

Again, the data reinforces the concept that fibromyalgia is not a homogeneous disease or process and that we have no understanding of what to target CBT interventions toward. Indeed, it is impossible to develop a thorough and comprehensive CBT program for fibromyalgia. After all, how can the provision of education be complete or satisfying when the question of what causes fibromyalgia can't be answered? How can specific behavioral intervention programs be devised when we don't know what drives symptoms in the individuals with fibromyalgia?

Complementary and Alternative Therapies Provide Inconsistent, Limited, or Temporary Benefit

Studies of complementary and alternative therapies are challenging to design and difficult to interpret due to the inherent methodological flaws related to the implementation of the various treatments. It is virtually impossible to perform blinded studies with regard to the patient and the treatment provider for non-medication interventions. The patient and provider obviously know the treatment being provided. Hands-on type treatments are subjective in their application and difficult to standardize. Further, they are prone to significant bias due the introduction of other uncontrolled but non-specific beneficial treatment elements as often ascribed to a placebo effect. These elements include: intended conscious healing efforts by the treatment provider; hopeful expectations by the patient; a supportive healing relationship with elements of compassion, caring, understanding, and support; the benefit derived from regular and intensive medical follow-up; providing attention and validation to the disease process; the relaxation that is attendant with many hands-on type treatments; and, most importantly, subconscious but intentional environmental accommodations and modifications of the surrounding environment by the patient.

Electromyography (EMG) biofeedback assisted relaxation training was assessed in one controlled study and was shown to improve pain and morning stiffness.

A study assessing the effectiveness of a program of hypnosis and relaxation training in fibromyalgia revealed improved pain, fatigue, sleep, and psychological state.

Meditation combined with relaxation techniques in fibromyalgia has revealed improvement in pain, depression, anxiety, and negative thoughts.

A study examining neck support in fibromyalgia suggested some benefit.

Acupuncture has been reported to demonstrate improvement in pain, pain threshold, sleep, morning stiffness, and global ratings of improvement in fibromyalgia patients. Electroacupuncture has similarly shown improvements in pain as well as depression.

Homeopathic treatment of Rhus toxicodendron, poison ivy, compared to placebo in fibromyalgia demonstrated reduction in tender point counts and improved pain and sleep in one study.

Nutritional interventions and dietary supplements have been assessed in fibromyalgia with no definite beneficial results. Magnesium supplementation was shown to improve tender point scores in one study but no improvement in tender point scores or pain was noted in another. SAMe has been studied in multiple trials, including controlled trials in fibromyalgia. Improved tender points and depression have been documented in multiple studies. This was not confirmed in a larger study, however. A study assessing the benefit of the green alga Chlorella pyrenoidosa showed reduction in tender points and improved function in fibromyalgia patients. A study of antioxidant supplementation with anthocyanidins revealed improvements in self-reported sleep ratings, fatigue, and general well-being.

Whirlpool baths with valerian have been reported to improve sleep and both valerian and pine oil baths improve reported well-being. Balneotherapy, warm mineral rich baths, may be of benefit to pain, fatigue, stiffness, tender points, and function.

Dietary modifications are carried out by 23% of patients with fibromyalgia in an attempt to control symptoms. Studies of diets composed of raw, vegan type foods reported improvement in pain, general health, and sleep.

Static magnet therapy was assessed in a trial involving sleeping on a magnetic mattress with fibromyalgia patients reporting improvements in pain, sleep, morning fatigue, and physical function. Another study of magnetic pads identified no significant improvement in pain and tender points.

Chiropractic intervention is frequently sought by individuals with a diagnosis of fibromyalgia with 19-49% of patients involved in chiropractic care. In a controlled study of soft tissue massage, stretching, spinal manipulation, and education provided to fibromyalgia patients three to four times weekly, no benefit was noted in pain or disability.

Massage therapy is sought by 17-75% of patients with fibromyalgia. One controlled study noted improvement in pain with reduction in analgesic use and improvement in depression and self-reported quality of life. Another study failed to find improvement in pain, depression, and overall well-being.

The results of studies using complementary and alternative treatment modalities are also dismally inconsistent and disappointing. The number of well designed study trials is exceedingly small and there are very few long term studies of efficacy. As with all the other treatment modalities reviewed, the treatment trial data clearly tell us that fibromyalgia is not a homogeneous disease or process and that we have no clue as to what to target our complementary and alternative therapies against.

Fibromyalgia Treatment is a Dismal Failure

The treatment of fibromyalgia as a whole is profoundly disappointing given the limited and inconsistent studies available as well as the frequently poor results from the data generated by these studies as reviewed. There are very few long term studies of efficacy and the results of those are not promising. Most recommendations for treatment are based on these limited data coupled with absolutely no understanding of what causes or drives the symptoms of fibromyalgia despite centuries of recognition of the disease and despite its common presence in the population as diseases go. Current treatment protocols emphasize multidisciplinary and individualized approaches. This is clearly done in the hope that if one blindly throws lots of different modalities at the process, something will stick and provide some benefit. The critical message from the treatment trials is that fibromyalgia is not a homogeneous disease or process and that we have no clue as to what to target any treatment against nor how to measure its benefit. Thus, if we are to ever find effective treatment, then we surely need a better understanding of what fibromyalgia is.

Third, Patients With Fibromyalgia Do Not Do Well In The Long-Term

As with everything else in fibromyalgia, the data regarding outcome also lacks uniformity and consistency. A long term study that assessed patients 14 years after the initial diagnosis found that 67% percent of patients felt better than when they were first diagnosed. It was further noted that 70% felt the fibromyalgia caused little or no interference in activities of daily living or work related activities. In that group, 9% noted they left their jobs because of fibromyalgia related symptoms. This study is contrasted by the results of a multicenter follow-up of over 500 patients followed for seven years in which there was no significant change in fibromyalgia related symptoms or functional ability. More than 50% of this group of patients rated their health status as poor or fair and 70% perceived themselves as being disabled. In this group, 26 % were receiving some type of disability benefit and 16% were receiving Social Security Disability benefits in contrast to 2.2% of the United States population. Dysfunction in activities of daily living in fibromyalgia patients has been reported to be comparable to that seen in rheumatoid arthritis.

Most fibromyalgia patients report that the chronic pain and fatigue adversely impacts their quality of life and impairs their ability to work. Disability rates, while highly variable, identify that disability is reported to occur in 9-44% of patients with fibromyalgia. Factors predicting the development of disability includes the patient's perception of disability and function, pain, psychological disruption with mood disturbances, coping skills, associated litigation, and educational achievement.

Healthcare utilization is also significant for patients with a diagnosis of fibromyalgia. A study from the mid-1990s identified an average of 10 medical visits per year by patients with fibromyalgia. The patients were noted to take an average of 3 medications per year to manage fibromyalgia symptoms. The annual cost of medical services was reported to be comparable to managing osteoarthritis at $2,274. Another study involving employees of a large manufacturer compared direct costs of medical care and medications and indirect costs including disability and absenteeism of individuals with at least one fibromyalgia health related administrative insurance claim and noted total annual costs for claimants at $5,945 compared to a random sample of the other insurance beneficiaries at $2,486 The study concluded that additional costs related to disability and illness other than fibromyalgia specific illness significantly add to the financial burden of fibromyalgia. Another study comparing patients with fibromyalgia to a group without pain, to another group with widespread pain but not meeting ACR criteria for the classification of fibromyalgia, and to a group of healthy controls revealed that the fibromyalgia group consumed healthcare services and medications in the highest frequency and incurred twice the healthcare costs compared to controls.

Despite the observation that patients with fibromyalgia constitute a heterogeneous population, no clinical strategies exist to stratify patients for purposes of treatment or determining prognosis. Indeed, no strategy can exist if there is no understanding of the cause or disease mechanism of fibromyalgia. Plainly, patients with fibromyalgia in general do not do well in the long term, although those with milder symptoms may do better because inherently they have less severe symptoms and involvement. However, the poor prognosis and increased healthcare utilization is really not surprising given the complete lack of understanding of what fibromyalgia is, the lack of knowledge as to its cause, and the lack of effective or specific treatment. Patients, in general have chronic, ongoing but variable symptoms with permanent remissions being rare and exceptional. Basically, fibromyalgia patients do not get better.

Something is Clearly Wrong

Clearly, what we really know about fibromyalgia is that we do not know very much about it, nor what to do for it. Indeed, we really don't know much more about fibromyalgia than we did 25-30 years ago other than developing an understanding that there is an abnormality of pain signal processing. Despite the sophisticated technology of modern medical science, the sum of all the research has failed to identify the source of pain in fibromyalgia, what causes it, why it develops, and how the symptoms evolve. Medications or strategies to effectively treat fibromyalgia remain desperately needed. Something is very wrong.

Chapter 3

Where Everything Went Wrong: The Shocking Truth

"Insanity: the belief that one can get different results by doing the same thing." —Albert Einstein

After nearly two hundred years of observation and description, fibromyalgia remains an unexplained syndrome characterized by pain from nowhere. Yet, in the medical office, a cognitive dissonance sets in whereby the doctor and patient simply suspend disbelief and, without basis, assume that all of the patient's symptoms and findings can be explained by the singular diagnostic label of fibromyalgia despite everything we do not know or understand about fibromyalgia and in the face what little we do know.

The Problems With Fibromyalgia as a Clinical Syndrome

The problems with fibromyalgia as a clinical syndrome are many:

1. The diagnosis is based on purely subjective characteristics of pain and tenderness of which tenderness is nothing more than a subjective response of pain to someone else looking for it.

2. Despite it being recognized for nearly 200 years, no known cause has been identified.

3. To date, fibromyalgia pain is pain from nowhere and nobody knows why an individual with fibromyalgia has pain.

4. No underlying pathologic abnormality has been identified that explains the symptoms.

5. There are no abnormal lab tests associated with fibromyalgia.

6. No theory of pathogenesis (disease mechanism) accounts for the wide constellation of symptoms and complaints.

7. Any symptom imaginable has been associated with fibromyalgia.

8. Any disease in the world can be associated with fibromyalgia.

9. Fibromyalgia syndrome follows no characteristic pattern.

10. Once diagnosed with fibromyalgia, all symptoms and findings are attributed to fibromyalgia without consideration to their independent significance. The possibility that they may identify another process is discounted or ignored.

11. There is no known specific treatment. Most treatment protocols are unsatisfactory or ineffective and despite pain and tenderness being the pre-eminent clinical features, treating pain is highly de-emphasized in the medical literature.

12. There is no consistent pattern of outcome, other than most patients do not get better.

The clinical entity of fibromyalgia is based on the assumptions that the widespread pain and tenderness of fibromyalgia: 1) are indeed unique; 2) that they are specifically related and linked to each other; 3) and, therefore, they comprise a unified, homogeneous disease. In view of these suppositions, in 1990, the American College of Rheumatology (ACR) undertook a muticenter study to develop standardized classification criteria to stratify patients with a common set of symptoms and findings for research into fibromyalgia. Table 3.1 describes the ACR classification criteria and Figure 3.1 shows the distribution of the fibromyalgia tender points defined by the criteria. However, through the subsequent misunderstanding and misapplication of the ACR classification study and the classification criteria, things went very wrong in the world of fibromyalgia.

I. HISTORY OF WIDESPREAD PAIN.

Definition: Pain is considered widespread when all of the following are present:

1) Pain in the left side of the body, pain in the right side of the body, pain above the waist, and pain below the waist.
2) In addition, axial skeletal pain (cervical spine or anterior chest or thoracic spine or low back) must be present.
3) In this definition, shoulder and buttock pain is considered as pain for each individual side.
4) "Low back" pain is considered lower segmental pain.
5) Widespread pain must have been present for at least 3 months.

IN COMBINATION WITH

2. PAIN IN 11 OF 18 TENDER POINT SITES ON DIGITAL PALPATION.

Definition: Subjectively identified pain on digital palpation with an approximate force of 4 kg. must be present in at least 11 of the following 18 tender point sites:

1) Occiput: bilateral, at the suboccipital muscle insertions.
2) Low cervical: bilateral, at the anterior aspects of the intertransverse spaces at C5-7.
3) Trapezius: bilateral, at the midpoint of the upper border.
4) Supraspinatus: bilateral, at origins, above scapula spine near the medial border
5) Second rib: bilateral, at the second costochondral junction, just lateral to the junction on upper surfaces.
6) Lateral epicondyle: bilateral, 2 cm. distal to the epicondyles.
7) Gluteal: bilateral, in upper outer quadrants of buttocks in anterior fold of muscle.
8) Greater trochanter: bilateral, posterior to the trochanteric prominence.
9) Knee: bilateral, at the medial fat pad proximal to the joint line.

Table 3.1: ACR criteria for the classification of fibromyalgia.

(adapted from Wolfe F, Smythe HA, Yunus MB et al. *The American College of Rheumatology 1990 criteria for the classification of fibromyalgia: report of the multicenter criteria committee. Arthritis Rheum 1990; 33: 160-172.* Reprinted with permission of Wiley-Liss, Inc., a subsidiary of John Wiley & Sons, Inc.)

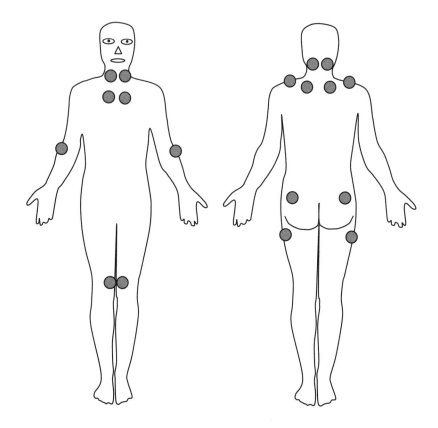

Figure 3.1: *The tender point sites identified in the ACR criteria for the classification of fibromyalgia.*

What The ACR Criteria for the Classification of Fibromyalgia Really Tell Us

First and foremost, it is critical to note that these criteria **are not and were never intended to be DIAGNOSTIC criteria** but simply classification criteria for the purpose of research studies to attempt to stratify patients with a common set of symptoms and findings. Thus, selected patients would be classified as having fibromyalgia for purposes of research study when they were found to have: I) widespread pain with pain in the left side of the body, pain in the right side of the body, pain above the waist, and pain below the waist as well as axial skeletal pain described as cervical spine, or anterior chest, or thoracic spine, or low back pain; 2) pain in eleven out of eighteen tender point sites on digital palpation with an approximate force of 4 kg; 3) and widespread pain having been present for at least three months. Unfortunately, over time and through misuse, these criteria have been subverted from research classification criteria to criteria used to make a clinical diagnosis of fibromyalgia in anyone who meets these criteria. Plain and simply, the ACR criteria for the classification of fibromyalgia are not validated as performance variables for the purpose of making a clinical diagnosis in an unselected, random population and this is clearly described in the study protocol used to establish these criteria. The performance characteristics of the ACR criteria only distinguish patients with fibromyalgia from patients with various localized regional pain conditions and some patients with rheumatoid arthritis, lupus, and other conditions with joint inflammation. The performance characteristics of the ACR criteria have not been studied or validated to distinguish patients with fibromyalgia from patients with widespread pain from many other well known and identified conditions. Specifically, they have not been shown to identify or distinguish patients who have diseases such as polymyalgia rheumatica, myositis, metabolic bone disease, malignancies, thyroid dysfunction, myelopathy, neuropathy, vasculopathy, psychological disorders, psychogenic rheumatism, malingering, primary generalized osteoarthritis, multiple syndromes of bursitis and tendinitis, and some patients with rheumatoid arthritis, lupus, and other conditions with joint inflammation. Further, the performance characteristics of the ACR classification criteria for fibromyalgia have not been studied or validated in populations in the setting of litigation and they have no established validity of this setting. Indeed, the criteria are not validated for use outside of research studies.

Research Makes Assumptions and Derives Statistics Based on Them

Basically, what the ACR criteria study looked at were multiple groups of patients from multiple centers who were felt by the individual doctors assessing them as having fibromyalgia and multiple groups of patients from multiple centers who were felt by the individual doctors assessing them as having certain conditions as noted above that were not fibromyalgia.

Thus, the presence or absence of fibromyalgia was assumed and predetermined at the outset by the individual opinion of each treating physician. Subsequently, the data from all the patients from all the centers was grouped to assess clinical features that were felt to be most unique or distinct to that group compared to a control group that was diagnosed as not having fibromyalgia. Importantly, the presence or absence of fibromyalgia hinged solely upon each individual investigator's opinion as to whether or not a specific patient had fibromyalgia and the diagnoses were assumed to be valid. There were no specific or special tests, measurements, or criteria to make or exclude the diagnosis, only the clinical impression of the investigator. The data from this kind of research is tabulated to obtain statistical information about the characteristics of the study population. Thus, this was a research study. The purpose of this study was to develop classification criteria that identify the minimum number of clinical features that exist within patients already diagnosed as having fibromyalgia by their doctors that would identify such patients fairly uniformly and would accurately distinguish them from those control patients who do not have fibromyalgia. Thus, if an individual has a diagnosis of fibromyalgia, that person would likely have the criteria and an individual who does not have a diagnosis of fibromyalgia would likely not meet the criteria.

The results of such a research study lead to two very important statistics. The first is the proportion of individuals who have an existing diagnosis of fibromyalgia who also demonstrate the clinical characteristics being screened. This is known as the sensitivity of the criteria, or the true positive rate. The sensitivity results of the ACR criteria study tell us that in a room filled with 100 individuals who are classified as having fibromyalgia 98 of them will have a widespread pain, 90 will have at least eleven out of eighteen painful tender fibromyalgia points and 88 will have a combination of widespread pain and at least eleven out of eighteen painfully tender fibromyalgia points. This is shown in Table 3.2.

The second important statistic is the proportion of individuals who do not have fibromyalgia and also do not have the clinical characteristics being screened. This is known as the specificity, or true negative rate. The specificity results of the ACR criteria study tell us that in another room filled with 100 individuals who do not have a diagnosis of fibromyalgia but do have various neck pain syndromes, low back pain syndromes, local tendinitis related pain syndromes, possible systemic lupus erythemato-sus, or rheumatoid arthritis (the control group): 31 of them will not have widespread pain, meaning 69 of them will have widespread pain; 78 of them will not have at least eleven out of eighteen painfully tender fibromyalgia points, meaning 22 of them will have at least eleven out of eighteen painfully tender fibromyalgia points; and 81 will not have a com-bination of widespread pain and at least eleven out of eighteen painfully tender fibromyalgia points, meaning 19 of them will have a combination of widespread pain and at least eleven out of eighteen painfully tender fibromyalgia points. This is also depicted in Table 3.2. Thus, the ACR criteria study tells us that 19 out of 100 (about one out of five) individuals who do not have fibromyalgia will be diagnosed in error as having fibromyalgia when relying on the ACR criteria to make that diagnosis. This is known as the false positive rate. This is a significant rate of misclassification considering treatment and prognosis are going to be ren-dered on the basis of an incorrect diagnosis.

	Sensitivity (If you have fibromyalgia, this is the prevalence of these features.)	Specificity (If you DO NOT have fibromyalgia, this is the prevalence of the ABSENCE of these features.)
Widespread Pain	98%	31%
At Least 11/18 Painful Tender Points	90%	78%
Widespread Pain For At Least 3 Months And At Least 11/18 Painful Tender Points	88%	81%

Table 3.2: Sensitivity and specificity data for widespread pain and painful tender points in patients characterized as having fibromyalgia.

Clinical Medicine Is Based on Probability
Looking at Facts, Not Assumptions

Unlike research, clinical medicine is not based on assumptions. It is based on the interpretation of clinical symptoms, signs, and findings leading to the highest likely possibility that a given diagnosis is correct. This is rooted in the understanding the clinical symptoms and signs are not sen-sitive or specific to any one particular disease or condition, except in very rare circumstances. For instance, widespread pain and tenderness are seen in a large number of medical conditions other than just fibromyalgia. Therefore, clinical medicine is based on probabilities. The clinical question always is: What is the likelihood that a particular set of symptoms and findings support a particular diagnosis? To answer this question, it is necessary to undertake a thorough and comprehensive medical assessment to catalog all the relevant symptoms and signs that are present as well as those that aren't. It is then necessary to know and understand preexisting knowledge and research using sensitivity and specificity data to understand how likely these symptoms and signs occur in the diagnoses under consideration. Finally, it is necessary to consider how likely the diagnoses under consideration are to occur in the specific clinical setting. For instance, the presence of a dry hacking cough and fever could indicate the presence of influenza or tuberculosis. Clearly, in the middle of a flu epidemic, the cough and fever most likely are diagnostic of influenza. Not 100%, but highly likely, nonetheless. On the other hand, if there is no influenza outbreak and the person comes from a community in which tuberculosis is known to exist, the same symptoms are more likely to be diagnostic of tuberculosis.

With regard to fibromyalgia, let's now apply the same probability principles to the clinical question: what is the likelihood that someone who has the ACR classification criteria of widespread pain for at least three months and pain in at least eleven out of eighteen tender point sites actually has fibromyalgia? To simplify things, let's look at 1000 people randomly selected from the community at large and look for ACR classification criteria of widespread pain for at least three months and pain in at least eleven out of eighteen tender point sites to make a diagnosis of fibromyalgia. Based on the data presented in Chapter 1, the prevalence of fibromyalgia in the community is about 2%. This means that of our random sample of 1000 people, 20 have fibromyalgia. We also have learned from the sensitivity data from ACR classification criteria study that 88% of these 20 have ACR classification criteria of widespread pain for at least three months and pain in at least eleven out of eighteen tender point sites. Thus, 18 of these 20 individuals with fibromyalgia actually meet the ACR classification criteria requirements. Two individuals with fibromyalgia do not meet these criteria. Importantly however, of the remaining 980 of the original 1000 who do not have fibromyalgia, the ACR specificity data tells us that 81% of them, or 794 people, do not fulfill the ACR classification criteria. However, the remaining 186 of the 980 people who do not have fibromyalgia actually have the ACR classification criteria of widespread pain for at least three months and pain in at least eleven out of eighteen tender point sites.

Armed with this information, we can display this data as shown in Table 3.3. Using Table 3.3, we can now answer the question: what is the likelihood that someone who has the ACR classification criteria of widespread pain for at least three months and pain in eleven out of eighteen tender point sites actually has fibromyalgia? The answer is derived by looking at the row "Widespread pain for at least 3 months and at least 11/18 painfully tender fibromyalgia points present" which shows the classification criteria are found in 18 individuals with fibromyalgia and in 186 individuals who do not have fibromyalgia. Thus, a total of 204 out of the original 1000 randomly chosen individuals has widespread pain for at least three months and pain in at least eleven out of eighteen tender point sites but only 18 of them actually have fibromyalgia. Thus, the probability of diagnosing fibromyalgia correctly using the ACR classification criteria exclusively is 18 divided by 204 (18/204) which is 8.8%. This is known as the positive predictive value or PPV. In other words, out of every 100 people who have widespread pain for at least three months and pain in at least eleven out of eighteen tender point sites, 8.8 have fibromyalgia, but most importantly, the other 91.2 people with widespread pain for at least three months and pain in at least eleven out of eighteen tender point sites do not have fibromyalgia.

We can also answer the question: what is the likelihood that someone who does not have the ACR classification criteria of widespread pain for at least three months and pain in at least eleven out of eighteen tender point sites actually does not have fibromyalgia? The answer is derived by looking at the row "Widespread pain for at least 3 months and at least 11/18 painfully tender fibromyalgia points absent" which shows the classification criteria are absent in 2 individuals with fibromyalgia and in 794 individuals who do not have fibromyalgia. Thus, a total of 796 out of the original 1000 randomly chosen individuals has an absence widespread pain for at least three months and pain in eleven out of eighteen tender point sites but only 2 of them actually have fibromyalgia. Thus, the probability of diagnostically excluding fibromyalgia correctly using the ACR classification criteria exclusively is 794 divided by 796 (794/796) which is 99.7%. This is known as the negative predictive value or NPV. In other words, out of 100 people who do not have widespread pain for at least three months and pain in eleven out of eighteen tender point sites, 99.7 do not have fibromyalgia. Thus, the absence of widespread pain for at least three months and pain in at least eleven out of eighteen tender point sites virtually excludes the diagnosis of fibromyalgia.

	1000 People Randomly Selected (2% of the population has fibromyalgia)		
	Fibromyalgia Present = 20 people	Fibromyalgia Absent=980 people	
	Sensitivity of ACR Fibromyalgia Criteria = 88%	Specificity of ACR Fibromyalgia Criteria = 81%	
Widespread pain for at least 3 months and at least 11/18 painfully tender fibromyalgia points **present**	18 (Sensitivity)	186	PPV= 18/(186+18) = 18/204 = 8.8/100
Widespread pain for at least 3 months and at least 11/18 painfully tender fibromyalgia points **absent**	2	794 (Specificity)	NPV=794/(2+794) =794/796 =99.7/100

Table 3.3: *Clinical fibromyalgia in the population at large looking at a random sample of 1000 people (PPV=positive predictive value, NPV=negative predictive value).*

Nearly 9 Out of 10 Patients Diagnosed with Fibromyalgia Do Not Actually Have Fibromyalgia

To summarize, what we learn from the analysis outlined in Table 3.3 is that when exclusively using the criteria of widespread pain and at least 11/18 painfully tender fibromyalgia points to diagnose fibromyalgia in an individual presenting to the medical office, for every 100 patients who have widespread pain for at least 3 months and at least 11/18 painfully tender fibromyalgia points, only 8.8 will actually have fibromyalgia. Therefore, in practical terms, approximately one out of ten individuals who have widespread pain for at least 3 months and at least 11/18 painfully tender fibromyalgia points have fibromyalgia. Most critically, the other nine out of the ten individuals who have widespread pain and at least 11/18 painfully tender fibromyalgia points do not have fibromyalgia. The ACR study clearly shows that the positive predictive value of the fibromyalgia criteria is extremely poor and cannot be relied upon to make an accurate diagnosis as it would incorrectly identify nine out of ten individuals with fibromyalgia when in fact they do not have fibromyalgia. It is precisely for this reason that the criteria were never intended to be diagnostic criteria and it is precisely the reason why they should never have been, nor ever be, used as diagnostic criteria. On the flip side, it is useful to note that if an individual does not have widespread pain and at least 11/18 painfully tender fibromyalgia points, it is with near absolute certainty that the individual does not have fibromyalgia given the powerful negative predictive value of 99.7%. This means that not having widespread pain and at least 11/18 painfully tender fibromyalgia points will correctly exclude the diagnosis of fibromyalgia in 99.7 out of 100 patients.

Of course this entire discussion is dependent upon the prevalence of fibromyalgia in the population being assessed is 2%. If the prevalence is higher, then the positive predictive value of the ACR criteria will subsequently be better. However, the ACR criteria are currently routinely being applied as diagnostic criteria to a general population setting to make a diagnosis of fibromyalgia exclusive of any other symptoms or findings that may point to another diagnosis, and therefore the 2% population prevalence probability is the most likely applicable probability. However, even if the population prevalence was increased tenfold up to a 20% prevalence of fibromyalgia, using the same analysis, the positive predictive value would be virtually no better than a coin toss in terms of being able to diagnose the presence of fibromyalgia.

The American College of Rheumatology Criteria for the Classification of Fibromyalgia DO NOT DIAGNOSE FIBROMYALGIA

Thus, it can be clearly seen that the widespread pain and tenderness seen with fibromyalgia is neither: unique, as widespread pain and tenderness occurs frequently in patients who do not have fibromyalgia; nor are they are closely related to each other, as widespread pain and the presence of at least 11/18 painfully tender fibromyalgia points do not consistently coexist in patients with fibromyalgia and are seen in significant frequency in patients without fibromyalgia.

What we also see is that the use of the ACR criteria of widespread pain and at least 11/18 painfully tender fibromyalgia points to DIAGNOSE the presence of fibromyalgia is in the terminology of logic, a tautology: a proposition which is always true and can never be false because it includes all possibilities. If 100% of individuals with widespread pain and tenderness are defined as having fibromyalgia, as is the case by misusing the ACR criteria for purposes of diagnosis, and 100% of individuals with fibromyalgia have widespread pain and tenderness then a tautology exists. Such a construct is of course meaningless as we are saying nothing more than everyone who has fibromyalgia has fibromyalgia.

Summarizing all of this, most individuals diagnosed with fibromyalgia, relying exclusively on the ACR fibromyalgia criteria to make the diagnosis, actually do not have fibromyalgia. This of course is a serious issue in the clinical setting, as physicians have come to rely upon the criteria exclusively to make the diagnosis of fibromyalgia. Most importantly, all research studies published subsequent to the introduction of the ACR fibromyalgia criteria have relied exclusively on the criteria to enter patients into the study protocols. The consequence of this is that the majority of individuals entered into fibromyalgia studies actually do not have fibromyalgia by definition. Indeed, a Pub Med review of the number of publications linked to the term fibromyalgia since the introduction of the ACR criteria reveals 3757 publications as of December 11, 2007 and most of these suffer from this methodological flaw.

Fibromyalgia Pain and Tenderness Are Subjective and Are Misinterpreted

One of the key issues in regard to the diagnosis of fibromyalgia is that the symptoms of pain are completely subjective as is the reporting of tenderness when assessed by an examiner. A very telling study reveals that when individuals without fibromyalgia are trained to intentionally fake symptoms and findings of fibromyalgia, experienced rheumatologists will misdiagnose 1 out of 3 of these individuals as having fibromyalgia. The powerful subjectivity of the pain related symptoms renders the interpretation of the pain and tenderness very difficult and makes them subject to significant observational error and leads to the misdiagnosis of patients.

Everybody Has Stopped Looking for the Cause of Pain in Fibromyalgia

The identification of abnormal pain processing strongly supports central nervous system sensitization as the mechanism by which individuals with fibromyalgia are sensitized to pain. However, abnormal pain processing is, in and of itself, insufficient to explain the pain in fibromyalgia, if indeed there is no source of pain to process. As the source or cause of pain in fibromyalgia has defied identification over nearly two hundred years, there has developed an unstated, unfounded, and unsubstantiated implication that the abnormality of central pain processing implies that the pain itself originates in the central nervous system. This is wrong. The typical causes of central nervous system originated pain such as vascular lesions in the brain and spinal cord, multiple sclerosis, traumatic spinal injury, syringomyelia and syringobulbia, brain tumors, brain inflammation and infections, epilepsy, and Parkinson's Disease are not identified in primary fibromyalgia syndrome. This tacit acceptance that the pain mysteriously arises in the central nervous system has contributed to the cessation in the search for the cause or source of the pain.

Fibromyalgia Remains Misunderstood

After seventeen years, the ACR classification criteria for fibromyalgia have really not brought us any closer to an understanding or explanation of what fibromyalgia is, where the pain comes from or why it occurs. Further, the ACR criteria have caused more harm than good by: being misused as diagnostic criteria; and by confounding the research into fibromyalgia by misclassifying large numbers of patients who were diagnosed as having fibromyalgia, but who in fact did not have fibromyalgia, into studies, thereby precluding meaningful interpretation of the results. Notably, the patients in these studies did have widespread pain and at least 11/18 painfully tender fibromyalgia points but, as discussed, the majority of these patients would not be classified as having fibromyalgia when relying on these two criteria to make the diagnosis of fibromyalgia. It certainly seems that the ongoing use of the ACR classification criteria is not destined to shed any further light upon understanding the issues related to fibromyalgia. All this, of course, leads to the question of what do these individuals with widespread pain and tender points really have and what does the presence of widespread pain and tender points really mean?

Part Two

The Key Question of Fibromyalgia Answered

Chapter 4

Uncovering The Source of Fibromyalgia Pain: A New Path

"If you want a better answer, ask a better question." — Jeff Sarkozi, M.D.

The hallmark features of individuals diagnosed with fibromyalgia are the presence of chronic widespread pain and at least 11/18 painfully tender fibromyalgia points. Yet, the majority of individuals having these characteristics, in fact, do not have fibromyalgia. Clearly then, if most of what is identified as fibromyalgia really isn't fibromyalgia, the issue about fibromyalgia isn't about fibromyalgia at all, but rather about the meaning of chronic widespread pain and tenderness from which fibromyalgia arises. Therefore, the key to understanding fibromyalgia pain resides in the understanding of what causes pain in individuals who have chronic widespread pain and at least 11/18 painfully tender fibromyalgia points. The challenge is to meticulously peel back the layers of widespread pain to identify where and how the pain originates.

A Study: What Patients Really Have

To answer the question "What do patients with chronic widespread pain and at least 11/18 painfully tender fibromyalgia points really have?", I undertook a clinical survey of patients in my fibromyalgia and chronic widespread pain specialty practice. All patients reported in this study participated in a program of extended assessment and care to better understand and manage the myriad of symptoms they presented with. They were assessed in detail regarding all musculoskeletal complaints, as well as issues related to sleep, fatigue, psychological, and psychosocial issues. Patients underwent a thorough and detailed general examination, neurological examination, and musculoskeletal examination. The musculoskeletal examination involved meticulous and comprehensive evaluations related to the joints and joint related structures such as ligaments, tendons, bursae, and fasciae including the assessment of pain, tenderness, redness, heat, swelling, alignment, deformities, range of motion, and hypermobility. Patients underwent a thorough and detailed soft tissue and pain threshold examination.

Patients included in this study were to have chronic widespread pain and painful tenderness in at least 11/18 fibromyalgia points as defined by the American College of Rheumatology (ACR) criteria for the classification of fibromyalgia (See Chapter 3). Patients in this study did not have rheumatoid arthritis, connective tissue diseases such as systemic lupus erythematosus, Sjogren's syndrome, mixed connective tissue disease, other overlap or undifferentiated connective tissue disease, reactive arthritis, infectious arthritis, polymyalgia rheumatica, vasculitis, metabolic bone disease, or active hypothyroidism.

A subject was considered to have diffuse tenderness when non-fibromyalgia soft tissue regions were reported to be painfully tender and of similar magnitude as the regionally located fibromyalgia point or points in three out of four soft tissue areas that included: the bilateral upper and lower half upper extremities; and the bilateral upper and lower half lower extremities.

Age, Sex, and Disease Duration Of Study Patients

As Table 4.1 shows, there were a total of 92 patients fulfilling the entry criteria of widespread pain for at least 3 months and at least 11/18 painfully tender fibromyalgia points who are reported here. There were 83 females and 9 males constituting 90% females and 10% males. Their mean age was 52.9 years with a range of 29 years to 86 years. The mean duration of symptoms related to the pain attributed to fibromyalgia was 17.6 years with a range as short as 0.5 years to as long as 48 years.

Characteristic	Demographic Data for 92 Patients
Age - Mean (Range)	52.9 years (29-86 years)
Sex - Female	83
- Male	9
Duration of Fibromyalgia Related Pain - Mean (Range)	17.6 years (0.5-48 years)

Table 4.1: Demographic data.

Where The Pain Comes From
What Patients Actually Would Tell Their Doctors If They Listened

The most common subjective complaints of aching, pain, and discomfort were symptoms of osteoarthritis and degenerative disc disease related to the neck and low back and their referred distribution sites, as noted in Table 4.2, each being noted in 97% of patients. Referred symptoms are symptoms that arise from a certain site but are felt away from that site. Typically, neck related symptoms may refer symptoms into the arms or chest and low back related symptoms may refer symptoms into the legs, buttock regions, or hip areas. The next most common symptom was cervical spine cephalalgia or neck related headache from the cervical spine osteoarthritis and degenerative disc disease noted in 83% of subjects. Cervical spine related headaches develop as a referred symptom from the cervical spine. The knees were symptomatic of osteoarthritis in 63% of individuals. The thoracic spine, or middle spine area between the neck and low back, was next most symptomatic with symptoms of osteoarthritis and degenerative disc disease being noted in 41% of subjects. Pain in the ball of the foot joints, or metatarsophalangeal joints, due to osteoarthritis was also noted in 40% of patients. While patients complained of pain in many joint specific or regional sites, when specifically asked, they noted in addition to their distinct localized symptoms, widespread, generalized head to toe to fingertip pain in 39% of the group. The remainder of the sites are as noted in Table 4.2. All these sites demonstrated symptoms of osteoarthritis. It is notable that involvement of many joint group or regions was noted at least in some patients and at least a few were noted in all, with the most predominant sites being that of the neck or low back and usually both.

Subjective Symptomatic Sites of Osteoarthritis and Degenerative Disc Disease	% Frequency of Occurrence in the 92 Patients
Cervical Spine and/or Referred Symptoms related to the Cervical Spine	97
Lumbar Spine and/or Referred Symptoms related to the Lumbar Spine	97
Cervical Spine related Cephalalgia (Headache)	83
Knee	63
Thoracic Spine and/or Referred Symptoms related to the Thoracic Spine	41
Metatarsophalangeal Joint (Ball of foot joint)	40
Generalized Widespread Pain (Head to toe to fingertip pain)	39
Ankle	37
Finger Proximal Interphalangeal Joint (Finger middle knuckle joint)	36
Anterior Chest	29
Elbow	27
Shoulder	26
Temporomandibular Joint (TMJ)	26
Wrist	25
Heel	25
First Carpometacarpal Joint (Thumb base joint)	25
Finger Metacarpophalangeal Joint (Finger back row knuckle joint)	22
Trochanter (Side of hip)	22
Sole	20
Inguinal (Hip crease)	16
Finger Distal Interphalangeal Joint (Finger end row knuckle joint)	12
Finger Diffusely	10
Midfoot	10
Toe Proximal Interphalangeal Joint (Toe middle knuckle joint)	7
Morning Stiffness (Average in Minutes)	57 minutes
Morning Stiffness (Range in minutes)	0-360 minutes
Patients with any morning stiffness	72%

Table 4.2: *Subjective osteoarthritis pain and stiffness based on self-reporting. (See Figure 4.1 for joint locations.)*

The average duration of morning stiffness from osteoarthritis for all sites noted to be stiff in the morning was 57 minutes. The range of morning stiffness was from none to as long as 360 minutes with 72% of patients noting any morning stiffness.

What Doctors Would Actually Find If They Looked

Distinct joint painful tenderness or pain with motion due to osteoarthritis identified objectively during the physical examination is shown in Table 4.3. The most characteristic finding was that all patients revealed distinct tenderness or pain with motion of the cervical spine due to osteoarthritis and degenerative disc disease. Osteoarthritis of the patellofemoral compartment of the knee was identified in 73% of the group followed by the first carpometacarpal (CMC) joint in the thumb at 63% and the metatarsophalangeal joints in the ball of the foot area at 51%. Osteoarthritis tenderness or pain with motion was noted at the finger proximal interphalangeal (PIP) joints in 25%, the toe proximal interphalangeal (PIP) joints in 25%, thumb metacarpophalangeal (MCP) joints in 22%, the finger distal interphalangeal (DIP) joints in 21%, the temporomandibular joints (TMJ) in 14%, and in lesser frequency in the remainder of the joints listed in Table 4.3.

Objective Symptomatic Sites of Osteoarthritis and Degenerative Disc Disease	% Frequency of Occurrence in the 92 Patients
Cervical Spine	100
Knee Patellofemoral Compartment	73
First Carpometacarpal (CMC) Joint	63
Metatarsophalangeal Joint	51
Finger Proximal Interphalangeal (PIP) Joint	25
Toe Proximal Interphalangeal (PIP) Joint	25
First Metacarpophalangeal (MCP) Joint	22
Finger Distal Interphalangeal (DIP) Joint	21
Temporomandibular (TMJ) Joint	14
Costochondral/Sternochondral Joint	10
Hip Joint	10
Thumb Interphalangeal Joint	9
Knee Joint – Medial/Lateral Compartment	9
Finger Metacarpophalangeal Joint	5
Thoracic Spine	4
Ankle Joint	3
Toe Distal Interphalangeal Joint	1

Table 4.3: Objective physical examination findings: distinct joint tenderness or pain with motion. (See Figure 4.1 for joint locations.)

Osteophytes are areas of new bone formation that develop in the joints as a result of osteoarthritis. They are identified as bony swelling in the joint area and in the more obvious form may be recognized, for instance in the fingers, as knobby knuckles. In the study group, osteophytes were noted most frequently in the thumb base joints, the first CMC joints, in 92% of the group as noted in Table 4.4. Osteophytes were detected in the finger end knuckle joints, the DIP joints, in 74%. The big toe joint as it attaches to the foot, the first MTP joint, revealed osteophytes in 58% of the patients. Osteophytes were detected in the finger middle knuckle joints, the finger PIP joints, in 27%. The presence of osteophytes was noted in other joints less frequently as noted in Table 4.4.

Joint alignment deformities due to the effects of osteoarthritis are described in Table 4.4 as well. Joint alignment abnormalities related to osteoarthritis were identified most frequently in the DIP joints, being seen in 95% of the group, followed closely by the first CMC joints at 92%, and the finger PIP joints at 88%. Deformities in the feet revealed reduced metatarsal arch in 95%, reduced longitudinal arch in 70%, and flat feet in 33%. Angular deformity of the big toe was noted in 86% and cock-up alignment of the toes was noted in 85% of the group. Knee valgus alignment describes a knock-knee position where the thigh bone comes inward toward the knee and the lower leg extends outward from the knee. Knee valgus alignment was seen in 93% of the group. Knee varus alignment, a bow legged alignment, was seen in 5%.

In addition to distinct joint involvement, distinct painful tenderness was identified in joint related structures, known as periarticular structures, such as bursae, tendon insertions, tendon sheaths, fasciae, and nodules as displayed in Table 4.5. The most common periarticular finding was trochanteric bursitis which was noted in 39% of the group. Plantar fasciitis was noted in 27% of the group, followed by subacromial bursitis/supraspinatus tendinitis in 21%, pes anserine bursitis in 19%, painfully tender flexor tendon nodules in 17%, deep Achilles bursitis in 10%, medial or lateral epicondylitis (golfer's or tennis elbow respectively) in 9%, de Quervain's tenosynovitis in 8%, Achilles tendon insertion tendinitis in 4%, and finger flexor tenosynovitis in 2%.

The joint and periarticular location sites described in the physical examination findings are displayed in Figures 4.1 and 4.2.

Osteophytes and Osteoarthritis Alignment Deformities	% Frequency of Occurrence in the 92 Patients
Osteophytes	
First Carpometacarpal (First CMC) Joint	92
Finger Distal Interphalangeal (DIP) Joints (Heberden's Nodes)	74
First Metatarsophalangeal (First MTP) Joint	58
Finger Proximal Interphalangeal (PIP) Joints (Bouchard's Nodes)	27
Thumb Metacarpophalangeal (MCP) Joint	8
Non-Thumb Metacarpophalangeal (MCP) Joint	7
Toe Proximal Interphalangeal (PIP) Joint	7
Talus	2
Knee	2
Acromioclavicular (AC) Joint	1
Osteoarthritis Alignment Deformities	
Finger Distal Interphalangeal (DIP) Joint	95
First Carpometacarpal (First CMC) Joint	92
Finger Proximal Interphalangeal (PIP) Joints	88
Reduced Metatarsal Arch in Foot	95
Reduced Longitudinal Arch in Foot	70
Pes Plano Valgus (Flat Foot)	33
Hallux Valgus	86
Cock-up Toes	85
Knee Valgus Alignment	93
Knee Varus Alignment	5

Table 4.4: *Objective physical examination findings: osteophytes, subluxation, and angular joint deformities. (See Figure 4.1 for joint locations.)*

Objective Symptomatic Periarticular Sites	% Frequency of Occurrence in the 92 Patients
Trochanteric Bursitis	39
Plantar Fasciitis	27
Subacromial Bursitis/Supraspinatus Tendinitis	21
Pes Anserine Bursitis	19
Finger Flexor Nodule Painful Tenderness	17
Deep Achilles Bursitis	10
Medial or Lateral Epicondylitis	9
DeQuervain's Tenosynovitis	8
Achilles Tendon Insertion Tendinitis	4
Finger Flexor Tenosynovitis	2

Table 4.5: *Objective physical examination findings: distinct periarticular structure painful tenderness. (See Figure 4.2 for periarticular locations.)*

Hypermobility, also known as loose or double-jointedness, was identified in many patients as noted in Table 4.6. The assessment for this was undertaken in 71 of the 92 patients. The most frequent finding was the ability to hyperextend the fingers at the MCP joints to 60° or more which was noted in 72% of the group. Almost as frequent, was the ability to extend the thumb through a closed fist, with this being noted in 62%. Apposing the thumb to the volar forearm by flexing the wrist to the palm side and pulling the thumb back to touch the palm side of the forearm was identified in 32% of the group. Twenty-seven percent of the group could touch the soles of their feet flat together while sitting with their knees held together. Further, 10% of the group could touch their palms flat to the ground while standing and bending forward without bending the knees.

Hypermobility Site	% Frequency of Occurrence in 71 Patients
Apposing the thumb to the volar forearm	38
Extending the thumb through a closed fist	62
Hyperextension of the metacarpophalangeal joints $\geq 60°$	72
Touching palms flat to the floor standing and bending	10
Touching soles flat sitting with knees touching together	27

Table 4.6: *Objective physical examination findings: joint hypermobility.*

Table 4.7 lists other findings that are associated with osteoarthritis, degenerative disc disease, or pain in the periarticular structures such as bursae, tendons, and fasciae. The presence of a thoracic rotoscoliosis, a scoliosis with a rotational component on flexing forward, was a highly characteristic finding being noted in 96% of the study population. Leg length discrepancies of greater that 0.5 cm. was noted in 48% of those for whom measurements were available, with 41% showing discrepancies of 0.5-1.0 cm., and 7% showing discrepancies greater than 1.0 cm.. The absence of a leg length discrepancy was noted in 27%. These figures may underestimate the true rate of leg length discrepancy as 25% of leg length measurements were indeterminate due to obesity or other difficulties ascertaining the measurement landmarks. Rolling the posterior thorax skin was reported to be painful by 57% of the group and reactive hyperemia with excess redness from skin rolling was also noted in 57% but not necessarily coexisting. Iliotibial band tightness, a predisposing factor to trochanteric bursitis, was present in a high frequency at 93%. Hyperextension of the low back, identified as lumbosacral hyperextension, was also present in high frequency at 88% with average lumbosacral hyperextension measuring on average 17.6 degrees in those with lumbosacral hyperextension being present.

Additional Findings Associated With Osteoarthritis, Degenerative Disc Disease, and Periarticular Pain (Number Assessed For Finding Noted)	% Frequency In Assessed Group	Quantity Mean (Range)
Thoracic Rotoscoliosis (92)	96	
Leg Length Discrepancy (92)		
0.5 cm. – 1.0 cm.	41	
Greater than 1.0 cm.	7	
None	27	
Indeterminate	25	
Skin Roll Painful Tenderness (67)	57	
Reactive Hyperemia Posterior Thorax (65)	57	
Iliotibial Band Tightness (44)	93	
Lumbosacral Hyperextension (92)	88	15.5 degrees (0-30 degrees)
Lumbosacral Hyperextension in those found to have Lumbosacral Hyperextension (81)		17.6 degrees (5-30 degrees)

Table 4.7: *Objective physical examination findings: additional findings associated with osteoarthritis, degenerative disc disease, and periarticular pain.*

As noted in Table 4.8, the presence of distinct painful fibromyalgia points without diffuse tenderness was noted in 49% of the study group with an average of 15.6 painful fibromyalgia points being present. Of more significance is that 51% of the group had diffuse, widespread soft tissue painful tenderness in all 4 extremities including the shoulder and hip girdle areas and the painful fibromyalgia point areas were not distinct or uniquely identified separately from the diffuse painful tenderness. In this group, an average of 17 painful fibromyalgia point sites were included, embedded within the diffuse painful tenderness. Diffuse soft tissue painful tenderness of the anterior and posterior thorax was noted frequently at 87% and 84% respectively. In a smaller subset of patients, diffuse soft tissue painful tenderness was noted in the scalp and face in 69% and 62% of the group respectively.

Objective Soft Tissue Painful Tenderness (Number Assessed For Finding Noted)	% Frequency In Assessed Group	Quantity Mean (Range)
Distinct Painful Fibromyalgia Tender Points Only (92)	49	
Number Painful Fibromyalgia Tender Points		15.6 (11-18)
Diffuse Non-Distinct Soft Tissue Painful Tenderness in all 4 extremities and shoulder and hip girdle areas (92)	51	
Number Non-Distinct Painful Fibromyalgia Tender Points		17.0 (11-18)
Diffuse Anterior Chest Soft Tissue Painful Tenderness (85)	87	
Diffuse Posterior Chest Soft Tissue Painful Tenderness (25)	84	
Diffuse Scalp Soft Tissue Painful Tenderness (13)	69	
Diffuse Facial Painful Soft Tissue Tenderness (13)	62	

Table 4.8: *Objective physical examination findings: soft tissue painful tenderness.*

The Cause of Fibromyalgia Pain

The predominant joint specific musculoskeletal symptoms and findings of osteoarthritis and degenerative disc disease related pain and painful tenderness are identified in Figure 4.1.

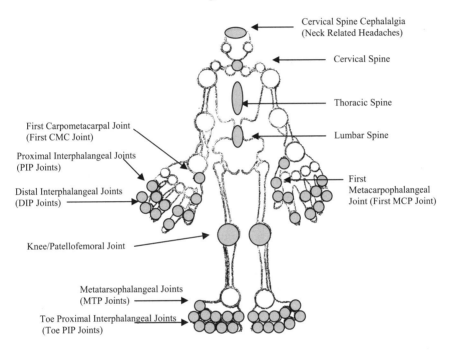

Figure 4.1: Joint specific symptoms and findings of osteoarthritis and degenerative disc disease related pain and painful tenderness.

The presence of symptoms and findings of joint specific pain and tenderness in patients who would otherwise be characterized as having fibromyalgia is noted in the cervical spine, thoracic spine, lumbar spine, thumb first CMC joints, thumb first MCP joints, finger DIP and PIP joints, knee and patellofemoral joints, and toe MTP and PIP joints. Other specific joint sites are noted in Tables 4.2, 4.3, and 4.4. The joint distribution pattern and presentation of symptoms is characteristic for the distribution of joint involvement in primary generalized osteoarthritis and accompanying spinal degenerative disc disease. Thus, patients who would be characterized as having primary fibromyalgia, that is fibromyalgia without an

identified cause, actually have symptoms and findings of primary generalized osteoarthritis and degenerative disc disease that are not recognized
or identified as a source of pain.

In addition to joint specific pain, many patients have periarticular
pain, which is pain in structures related to joint function but not the joint
itself. Figure 4.2 demonstrates the periarticular sites identified in the study
as noted in Tables 4.2 and 4.5. The commonest periarticular finding is
trochanteric bursitis followed by plantar fasciitis, subacromial bursitis/
supraspinatus tendinitis, pes anserine bursitis, flexor nodule painful tenderness, deep Achilles bursitis, epicondylitis, de Quervain's tenosynovitis, Achilles insertion tendinitis, and finger flexor tensynovitis.

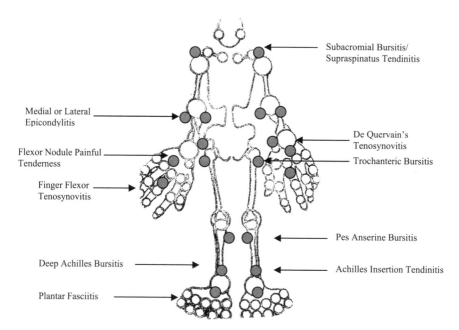

Figure 4.2: Periarticular symptoms and findings of pain and painful tenderness.

In addition to having identifiable spine, joint, and periarticular causes
of pain, patients with fibromyalgia characterized with widespread pain
and painful tenderness in at least 11/18 fibromyalgia points have a variable
pattern of tenderness with increased sensitivity to painful and non-painful
stimulation ranging from the minimum definition of 11/18 painful

fibromyalgia points to diffuse non-distinct tenderness involving all the extremities, chest, scalp, and face in which the painful fibromyalgia tender point tenderness cannot be distinguished from the adjacent and remote soft tissue. This is shown in Figure 4.3.

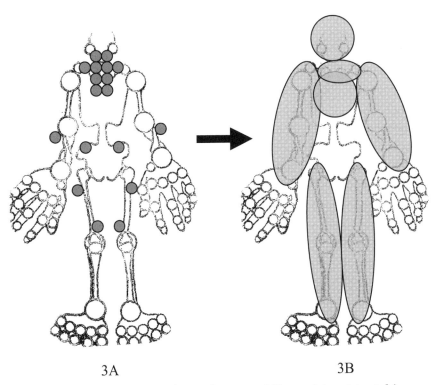

3A   3B

Figure 4.3: *Range of painful tenderness from typical fibromyalgia point painful tenderness as shown in Figure 3A to diffuse non-distinct painful tenderness as shown in Figure 3B.*

The results of this study shed significantly important new light on the cause of pain in fibromyalgia and provide the answer to the missing link of what the cause of pain is in patients with fibromyalgia. For the first time, the source of pain in fibromyalgia is identified and defined. All patients with widespread pain, defined as pain on the left side of the body, the right side of the body, above the waist, below the waist, and involving the axial skeleton for at least 3 months with at least 11/18 painfully tender fibromyalgia points who have no evidence of rheumatoid arthritis, connective tissue diseases such as systemic lupus erythematosus, infection related arthritis, metabolic related arthritis, or crystal related arthritis have primary generalized osteoarthritis predominantly involving the neck and back with associated degenerative disc disease and a variable combination of associated tendinitis, bursitis, and fasciitis and increased nociception (nociception is the sensing of painful sensation and increased nociception is the increased sensitivity or sensation that a stimulus is in fact perceived as painful) to these painful sources, triggers, and drivers.

In order to recognize the polyregional sources of osteoarthritis, degenerative disc disease, and periarticular sources of pain in addition to the increased sensitivity to that pain as well as other painful or non-painful stimulation, I will refer to this symptom complex as fibromyalgia polypain, or simply polypain. Polypain is an acronym standing for polyregional pain and increased nociception. All patients diagnosed as having fibromyalgia by the ACR criteria have polypain. Unlike fibromyalgia, it defines all individuals with chronic widespread pain and painful tenderness including everyone diagnosed with fibromyalgia. Polypain identifies the 2 major components related to the production of pain and its appreciation. First, it identifies the sources and causes of the pain. Second, it identifies increased sensitivity to that pain. Thus, the origin and distribution of pain can be quantified and qualified as can the factors that regulate pain awareness or pain sensitization. This provides the opportunity to appropriately categorize and classify patients in terms of site specific pain to optimize treatment and for further study by providing more homogeneous and well-defined groups.

What Else Patients with Chronic Widespread Pain and at Lease 11/18 Painfully Tender Fibromyalgia Points Really Have

Sleep Disturbances and Fatigue

As Table 4.9 shows, sleep disruption is very common in this group of patients, being noted in 90%. The average sleep latency, or time it takes to fall asleep, is 51 minutes ranging from no noticeable time at all up to 360 minutes. It took 15 minutes or longer to fall asleep in 76% of the respondents. The average frequency of wakening is 2.4 times nightly. The commonest reasons for wakening are nocturia (getting up at night to urinate) noted in 57% and pain noted in 51%. Other reasons for wakening include reasons unknown, noise/light, flush/sweat, nightmare/dream, psychological stress, intruding thoughts, and cough. The duration of sleep time was greater than 8 hours in 50% of the patients, between 6-8 hours in 41% of patients, and less than 6 hours in 9% of patients. The average duration of morning fatigue of the entire group is 67 minutes, but in the subgroup that had any morning fatigue and excluding those with no morning fatigue, the average duration was 138 minutes. Daytime fatigue was reported by 82% of respondents with 63% noting constant all day fatigue. Fatigue was noted to develop or worsen in the evening in 51% and develop or worsen in the morning in 39%. Daytime napping was undertaken by 53% for an average duration of the entire responding group of 44 minutes at an average frequency of approximately every other day.

Psychological Issues

Table 4.10 shows that the subjective reporting of stress or anxiety was highly prevalent with 91% of the responding group having a subjective awareness of stress and anxiety. Depression was almost as frequently reported, with subjective depression being reported by 89% of the group.

Subjective Sleep and Fatigue Symptoms (Number Assessed For Symptom Noted)	% Frequency In Assessed Group	Quantity Mean (Range)
Sleep		
Latency to Fall Asleep (74)		51 minutes (0-360)
Latency 15 minutes or longer to Fall Asleep (74)	76	
Disruption (91)	90	
Disruption – Wakenings/night (91)		2.4/night (0-20)
Nocturia	57	
Pain	51	
Reason Unknown	16	
Noise/Light	8	
Flush/Sweat	5	
Nightmare/Dream	4	
Psychological Stress	3	
Intruding Thoughts	1	
Cough	1	
Sleep Duration (56)		
Less than 6 hours	9	
6-8 hours	41	
More than 8 hours	50	
Morning Fatigue Duration (91)		67 minutes (0-660)
Morning Fatigue in those Reporting the Presence of Morning Fatigue (44)	48	138 minutes (0.5-660)
Daytime Fatigue (87)	82	
Constant All Day Fatigue	63	
Fatigue noted in the morning or Increased in the morning	39	
Fatigue noted in the evening or Increased in the evening	51	
Napping (73)		
None	47	
Yes	53	
Duration (73)		44 minutes (0-360)
Frequency (73)		0.45/day or every 2.2 days (0-2.5 per day)

Table 4.9: *Sleep disturbances and fatigue based on self-reporting.*

Subjective Psychological Symptoms (Number Assessed For Symptom Noted)	% Frequency In Assessed Group
Stress/Anxiety (55)	91
Depression (56)	89

Table 4.10: *Psychological issues based on self-reporting.*

Cognitive Function

Subjective cognitive impairment was reported often in the subgroup that was assessed for this, as noted in Table 4.11. Short term memory relates to holding information for one minute or less and relates to immediate recall and attention. Recent long term memory relates to holding information longer than one minute and relates to new learning. Remote long term memory refers to retrieval of established information. Patients reported subjective impairment or reduction in short term memory or recent long term memory in 77% of the respondents. Subjective impairment of remote long term memory was reported by only 19% of the group. Subjective difficulties in word and/or name finding such as correctly naming objects or people was reported in 68% of the group responding. Subjective difficulties with concentration such as being able to concentrate in reading, completing multi-step tasks, or writing for more than a few minutes or a few paragraphs was reported by 75% of the responding group. It is important to emphasize that this reporting is totally subjective and there is no objective data such as neuropsychological testing to assess the accuracy of the subjective observations nor to determine if any change in cognitive ability has occurred. It is also of note that all patients were able to provide a complex, long standing, detailed, first hand medical history and did not demonstrate any objective cognitive impairment during the assessments.

Subjective Cognitive Symptoms (Number Assessed For Symptom Noted)	% Frequency In Assessed Group
Impaired Short Term and/or Recent Long Term Memory (22)	77
Impaired Remote Long Term Memory (21)	19
Impaired Word and/or Name Finding (22)	68
Impaired Concentration (24)	75

Table 4.11: *Cognitive impairment based on self-reporting.*

Weight and Libido

As shown in Table 4.12, of the 81 patients responding to questions about changes in weight, 42% of them noted a weight gain averaging 22.8 pounds. The period of time for the weight gain was the interval from when the weight was last stable from a subjective standpoint. No change in weight was noted by 40% and weight loss was reported in 18%. Reduced libido was reported in 66% of the responding group.

What Patients with Chronic Widespread Pain and At Least 11/18 Painfully Tender Fibromyalgia Points Really Have

Based on the results above, we can now derive a composite picture of what an individual with widespread pain and at least 11/18 painfully tender fibromyalgia points, someone who would otherwise be diagnosed as having primary fibromyalgia by the ACR criteria, really has.

Typically she or he is between 30-60 years old and has a longstanding history of musculoskeletal pain related to the current presenting pain symptoms. The symptoms and findings are consistent with: the presence of primary generalized osteoarthritis involving the cervical spine, thoracic spine, lumbar spine, thumb first CMC joints, thumb first MCP joints, finger DIP and PIP joints, knee and patellofemoral joints, toe MTP, PIP joints, and other specific joint sites as noted; and degenerative disc disease involving the spine, predominantly the cervical and lumbar spine. Headaches related to the osteoarthritis of the cervical spine, cervical spine cephalalgia, are noted by the majority. There are frequent physical find-

Subjective Weight and Libido Changes (Number Assessed For Symptom Noted)	% Frequency In Assessed Group	Quantity Mean (Range)
Weight Change (81)		
Increase	42	
Average Reported Increase		22.8 pounds
Decrease	18	
No Change	40	
Reduced Libido (41)	66	

Table 4.12: *Subjective reporting of weight and libido changes.*

ings of osteoarthritis as well including the presence of osteophytes and joint deformities related to the osteoarthritis such as angular deformities and loss of arches in the feet. Stiffness on wakening in the morning is present in the majority. A thoracic rotoscoliosis is almost always present with leg length discrepancy noted in a large number of individuals. The thoracic rotoscoliosis is associated with secondary osteoarthritis changes related to the rotoscoliosis. Lumbosacral hyperextension is present in most and is a risk factor for the low back related symptoms. Iliotibial band tightness is present in most and is a risk factor for low back related symptoms and trochanteric bursitis. Periarticular symptoms and findings are also noted in many individuals with the most frequent findings being that of trochanteric bursitis followed by plantar fasciitis, subacromial bursitis/ supraspinatus tendinitis, pes anserine bursitis, flexor nodule painful tenderness, deep Achilles bursitis, epicondylitis, de Quervain's tenosynovitis, Achilles insertion tendinitis, and finger flexor tenosynovitis. Joint hypermobility may be noted with the hands most likely involved.

Increased nociception, as defined by painful tenderness in the soft tissues, is expected given the requirement that all patients have at least 11/ 18 painful fibromyalgia tender points. The range of increased nociception varies with basically two extremes being identified. The group at one end has distinctly painful fibromyalgia points, on the average having about 16/ 18 points positive. The group on the other end has widespread painful tenderness involving the soft tissues of all the extremities with most having involvement of the anterior and posterior chest as well as scalp and face and the painful fibromyalgia points are not distinct from the adjacent and remote soft tissue painful tenderness.

Sleep disturbances are noted by most individuals. The majority have difficulty falling asleep, taking an average of 51 minutes to do so. Almost all individuals waken from their sleep, averaging 2–3 times nightly. They

The Composite Polypain Individual:
Age: average range 30-60 years
Primary generalized osteoarthritis involving the cervical spine, lumbar spine, thoracic spine, thumb first CMC joints, thumb first MCP joints, finger DIP and PIP joints, knee and patellofemoral joints, toe MTP and PIP joints and other specific joint sites as noted; and degenerative disc disease involving the spine
Headaches related to the osteoarthritis of the cervical spine (cervical spine cephalalgia)
Physical findings of osteoarthritis including osteophytes and joint deformities related to the osteoarthritis
Stiffness on wakening
Thoracic rotoscoliosis with leg length discrepancy associated with secondary osteoarthritis
Lumbosacral hyperextension
Iliotibial band tightness
Periarticular symptoms and findings including trochanteric bursitis, plantar fasciitis, subacromial bursitis/supraspinatus tendinitis, pes anserine bursitis, flexor nodule painful tenderness, deep Achilles bursitis, epicondylitis, de Quervain's tenosynovitis, Achilles insertion tendinitis, and finger flexor tenosynovitis
Joint hypermobility
Increased nociception with painful tenderness in the soft tissues
Sleep disturbances with prolonged sleep latency and wakening from sleep
Fatigue
Psychological impairment with stress, anxiety, and depression
Subjective cognitive impairment
Reduced libido

Table 4.13: *The composite polypain individual that includes all individuals diagnosed with fibromyalgia by the ACR classification criteria for fibromyalgia.*

waken most frequently with a need to urinate, and/or with pain, or for reasons unknown.

Morning fatigue, defined as fatigue on wakening, is only noted by half of the individuals. However, daytime fatigue, defined as fatigue through the day, is noted by most with constant fatigue being noted most frequently and fatigue worsening as the day goes on noted next most frequently. About half the individuals undertake napping through the day which occurs on the average about every other day for 44 minutes.

Psychological impairment, with subjectively noted stress, anxiety, and depression is noted in almost all individuals.

Cognitive impairment, with subjectively noted impairment in short term and/or recent long term memory, word and/or name finding, and/or impaired concentration is noted by the majority.

Weight gain is noted in 42%. Reduced libido is noted in the majority.

Thus, the composite patient with widespread pain and tenderness has many features seen in patients with fibromyalgia, but most importantly and contrary to the existing knowledge in fibromyalgia, the source of pain in this group of patients is clearly identified and defined.

Part Three

The Fibromyalgia Polypain Model Explains Everything

Chapter 5

Fibromyalgia Polypain: A Model of Fibromyalgia and Chronic Widespread Pain With Tenderness

"Know what you don't know." — Jeff Sarkozi, M.D.

Polypain is an acronym standing for polyregional pain and increased nociception. It accurately identifies, describes, and defines the polyregional sources of osteoarthritis, degenerative disc disease, and periarticular sources of pain in addition to the increased sensitivity to that pain as well as other painful or non-painful stimulation seen in patients with widespread pain defined as pain on the left side of the body, the right side of the body, above the waist, below the waist and involving the axial skeleton for at least 3 months with at least 11/18 painfully tender fibromyalgia points who have no evidence of rheumatoid arthritis, connective tissue diseases such as systemic lupus erythematosus, infection related arthritis, metabolic related arthritis, or crystal related arthritis. In these individuals, polypain identifies: 1) the pain caused by primary generalized osteoarthritis predominantly involving the neck and back with associated degenerative disc disease and a variable combination of associated tendinitis, bursitis, and fasciitis; 2) and the tenderness with increased nociception (increased appreciation or sensitivity to a sensation being perceived as painful) to these painful sources, triggers, and drivers. All individuals with fibromyalgia have polypain.

The Polypain Model of Fibromyalgia and Chronic Widespread Pain With Tenderness

Polypain identifies the two major components related to the production of pain and its appreciation. First, and most importantly, unlike the situation with fibromyalgia to date in which there is no identified cause of pain, polypain clearly demonstrates identifiable and specific sources of polyregional pain. Second, the tenderness component identifies increased sensitivity to that pain as well as any other induced pain, consistent with what is seen in fibromyalgia. This increased sensitivity to pain is due to abnormal pain processing producing lowered pain thresholds. Thus, polypain provides the basis for a more accurate, specific, and appropriate two component model of chronic widespread pain and tenderness as seen in fibromyalgia and fibromyalgia-like syndromes. The basic two component polypain model is shown in Figure 5.1.

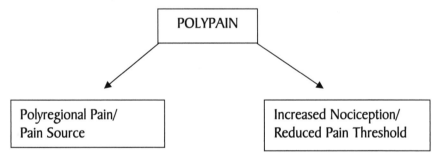

Figure 5.1: *Basic two component polypain model.*

Pain Begets Pain

The pain in polypain arises from polyregional pain occurring in multiple widespread areas. It is due to a combination of symptoms related to primary generalized osteoarthritis, degenerative disc disease, and a variable combination of periarticular pain symptoms associated with tendinitis, bursitis, and fasciitis. This causes mechanical and inflammatory mediators of pain to stimulate the pain process at the affected local sites. The chronic nature of these musculoskeletal conditions allows this pain stimulation to be sustained. In addition, these sites of local pain may generate referred pain, a process by which a local pain is sensed away from the site of origin.

The increased nociception or sensitivity to pain in polypain has been studied in patients with fibromyalgia. As discussed in Chapter 2, the evidence in the medical literature is strongly supportive of abnormal processing of pain in the central nervous system to physically induced pain such as pressure, heat, cold, or electrical stimulation resulting in generalized lowered pain thresholds in fibromyalgia. This leads to hyperalgesia, an increased pain response to a noxious stimulus; and allodynia, a pain response to what would normally be perceived as a non-painful stimulus. The best evidence supports central nervous system sensitization, or central sensitization for short, as the explanation for this process. Central sensitization is process that develops in the spinal cord pain pathways and spinal cord dorsal horn pain message areas whereby a repetitive or ongoing painful stimulus sensitizes these pathways. The result of this sensitization is the development of reduced pain thresholds, increased sensitivity to painful stimuli, spreading of the pain sensitivity field, and longer duration of pain after stimulation stops. Thus, in the face of central sensitization, stimulated pain is felt more readily, more severely, more broadly, and persists for a longer period of time after the stimulus is discontinued. This leads to the well recognized phenomena of pain magnification and pain amplification in fibromyalgia. Referred pain with pain felt far away from the site of the original pain stimulus is also, in part, explained by this phenomenon of central sensitization.

It is important to take note, however, that the development of central sensitization requires a repetitive or ongoing painful stimulus. Absent a pain stimulus, the central sensitization state eventually returns to normal. It is here that the concept of fibromyalgia has fallen apart. If there is no source of pain, as we have been led to believe with fibromyalgia, there can be no central sensitization, and there can be no increased sensitivity to pain. Polypain, on the other hand, clearly and unequivocally identifies the repetitive or chronic source of musculoskeletal pain and provides the basis through which central sensitization evolves and may persist. Fibromyalgia does not. Polypain and central sensitization also explain the phenomenon of wind-up, a process whereby pain sensitivity progressively increases with repeated exposure to a painful stimulus through a process called temporal summation. In essence, pain begets pain.

There is also another mechanism of pain that has not been recognized in fibromyalgia due to the absence of evidence for a cause of pain in fibromyalgia that also addresses a component of pain appreciation in polypain. This is known as primary hyperalgesia or peripheral sensitization and is a process that develops directly at the site of pain causing sensitization of the pain sensor area. This results in reduced pain thresholds and increased sensitivity to pain at the local site of pain. The local painful areas identified in polypain are subject to this process. Again, pain begets pain.

The Polypain Model Explains The Interaction of Sleep and Pain

Another important factor affecting sensitivity to pain in polypain has also been richly studied in fibromyalgia. There is an abundance of supportive evidence in the medical literature correlating sleep disturbances with reduced pain thresholds and increased pain sensitivity. Indeed, there are studies clearly showing the experimental induction of increased pain sensitivity by introducing sleep disruption to normal individuals. Disruption of slow wave, stage 3 and stage 4 Non-Rapid Eye Movement (NREM) sleep has been strongly correlated with the symptoms of fibromyalgia. The poorer the sleep quality and architecture, the more the sleep disruption, the greater the pain felt, and the lower the pain thresholds. Sleep disruption in polypain is noted in 90% of the patients and clearly plays a significant role in affecting pain sensitivity and thresholds. It appears the facilitation of pain by sleep disturbances arises somewhere in the brain and heightens pain sensitivity and reduces pain thresholds by sending signals through spinal cord pain pathways to the spinal pain message areas to reduce pain thresholds.

The Polypain Model Explains the Interaction of Psychological Disturbances and Pain

In assessing the psychological components of pain perception in individuals with fibromyalgia, there is strong evidence for a higher prevalence of psychological symptoms in those with fibromyalgia compared to controls. Patients with fibromyalgia have a greater number of lifetime psychiatric diagnoses compared to controls. The most frequent psychiatric disorders in these patients are anxiety, stress, and depression. Amongst patients with chronic musculoskeletal pain, there is an increased prevalence of depression. The psychiatric symptoms correlate directly with health-care seeking behavior and the perceived severity of the symptoms of pain. In chronic musculoskeletal disease, psychological status is a major determinant of health status along with physical functioning and the pain itself. Clearly, anxiety, stress, and depression significantly affect the appreciation of pain and its presentation in fibromyalgia.

The mechanism of how stress, anxiety, and depression modulate pain is not precisely known. As noted in Chapter 2, fibromyalgia patients display impairment in diffuse noxious inhibitory control, a central nervous system mechanism that mediates the severity of a painful stimulus. It appears the facilitation of pain by psychological disturbances such as anxiety, stress, and depression and the associated cognitive behavioral responses arises somewhere in the brain to heighten pain sensitivity and reduce pain thresholds by sending signals through spinal cord pain pathways to the spinal pain message areas to lower pain thresholds.

As noted, the individuals with polypain have a high prevalence of self-reported stress and anxiety in 91% and depression in 89%. My own experience with polypain patients clearly shows a relationship between pain quality and quantity that correlates with the presence and severity of the psychological disturbance. This relationship holds for the other symptoms of polypain as well. In addition, psychological disruption may have other effects that impact pain processing such as disrupting sleep and affecting physical functioning such as producing muscle tension or inappropriate physical posturing that may directly impact the pain arising from the musculoskeletal symptoms.

The Polypain Model Explains Fibromyalgia and Chronic Widespread Pain With Tenderness

Thus, the basic polypain two component model above can be broadened to include these factors to create the Polypain Model as shown in Figure 5.2. The Polypain Model is a two component model that identifies the sources by which pain is generated and the mechanisms by which tenderness and increased nociception with increased sensitivity to pain develops in individuals with polypain. The Polypain Model consists of: 1) pain caused by primary generalized osteoarthritis predominantly involving the neck and back with associated degenerative disc disease and a variable combination of associated tendinitis, bursitis, and fasciitis; 2) and tenderness with increased nociception, increased sensitivity with reduced pain thresholds, to these painful sources, triggers, and drivers modulated by the pain sources themselves, sleep disturbances, and psychological disturbances. All individuals with fibromyalgia have polypain.

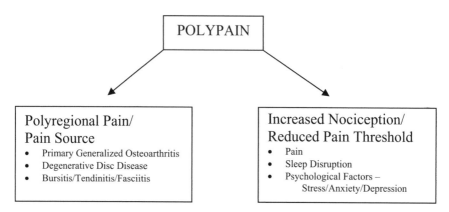

Figure 5.2: The Polypain Model.

The appreciation of pain itself or the degree of pain perceived is an interplay between the pain stimulus itself and the pain threshold. The Polypain Model accounts for the variation of pain experienced by individuals with polypain and serves well in understanding pain and its management in my polypain patients. The appreciation or perception of pain is dependent upon the severity or intensity of the pain generated by the pain source relative to the set level of the pain threshold. If the pain severity or intensity being generated is below the given pain threshold, then no pain is appreciated or perceived. If pain severity or intensity being generated is above the given pain threshold, then pain is felt. Figures 5.3 and 5.4 graphically display these circumstances. Basically, if the pain threshold level is set, for example at level 5 pain perception, any pain intensity generated by a pain source below level 5 will not be felt and any pain intensity generated by a pain source above level 5 will be.

Similarly, the other significant component impacting the appreciation or perception of pain is the set level of the pain threshold relative to the severity of pain. Thus, if the pain threshold is above the intensity set level of the pain source, no pain is felt by the individual. However, if the pain threshold falls below the intensity set level of the pain source due to factors related to pain related central sensitization, sleep disruption, and psychological factors, then the individual will note pain. This information is graphically displayed in Figures 5.5 and 5.6. In these examples, the pain intensity generated by the pain source is at a severity of level 5 and the

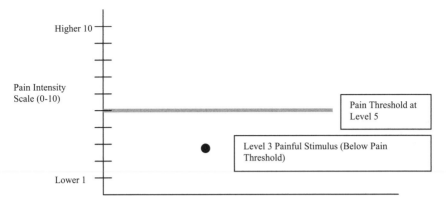

Figure 5.3: *Low level painful stimulus intensity below pain threshold. No pain felt by the individual.*

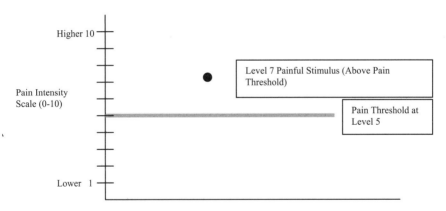

Figure 5.4: *High level painful stimulus intensity above pain threshold. Pain felt by the individual.*

pain threshold varies (compared to Figures 5.3 and 5.4 in which the pain intensity generated by the pain varies and the pain threshold set at level 5). As seen in Figure 5.5, if the pain threshold is above the pain source intensity of level 5, then no pain is felt as the pain source severity is below the perception level for pain. In Figure 5.6, the pain threshold falls below the level 5 pain intensity being generated by the pain source causing pain to be noted by the individual.

Therefore, the Polypain Model provides for the dynamic interaction between the pain source itself and the factors that influence the processing of this pain information by altering nociception and pain thresholds. Individuals, including patients with polypain, have no way of gauging their pain in an absolute manner. All pain is subjective and, therefore, all pain is relative to one's own framework. Basically, one person's severe pain may be someone else's mild pain despite the exact same musculoskeletal symptoms and findings. Assuming the same drivers and generators of pain exist in two individuals, then the subjectivity of interpretation lies in the pain thresholds. This is in part due to the genetic inheritance of pain sensitivity with evidence that women

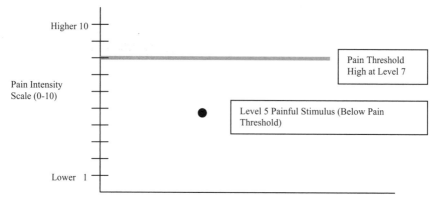

Figure 5.5: High pain threshold above pain stimulus intensity level. No pain felt by individual.

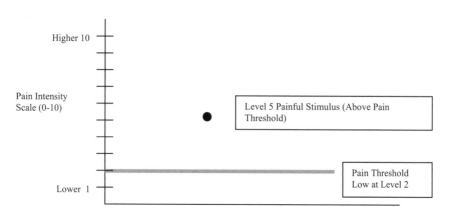

Figure 5.6: Low pain threshold below pain stimulus intensity level. Pain felt by the individual.

with fibromyalgia have more tenderness and lower pain thresholds compared to men with fibromyalgia and increased tenderness and lowered pain thresholds are noted in first degree female relatives of individuals diagnosed with fibromyalgia. In other part, it is due to modulation of pain thresholds by the exposure to pain as well as sleep disturbances and psychological factors. Patients cannot distinguish the independent contributions of the sources of pain and pain thresholds that create the perception of pain and its severity. Ultimately, it is the relative relationship of pain stimulus to pain threshold that determines not only the presence of symptoms but also the severity of symptoms. Thus, the subjective recognition of pain and its severity is identified by the size of the pain gap between the severity of the pain stimulus and the threshold to sense that pain. When the level of pain generated by the sources of pain exceeds the pain threshold level, a pain gap develops. The pain gap between the level of the pain stimulus generated and pain threshold level serves as a marker to gauge the severity of pain appreciated by the individual. The larger the gap between pain and pain threshold, the more severe the symptoms. This is depicted in Figure 5.7. Similarly, when the pain threshold level is higher than the level of pain generated by the sources of pain, a pain free gap develops. If this pain free gap develops by virtue of treatment, then this leads to therapeutic reserve. This is shown in Figure 5.8. In the presence of a therapeutic reserve, activities that would have otherwise caused pain would generate increased pain drive and raise the pain stimulus level, but the stimulation would not be perceived as painful as long as the increased pain stimulus fails to reach the pain threshold. Thus, the larger the pain free gap, the more therapeutic reserve is available to draw on before pain symptoms appear.

The Polypain Model Explains Why Today's Pain Is The Worst Pain

Another concept the Polypain Model helps explain is the concept of chronic pain memory. Just as patients are unable to gauge their current symptoms relative to others in an absolute manner due to the subjectivity of pain, they also have difficulty gauging their current symptoms relative to their past appreciation of symptoms of their pain. There is good evidence to show that individuals suffering chronic pain, especially chronic nociceptive pain, do not recall the severity of their prior chronic pain accurately. Generally, today's pain is the worst pain. Some of the factors contributing to this have been attributed

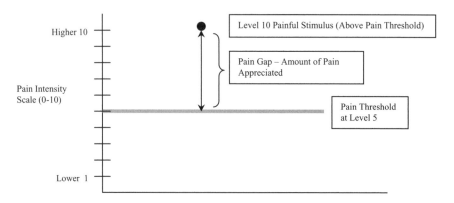

Figure 5.7: *Pain gap.*

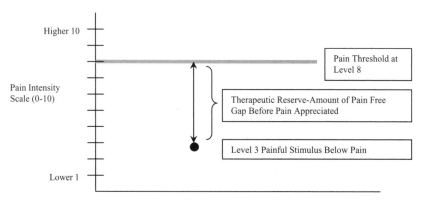

Figure 5.8: *Therapeutic reserve/Pain free gap.*

to the fundamental issues of recalling past events. This process of recall is biased by the fact that more recent experiences influence recall, individuals are prone to post-hoc analysis whereby past events are selectively reconstructed to explain the current circumstance, more intense or more salient experiences are better recalled, more recent events are more easily recalled and are disproportionately remembered, and background psychological state influences recall of certain events such that an individual in a bad mood is more likely to recall bad or negative events. The components of this memory effect are also related to the relationship of pain and pain thresholds over time. To understand this concept, we need to consider the factor of functional activity and

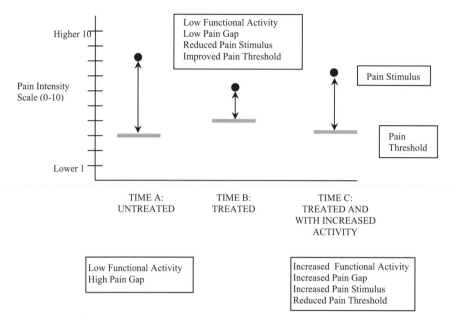

Figure 5.9: *Time-related changes in pain appreciation.*

the effect of usage, biomechanics, ergonomics, and posture on the sources of pain in polypain. In essence, interpretation of pain appreciation over time is strongly affected by the functional activity level of the individual. The patient will, as best as possible, avoid activities that trigger or worsen the osteoarthritis, bursitis, tendinitis, and fasciitis. The decrease in activity will result in lesser pain being driven by the sources of pain reducing the pain level, improving pain thresholds, and improving the relationship of pain stimulus to pain threshold. Figure 5.9 depicts this change from Time A to Time B. However, as pain improves whether by avoidance or by treatment, the natural tendency of the individual will be to increase the activity level. This increased activity will cause an increase in joint and periarticular related symptoms that are not adequately controlled and worsen the relationship of pain stimulus to pain threshold. This is depicted in Figure 5.9 as the change from Time B to Time C. This relative recent change in symptoms over time is what will be recalled as the time-related recall of change in symptoms. Patients will report that they feel worse for the interval from time A to time C despite still having a lesser pain gap at time C compared to time A and being overall better at time C compared to time A. As patients will always try to do more, especially as they improve, the natural tendency is to have a relative worsening of appreciated pain over time despite improvements in pain and pain threshold. Thus, the Polypain Model provides a basis by which to understand and evaluate changes in pain appreciation over time.

The Polypain Model Explains How True Improvement May Occur But Not Be Felt

In addition to the issue of pain memory, the Polypain Model also provides for a basis of understanding as to why seemingly reasonable interventions may produce objective signs of improvement but no subjective sense of improvement. If the pain gap, the difference between the pain stimulus and the pain threshold is very large in the presence of a very low pain threshold, the patient may not sense objectively measurable decreases in pain source intensity and effective, but not optimized, therapies may be discarded. For instance, as Figure 5.10 depicts, if the pain threshold is at level 1 and pain stimulus is at level 10, a 20% improvement in pain stimulus by the use of appropriate pain treatment would reduce the pain stimulus level to 8. Yet, despite the improvement in pain stimulus, a considerably large gap still exists and the patient might not be sensitive to that clinically significant change because the residual pain threshold remains low and the gap still remains large.

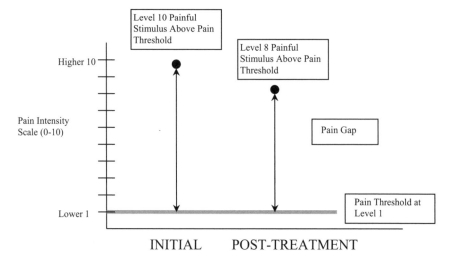

Figure 5.10: Pain gap after treatment of the pain stimulus.

The Polypain Model Explains
Why Symptoms Vary Over Time

Of course these descriptions are simplistic as they are limited to single measures of the relationship of pain stimulus to pain threshold. Pain generation and pain threshold are in constant flux in polypain. Polypain, and thus fibromyalgia, does not exist in a vacuum. As such, there are numerous factors impacting the generation of pain at the polyregional pain sites involved with active primary generalized osteoarthritis, degenerative disc disease, bursitis, tendinitis, and fasciitis. Joint and joint related structures exist for one reason and one reason only: to allow movement of the joint. Unfortunately, the presence of joint and joint related disease can be adversely impacted by use and movement and symptoms are affected by usage, adverse biomechanics, adverse ergonomics, and posture from moment to moment. Similarly, nociception and pain thresholds are affected not only by the severity of pain and how it varies but also by the highly situation specific factors that affect psychological well-being and sleep. Thus, symptoms vary moment to moment, throughout the day, day to day, and gradually over longer periods of time measured in years as primary generalized osteoarthritis, degenerative disc disease and the chronic sequelae of periarticular disease progress.

While the relationship of pain to pain threshold identifies the symptoms experienced by the individual, this relationship is not static over time. As Figure 5.II depicts, the course of primary generalized osteoarthritis and related polyregional pain is a variable but progressive process over a lifetime. The course of pain threshold is also variable and plastic in relationship to the factors that modify it, predominantly pain itself, sleep related factors, and psychological disturbances. Thus, up until point A in Figure 5.II, despite the presence of established osteoarthritis and degenerative disc disease at a subclinical but pathologically identifiable level, the disease course to that point does not produce discernable symptoms as the pain stimulus does not exceed the pain threshold. It is subclinical and without physical symptoms. The graph clearly identifies the concept that the absence of symptoms does not imply the absence of disease. At point A, the pain generation exceeds the pain threshold and becomes symptomatic. At point B, the pain stimulus continues to exceed the pain threshold with ongoing perceived pain. At point X, the relationship between pain stimulus and pain threshold improves with pain threshold being higher than the pain stimulus. This occurs as a result of reduced pain stimulation from reduced movement and loading of the affected joint areas and/or treatment interventions directed at the pain. The improved pain thresholds are a result of improvement in pain, sleep, and psychological factors in some combination. Subsequent to point X, the pain stimulus and pain threshold vary in relation to these factors, producing varying intensities of symptoms that an individual with polypain would sense including symptom-free periods. Due to disease progression however, subsequent to point C, despite the variation in pain stimulus and pain threshold, the pain stimulus always exceeds the pain threshold with constant but variable symptoms.

This "polypain effect" also explains why the absence of symptoms is not the absence of musculoskeletal disease such as primary generalized osteoarthritis, degenerative disc disease, chronic tendinitis, bursitis, and fasciitis. It explains why the symptoms of pain in the presence of underlying musculoskeletal disease as identified by other means such as lab tests, radiographic studies, or provocative clinical examination do not necessar-

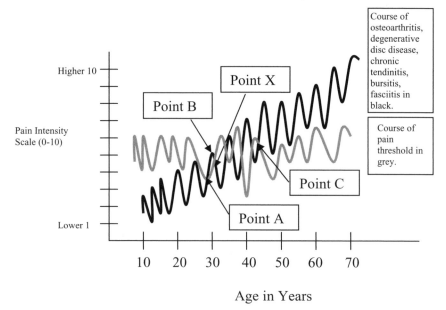

Figure 5.II: *The relationship of primary generalized osteoarthritis and chronic polyregional pain to pain threshold over a lifetime.*

ily correlate with each other and why there can be underlying progressive disease that is subclinical and without any symptoms. It further underscores the critical importance of early disease recognition for earlier treatment intervention to minimize the symptomatic impact of progressive musculoskeletal disease by keeping the pain stimulus as far below as possible from the pain threshold and maintaining optimal joint and joint related health and function.

The Polypain Model Explains Why Placebo Treatment Works and Why Symptoms May Worsen With Effective Treatment

Polypain additionally explains two other well known phenomena of any chronic widespread musculoskeletal pain process. No matter how bad one feels, one will always feel better even absent direct medical intervention. Similarly, no matter how good one feels, even absent any obvious effort, one is bound to be worse. This is depicted in Figure 5.II by point B, where in that time frame there is a peak in symptoms. Even absent specific treatment, the underlying factors that impact musculoskeletal pain such as usage, adverse biomechanics, adverse ergonomics, and posture as well those impacting pain thresholds such as highly situation specific factors that affect psychological well-being and sleep will be subconsciously and self-protectively optimized by the patient. Such accommodations and modifications result in reduced pain stimulation and improved pain thresholds as denoted by point X. The end result is that lesser pain is sensed. This, in part, accounts for the well known phenomenon of the placebo effect with regard to widespread musculoskeletal pain. The same process applies when symptoms are at a nadir. As one feels better, the natural tendency is to do more, thereby introducing more usage, adverse biomechanics, adverse ergonomics, and unfavorable posture on the joints and joint related structures in addition to adversely impacting pain threshold issues such as psychological well-being and sleep. The outcome will then result in increased pain generation and reduced pain thresholds with resultant increased pain being sensed. In statistical terms, this is known as regression to the mean. However, because the pain stimulus curve is up-sloped, the mean constantly rises over time with ongoing, progressive generalized osteoarthritis, degenerative disc disease, chronic tendinitis, bursitis, and fasciitis.

The Polypain Model Explains Why Symptoms Vary Through The Day

The same consideration applies even when considering the variable severity of symptoms throughout an average day. Figure 5.12 depicts an example of the frequently reported worsening of symptoms as the day progresses in individuals with polypain. At point B, after a day of use and movement of affected joint and perarticular sites, there is increased pain stimulation coupled with increased sensitivity to pain with reduced pain thresholds at that later point in the day compared to point A earlier in the day. Point A demonstrates the beneficial effect of sleep on reducing pain and improving pain thresholds which are adversely impacted through the day from joint use and movement. Day to day variation is highly individualized and is affected by multiple factors associated with joint use and movement including extent and degree of usage, biomechanics, ergonomics, and posture from moment to moment as well as the factors affecting pain thresholds including the severity of pain and how it varies and the highly situation specific factors that affect psychological well-being and sleep.

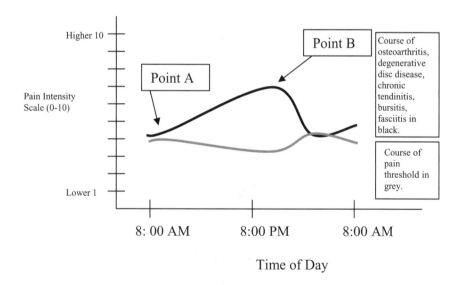

Figure 5.12: *Example of the relationship of primary generalized osteoarthritis and chronic polyregional pain to pain threshold over the time span of one day.*

The Polypain Model Explains Other Sensitivities

Additionally, the Polypain Model fully confirms an obvious experience we are all innately aware of. Namely, any pleasant or non-specific sensory experience can become unpleasant depending on the level of sensory input and the threshold for receiving that sensation. Patients with fibromyalgia are reported to have multiple sensitivities such as to temperature, medications, sounds, lights as well as irritability of the bowel and bladder. This is consistent with the Polypain Model generalized to any sensory input with reduced threshold for that sensation as depicted in Figure 5.13.

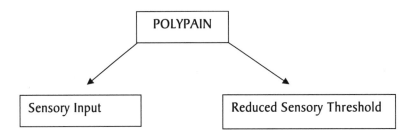

Figure 5.13: *The Generalized Polypain Sensory Model*

The Polypain Model Explains Fatigue

The Polypain Model also likely accounts for the most of the variation of the fatigue experienced in polypain. Fatigue, in essence is an interplay between the available energy to do things and the threshold at which the energy is expended. The factors that affect the energy threshold are the same as those affecting pain thresholds, namely pain, sleep disturbance, and psychological factors of stress, anxiety, and depression. This is consistent with the evidence regarding fatigue noted in fibromyalgia which has been attributed to sleep disruption, psychological stressors including depression, deconditioning related to symptoms, and endocrine dysfunction. One other important factor impacting fatigue may be that of medication side effect.

The Polypain Model Explains Chronic Widespread Pain and Tenderness in Other Rheumatologic Conditions

While not specifically studied herein, patients with features of fibromyalgia who have other rheumatologic conditions such as associated rheumatoid arthritis, connective tissue diseases such as systemic lupus erythematosus, infection related arthritis, metabolic related arthritis, or crystal related arthritis likely have polypain with a contribution of pain from the associated arthritis condition. The Polypain Model remains completely consistent and applicable with the additional understanding that the source of pain arises from the accompanying active arthritis. The Polypain Model can be used to categorize any widespread pain and tenderness syndrome by categorizing the source of pain and the factors contributing to increased nociception and reduced pain thresholds.

The Need for Thorough, Comprehensive Assessment

The evaluation of where an individual is in regard to pain stimulus sources relative to pain threshold requires a detailed historical and physical evaluation of each individual site and region of pain to determine the contribution of each to the overall presence of pain. Similarly, a detailed evaluation of the pain, sleep, and psychological factors along with measurements of tenderness is required to determine the contribution of the pain threshold level to the overall pain. Such an assessment provides the ability to classify polypain patients in a manner similar to what we do with patients with rheumatoid arthritis or systemic lupus erythematosus. For instance, patients with rheumatoid arthritis are defined by whether they are rheumatoid factor positive, whether they have erosive joint disease, whether they have joint deformities or destruction, whether they have extra-articular features such as nodules, Sjogren's syndrome or Felty's syndrome, by the total active joint count and damaged joint count, and other factors. Similarly, patients with systemic lupus erythematosus are categorized by virtue of their major clinical organ involvement such as subacute cutaneous lupus, renal lupus, or neuropsychiatric lupus and other clinical features, as well as by their autoantibodies such as being anti-SSA (anti-

Ro) antibody positive or anticardiolipin antibody positive and others in addition to markers of disease activity such as levels of anti-double-stranded DNA and complement levels. In similar way, polypain patients should be categorized as to the distribution of joint involvement, the presence of osteophytes, joint deformity, hypermobility, the presence of rotoscoliosis, the presence of leg length discrepancy, the distribution of periarticular involvement, the distribution and degree of soft tissue tenderness, the nature of the sleep disruption and psychological factors, and other associated factors impacting the presentation of polypain. This type of evaluation and synthesis provides for an understanding of the factors contributing to the patient's symptoms, provides for an understanding of the patient's perception of pain, and provides more specific targeted avenues for interventions needed to control pain and pain threshold issues.

Chapter 6

Fibromyalgia Polypain Management Principles: The Basis of Effective Integrated Treatment

"You can't always get what you want, you can't always get what you want, you can't always get what you want...but if you try sometimes...you might find... you get what you need."
—The Rolling Stones, You Can't Always Get What You Want, 1969

By understanding the sources from which pain is generated and how such pain message is modulated, specific and targeted treatment can be developed. Such treatment must be considered in the context that polypain is a chronic disease process influenced by: 1) pain caused by primary generalized osteoarthritis predominantly involving the neck and back with associated degenerative disc disease and a variable combination of associated tendinitis, bursitis, and fasciitis; 2) and the interaction of the pain sources, sleep disturbances, and psychological disturbances on pain perception modulation resulting in the increased nociception and tenderness.

The General Polypain Treatment Principles

1. It's about the polyregional musculoskeletal pain first, and then the pain threshold.

a. Treat the source of pain first, then the pain thresholds.

The entire cascade of events occurring in polypain develops primarily as a result of polyregional musculoskeletal pain. The pain stimulus of polypain is neither vague nor non-specific as described in Chapters 4 and 5. Absent the polyregional musculoskeletal pain stimuli from primary generalized osteoarthritis predominantly involving the neck and back with associated degenerative disc disease and a variable combination of associated tendinitis, bursitis, and fasciitis there would be no pain. If there is no pain source, there is no pain. Like a tuner in a sound system, pain thresholds are the volume control and determine the intensity of the pain; the pain itself is like the radio station signal, waiting to be received and converted into sound. No matter how loud the volume is adjusted, there is no sound if the system is not tuned to a station signal. Thus it is with polypain. The symptoms of polypain are driven by the pain signal of polyregional musculoskeletal disease which is converted by the mind and body to produce the symptoms and findings of polypain. A strong signal is easier to tune into and receive than a weak signal and thus it is in regard to the musculoskeletal pain sources identified in polypain. The more painful the stimulus, the more likely it will be felt, and when sensed, the more intensely it will be felt with a larger pain gap. On the other hand, independent of pain threshold, the lesser the polyregional pain stimulus the less intense the pain appreciated with a smaller pain gap. Once the pain stimulus falls below the pain threshold, pain indeed will not be sensed and there will be a therapeutic reserve/pain free gap. Pain gap and theraputic reserve/pain free gap are described in Chapter 5. Ultimately, regardless of pain thresholds: no pain source – no pain. Thus, the issue of pain thresholds is relevant only in the face of a pain stimulus.

Continuing with the analogy of the tuner and the sound system, if the sound system is tuned to a particular radio station, then the volume control determines the intensity of the sound. The symptoms of polypain are driven by the pain signal of polyregional musculoskeletal disease which is converted by the mind and body to produce the symptoms and findings of polypain. Pain thresholds are the volume control which determine the intensity of the pain signal after the pain stimulus is processed. Just like turning up the volume on the sound system, the lower the pain threshold, the more likely pain will be felt, and when sensed, the more intensely it will be felt with a larger pain gap. On the other hand, independent of the level of pain stimulation, just like turning down the volume on the sound system, the higher the pain threshold, the less intense the pain appreciated with a smaller pain gap. Once the pain threshold rises above the pain stimulus, just like turning the volume off on the sound system, pain will not be sensed despite the ongoing pain signal, and there will be a therapeutic reserve/pain free gap. This is described in Chapter 5, Figures 5.5, through 5.8.

These concepts lead to two critical management principles. First, there is an underlying disease process that causes pain. It can be identified clinically, radiographically, and pathologically. Thus, treatment must primarily be directed toward the management of primary generalized osteoarthritis predominantly involving the neck and back with associated degenerative disc disease and the variable combination of associated tendinitis, bursitis, and fasciitis. Second, there are abnormalities in the processing of pain generated by these pain drivers which relate to altered pain thresholds. The treatment of polypain clearly requires the management of the disease elements generating the pain as well as the management of the components that are independent of the pain source and related to the issues of pain processing that directly impact pain thresholds. In other words, there is a need for pain source specific pain management and pain source independent pain management related to pain message processing. Most crucially however, failing to attend to the disease specific components as is the current paradigm in fibromyalgia, leads to the mostly unsuccessful treatment of fibromyalgia as reviewed in Chapter 2.

b. Reduce the variability in the pain drivers and pain thresholds, then reduce the baseline pain intensity level and raise the baseline pain threshold level to eliminate the pain gap and develop a pain free reserve.

As discussed in Chapter 5, the relationship between pain stimulus and pain threshold is a dynamic one. Symptoms vary moment to moment, day to day, and over years due to the progressive and chronic disease course of primary generalized osteoarthritis, degenerative disc disease, and the chronic sequelae of periarticular disease. The course of pain threshold is also variable and plastic in relationship to the factors that modify it: predominantly pain itself, sleep related factors, and psychological disturbances. This is depicted graphically in Chapter 5, Figures 5.11 and 5.12. This understanding lends itself to two more important treatment concepts with respect to managing the sources of pain and the pain thresholds. In the short term, treatment should be directed at reducing the variability of the pain itself and the pain thresholds. By flattening the two curves, the pain gap diminishes overall and lesser pain is sensed and appreciated. In the long term, treatment must be directed to lowering the baseline intensity of the pain generated by the polypain sources and raising the overall pain threshold baseline. As depicted in Figure 6.1, at point A, the pain

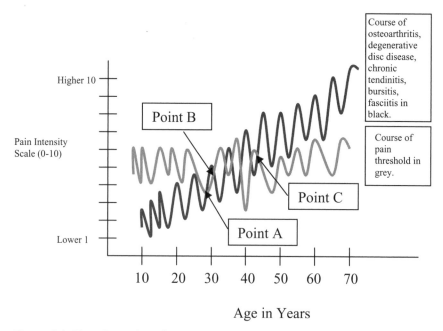

Figure 6.1: *The relationship of primary generalized osteoarthritis and chronic polyregional pain to pain threshold over a lifetime.*

generated by the sources of pain stimulation in polypain exceeds the pain threshold and becomes symptomatic. At point B, the relationship between pain stimulus and pain threshold improves with pain threshold being higher than the pain stimulus and the patient does not sense the ongoing disease processes of polypain as being painful. This occurs as a result reduced pain stimulation from reduced movement and loading of the affected joint areas and/or treatment interventions directed at the pain. The improved pain thresholds are a result of improvement in pain, sleep, and psychological factors in some combination. Subsequent to point B, the pain stimulus and pain threshold vary in relation to these factors, producing varying intensities of symptoms that an individual with polypain would sense coupled with pain free periods. Due to disease progression however, subsequent to point C, despite the variation in pain stimulus and pain threshold, the pain stimulus always exceeds the pain threshold with constant but variable symptoms.

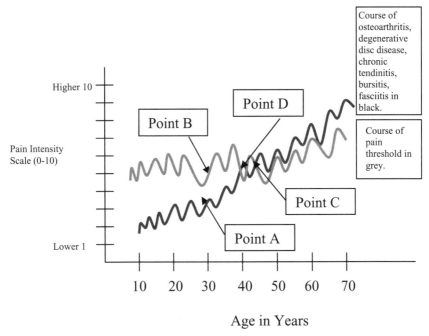

Figure 6.2: *The relationship of primary generalized osteoarthritis and chronic polyregional pain to pain threshold with treatment reducing the variability of the pain sources and pain thresholds.*

Figure 6.2 depicts the effect of treatment that **reduces the variability** of the sources of pain as well as the pain thresholds through the short term. At point A, where previously the patient became symptomatic in Figure 6.1, with treatment to reduce the variability, the patient remains asymptomatic and without pain. Indeed, in this example, the onset of the sensing of symptoms of pain is delayed by many years until point D by controlling the moment to moment, day to day, and long term variability of the sources of pain and pain threshold factors. In this example, subsequent to point C, the pain stimulus always exceeds the pain threshold with constant but variable symptoms. Note, however, that with tighter control of the pain stimulus variability and pain threshold variability, the pain gap is much smaller with overall less severe pain being sensed than the situation in Figure 6.1 when pain stimulus exceeds the pain threshold.

Figure 6.3 depicts the results of **therapeutically shifting the**

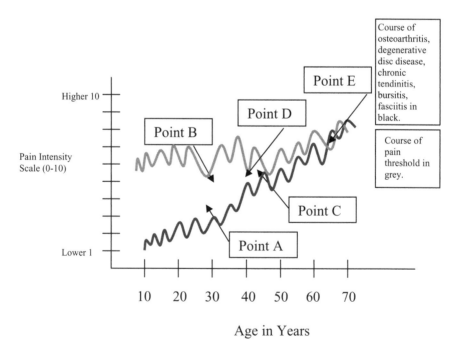

Figure 6.3: *The relationship of primary generalized osteoarthritis and chronic polyregional pain to pain threshold with treatment reducing the baseline pain stimulus and increasing the baseline pain threshold.*

baselines by lowering the baseline intensity of the pain generated by the polypain sources and raising the overall pain threshold baseline. Compared to Figure 6.2, in this example, the onset of the sensing of symptoms of pain is delayed further than point D until point E by additionally lowering the baseline pain stimulus level and raising the baseline pain threshold. In this example, subsequent to point E, the pain stimulus exceeds the pain threshold with the development of pain symptoms. Subsequent to point E, the pain stimulus and pain threshold vary in response to the factors impacting the intensity of symptoms that an individual with polypain would sense producing periods during which pain is sensed coupled with symptom free periods. Note again, however, that with tighter control of the pain stimulus variability and pain threshold variability, the pain gap is much smaller with overall less severe pain being sensed than the situation in Figure 6.2. There is also a longer period of therapeutic reserve/pain free gap lasting until point E in Figure 6.3 with larger therapeutic reserves overall prior to point E compared to the prior point A of Figure 6.1 and the prior point D of Figure 6.2.

Thus, by directing therapy at reducing the baseline variability of pain stimulus and pain threshold as well as reducing the overall intensity of pain stimulus and raising overall pain thresholds, pain symptoms are significantly reduced or eliminated in the short term. The onset of pain symptoms and the progression of polypain symptoms is subsequently delayed with less severe and less persistent symptoms developing in the long term.

c. Effective treatment requires an understanding of nociception and nociceptive pain processing.

The International Association for the Study of Pain defines pain as "an unpleasant sensory and emotional experience associated with actual or potential tissue damage or described in terms of such damage". The purpose of pain is protective to warn the individual of the presence of physical injury with tissue damage or the threat of such injury accompanied by the psychological and emotional components associated with the experience of pain even absent tissue injury. As discussed extensively, the appreciation of an identical painful stimulus is not homogeneous between individuals. Indeed, not all interactions with the environment are painful.

Most such interactions are bland and non-painful and some are pleasurable. Unfortunately, some interactions are painful. Even a bland or pleasurable stimulus can be stimulated sufficiently to become painful. On the other hand, many bland sensory interactions are readily adapted and incorporated into a new sensory state whereby such interactions are no longer recognized, such as not sensing a watch, ring, necklace, or glasses despite its ongoing presence. The polypain model accounts for the individual appreciation of pain as well as the degree of stimulation that produces a sense of pain by addressing the relationship between pain stimulus and pain threshold. To understand nociception and nociceptive pain processing in polypain, it is crucial to understand at what levels of the nervous system pain sources and pain thresholds are expressed and modified and how such pain transmission and modifications evolve neuroanatomically and neurophysiologically at a molecular level.

Nociception is a process that develops as a response to a noxious or tissue damaging stimulus with activation of nerve receptors known as primary afferent neurons. They respond to thermal, chemical, and mechanical pain stimuli and transduce these energies into electrical nerve impulses that send a message of pain to the central nervous system. These nerve receptors also respond to pain caused by inflammation in the area. In the case of polypain, the source of pain is polyregional musculoskeletal pain related to primary generalized osteoarthritis, degenerative disc disease, fasciitis, bursitis, and tendinitis. Pain from osteoarthritis derives from multiple sites including stress on the bone adjacent to the joint, inflammation in the joint, stress and stretch on the joint capsule, stress and stretch on the joint ligaments and tendons, inflammation of the joint related periarticular structures, the joint related muscles with stretch or spasm, and torn meniscal cartilage. Similar sources of pain are noted in degenerative disc disease. The pain from fasciitis, bursitis, and tendinitis is due to inflammation. Thus, the pain stimulus of polypain stimulates nociception directly as well as indirectly through the process of inflammation. This is depicted in the top portion of Figure 6.4.

In response to the tissue changes and inflammation, the nociceptor threshold for stimulation decreases. This occurs due to changes in the transducers themselves or to increased receptor sensitivity. The injured tissue releases inflammatory mediators which results in the increased production of the inflammatory mediators classified as prostaglandins. The prostaglandins and other inflammatory mediators act on receptors on the nerves stimulating signal transduction to produce sensitization of the nociceptive receptors with reduced pain stimulus thresholds. This process is known as peripheral sensitization. Thus, the initial pain and inflammation of polypain causes increased sensitivity to the ongoing pain and inflammation of polypain in an ongoing cycle where pain begets pain. See Figure 6.4.

The pain signal is then propagated through the process of conduction to the pain processing area in the spinal cord known as the dorsal horn.

The dorsal horn is an area of rich nerve cell or neuronal intercommunication and it is at the dorsal horn where significant components of pain signal processing occurs prior to the upward conduction of this modulated pain information through the spinothalamic tract to the brain. The primary afferent neurons carrying the pain signal interact with: 1) local interconnecting neurons related to modulating pain message; 2) projecting neurons that directly conduct pain message through the spinal cord via the spinothalamic tract; 3) wide dynamic range neurons thorough which convergent sensory information from other structures innervated by that spinal cord level but not necessarily involved in the pain process is simultaneously conducted and through which referred pain, pain felt in sites and tissues that are otherwise normal and not involved in pain generation, develops; 4) and descending modulation neurons that transmit signals from various areas of the brain to the dorsal horn to regulate and modify by inhibition or facilitation the incoming pain message before it is conducted upward to the brain and are responsible for increased pain sensitivity due to psychological disturbances, fear induced pain tolerance, and, at least in part, for the placebo effect. Multiple neurotransmitters and amino acids are involved in these nerve signal transmission pathways. It is at the dorsal horn site that central sensitization evolves. Central sensitization is a process whereby pain thresholds are modulated and reduced in response to repetitive painful stimulation to result in increased sensitivity to nociceptive pain. In addition to increased responsiveness and sensitivity to nociceptive pain stimuli with attendant pain amplification and magnification, the process of central sensitization leads an enlarged receptor field size of the dorsal horn cells as well as interaction with wide dynamic range neurons resulting in the development of referred pain with pain felt far away from the site of the original pain stimulation in normal tissues that are not exposed to any painful stimulus. Central sensitization also explains the phenomenon of wind-up, a process whereby pain sensitivity progressively increases with repeated stimulation by pain through a process called temporal summation. Again, pain begets pain. The dorsal horn is also highly plastic and changeable absent actual damage to the nervous system. Thus, absent an ongoing, repetitive pain stimulus and absent actual damage to the nervous system, the central sensitization state eventually returns to its normal baseline.

Central sensitization occurs through a complex interaction of multiple neurotransmitter and amino acids interacting with cell surface receptors in two phases. First, there occurs an immediate, nociceptor driven phase of central sensitization. This phase is similar to the process of peripheral sensitization with the release of neurotransmitter stimulated release of chemicals and inflammatory mediators that produce enhanced responsiveness. Subsequently, there is a delayed second phase with the development of central nervous system inflammation with endogenous production of prostaglandins in the central nervous system.

The processed pain signal is subsequently conducted upward through the spinothalamic tract in the spinal cord to various levels of the brain where further modification takes place and results in what is interpreted as the perception of pain. It is at this level that that affective, behavioral, and cognitive components modify the pain message resulting in pain responses manifested as pain behavior and suffering. In addition, it is also from the brain that the descending modulation pathway originates to send signals to the dorsal horn impacting pain message processing through inhibition or facilitation. See Figure 6.4.

The clinical model of polypain is consistent with and completely comports to the process of nociceptive pain processing. In polypain, the source of pain is polyregional musculoskeletal pain related to primary generalized osteoarthritis, degenerative disc disease, fasciitis, bursitis and tendinitis. The pain generated by these processes is clearly due to mechanical, chemical, and possibly thermal nociception as well as inflammation in the joint and joint related structures. There is chronic but variable

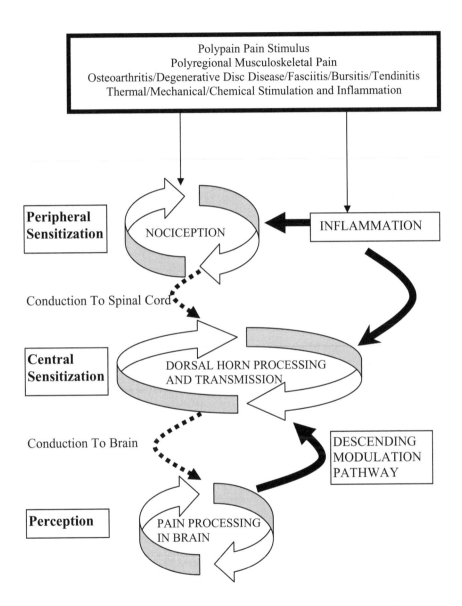

Figure 6.4: Nociception and nociceptive pain processing.

pain arising at the involved sites which are affected moment to moment, day to day, and over longer periods of time by multiple factors associated with joint use and movement including extent and degree of usage, biomechanics, ergonomics, and posture. Thus there is a chronic, repetitive pain stimulus generating nociceptive and inflammatory pain. The ongoing nociception and inflammation generates lowered pain thresholds through peripheral sensitization. The ongoing nociceptive and inflammatory pain message is conducted to the dorsal horn where this chronic and repetitive pain message is processed. As a result of this processing, central sensitization develops whereby pain thresholds are further reduced and the pain sensitivity fields are broadened. This results in pain amplification and magnification, referred pain, and wind-up. This processed pain message is then conducted to various sites in the brain where perception of pain occurs with further reduction of pain threshold as well as the development of the affective, behavioral, and cognitive responses to it. In addition, various areas of the brain generate a response to pain that is conducted through the descending modulation pathway back to the dorsal horn to impact pain thresholds through central sensitization. It is through this latter mechanism that impaired sleep and psychological disturbances such as stress, anxiety, and depression act to reduce pain thresholds in addition to the ongoing and repetitive pain message itself. It is also through this pathway that beliefs and expectations act to modulate pain thresholds such as increasing pain thresholds as seen in the placebo effect.

The clinical model of polypain also accounts for the biopsychosocial concept model of pain. This model brings together the concepts of the biologic aspects of pain with the cognitive, perceptual, psychological, and sociologic components of pain. This pain model incorporates the biological factors accounting for symptoms, including in the case of polypain, polyregional nociceptive and inflammatory pain. It also incorporates: 1) the impact of psychological disturbances such as anxiety, stress, and depression; 2) the cognitive perceptual effect of pain on the individual; 3) and the interpersonal interaction of the individual with others in relation to such factors as pain behavior, pain coping, self-efficacy, helplessness, cognitive distortion, and personality. In the case of polypain, these issues relate directly to the polyregional pain due to primary generalized osteoarthritis, degenerative disc disease, fasciitis, burstis, tendinitis, and the issues of pain processing. Finally, the biopsychosocial model considers interpersonal interactions and social factors associated with socioenvironmental function in related work, home, and recreation. In the case of polypain, again these issues relate directly to the polyregional pain due to primary generalized osteoarthritis, degenerative disc disease, fasciitis, burstis, tendinitis, and the issues of pain processing with reduced pain thresholds.

The clinical model of polypain further accounts for the process of neurogenic inflammation whereby the process of an inflammatory pain stimulus generating nociception and subsequent pain processing induces the release of neurotransmitters at the site of inflammation which themselves induce further inflammation. Basically, the musculoskeletal pain generated by the inflammation related to the primary generalized osteoarthritis, degenerative disc disease, fasciitis, bursitis, and tendinitis of polypain induces further inflammation. Thus, not only does inflammation generate pain, but pain generates further inflammation and pain not only begets pain unto itself, but also pain begets inflammation which in turn begets further pain and further inflammation.

d. Pain can be felt in sites remote from which the pain stimulus originates.

 Patients with polypain frequently feel pain in areas remote to joints and joint related structures. They may be painfully tender in areas that were otherwise not recognized to be painful subjectively and where there is no obvious joint, joint related structure, or other pain source. Such remotely perceived pain and painful tenderness occurs via two mechanisms. First, both peripheral and central sensitization produce referred pain. This develops through an enlarged receptor field size of primary afferent neurons and the dorsal horn cells resulting in a much larger area of pain sensitization and reduced pain thresholds than the original pain stimulus. Second, the interaction of nociceptive and inflammatory pain message with wide dynamic range neurons in the dorsal horn provides for the opportunity of convergent sensory input from other tissues and structures not affected by the pain stimulus to be essentially mixed with the pain signal and be perceived as being painful when in fact there is no pain stimulus present at those sites. In addition, the pain thresholds at those otherwise unaffected sites are reduced rendering those areas more tender to any pain stimulus that may occur at that site. This is exemplified by the soft tissue tenderness noted in fibromyalgia polypain.

Additionally, the normal innervation of the skin and deeper tissues does not always follow an obvious distribution. Figure 6.5 depicts the the cutaneous dermatomal nerve root distribution. Clearly, upper cervical spine involvement in polypain can lead to head pain, headaches, and tenderness known as cervical cephalalgia. Mid through lower cervical spine involvement may result in shoulder area pain, arm pain, chest pain and tenderness, or pain and tenderness between the shoulder blades. Thoracic spine involvement may cause chest pain and chest wall tenderness or abdominal pain and abdominal wall tenderness. Lumbar spine involvement may cause pain and tenderness in the hip areas, buttocks, legs or feet. In addition, the sensory nerves at any particular site in the body transmit sensory messages that are eventually processed at their respective nerve root origins and may similarly generate referred pain and tenderness in the dermatomal distribution of that nerve root level. For instance, shoulder pain refers pain to the upper outer arm, tennis elbow (lateral epicondylitis) and golfer's elbow (medial epicondylitis) refer pain to the forearm, hip joint pain refers to the groin, inner or outer thigh, knee, or buttock, and trochanteric bursitis refers to the outer thigh or buttock.

e. Pain is widespread because the pain stimulus of polypain arises in multiple sites and pain processing occurs at all sensory nerve root levels that receive pain message.

The above discussion regarding pain processing relates to one sensory nerve root level. A sensory nerve root level comprises the sensory input from the nerves in those parts of the body that are served and processed by a particular level of the spinal cord. The nerve roots exit the spinal cord between the vertebra. Thus, there are spinal sensory nerve roots receiving and processing information at 8 levels of the cervical spine, 12 levels of the thoracic spine, 5 levels of the lumbar spine, and the 5 levels of the sacral spine. Further, the pain stimulus of polypain is generated by primary generalized osteoarthritis including spinal osteoarthritis predominantly involving the cervical spine and lumbar spine, degenerative disc disease of the spine with predominant involvement of the cervi-

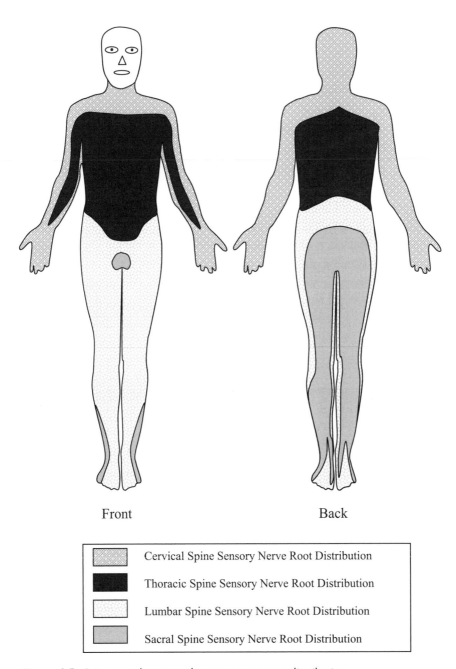

Front　　　　　　　Back

	Cervical Spine Sensory Nerve Root Distribution
	Thoracic Spine Sensory Nerve Root Distribution
	Lumbar Spine Sensory Nerve Root Distribution
	Sacral Spine Sensory Nerve Root Distribution

Figure 6.5: Cutaneous dermatomal sensory nerve root distribution.

cal spine and lumbar spine, and multiple areas of fasciitis, bursitis, and tendinitis. Thus, numerous levels of sensory nerve root pain information on both sides of the body are being processed simultaneously at their sites of origin as well as in their respective dorsal horn nerve root levels with attendant pain amplification and magnification, wind-up, and referred pain messages. Thus, it is easy to see how discrete and identifiable musculoskeletal pain due to the joint and joint related processes of polypain coupled with factors the alter pain thresholds such as sleep disturbances and psychological disturbances induces widespread pain and tenderness and becomes lost and indistinct in the widespread pain and tenderness that it generates.

2. The assessment is key.

Given that the pain stimulus and the pain threshold are the primary issues related to pain perception, the most critical component related to treatment is the patient assessment, especially in regard to the polyregional musculoskeletal assessment and the components related to pain thresholds. The assessment must be thorough and complete. The history taking component should include a detailed chronological review of the course of symptoms and interventions from the earliest presence of any pain symptoms. This chronology provides for an understanding of the natural history and progression of symptoms, functional ability, and the impact of factors affecting the symptoms including ergonomic and environmental influences as well as treatment interventions. This should be followed by a detailed, site specific joint and musculoskeletal regional review of all joint and joint related areas as well generalized, widespread symptoms to ascertain the nature and severity of site specific and widespread involvement, the impact on function, and the factors influencing symptoms. The degree of morning stiffness should be ascertained. Details regarding sleep including times, durations, disruptions, the nature of disruptions, sleep mechanics such as posture and support, and sleep quality including morning fatigue should be determined. Characteristics of daytime fatigue, daytime sleepiness, and napping are important to elucidate. A thorough review of functional ability is absolutely necessary given the treatment goals include not only symptom reduction but functional improvement as well. Functional items to assess include a thorough work history including work duties performed as well as work related disability, exercise and recreational sports activities, hand and upper extremity function, lower extremity function including walking ability, ability to get dressed, ability to bathe or shower, ability to drive, ability to participate and perform household duties and activities, hobbies, and recreational activities. A complete and detailed rheumatologic systems review is mandatory to assess for other underlying rheumatologic or general medical conditions causing or contributing to the pain or dysfunction reported by the patient and this should include any concerns or changes in sexual functioning in sexually active individuals as well as the use of recreational drugs. A detailed psychological and psychosocial history is mandatory. A review of cognitive abilities, impairments, and changes is required. A thorough and complete review of all current medications is mandatory including prescribed medications, over-the-counter medications, alternative medications, and supplements. A review of allergies and adverse drug reactions is mandatory. History of past health including surgeries, fractures, other medical illnesses, pregnancies, and the attendant details should be reviewed. Family medical history should noted for significant medical issues. Social history including family status, living conditions and arrangements, and the use of tobacco and alcohol should be described. A residual review of systems should be made for health matters not covered otherwise.

Similarly, the physical examination must be thorough and complete. It should include a general physical examination assessing the skin and extremities, head and neck, respiratory system, cardiovascular system, and abdominal sites. A complete neurological exam including a thorough determination of motor strength, sensation to different modalities, reflexes, gait, and coordination is necessary. The musculoskeletal exam must be thorough and complete. It must include a thorough and detailed examination of all joints as well as the cervical, thoracic, and lumbosacral spine. Sites must be assessed for issues of alignment, deformity, range of motion, tenderness, pain with motion, swelling, redness, warmth, and integrity of ligaments. The exam must include a thorough and detailed examination of periarticular sites including tendon sheaths, tendon insertions, bursa areas, and fascia areas. A detailed assessment of soft tissue, bone, and joint related tenderness is mandatory. Leg length discrepancy should be measured. The presence of hypermobility should be ascertained.

The role of laboratory investigation in polypain is fivefold. First it is done to assess, as clinically indicated, for the presence of other conditions that co-exist with polypain that contribute to pain. Second, it is done to determine, if the clinical picture is suggestive, if there is a musculoskeletal disease process that follows the polypain model but whose widespread pain is due to a process other than generalized osteoarthritis such as rheumatoid arthritis or systemic lupus erythematosus. Third, studies such as radiographic studies like X-rays and MRI help determine the degree of damage change in joints and the spine that may not be amenable to being reversed by treatment. Fourth, studies such as neurodiagnostic studies may help determine complications of osteoarthritis and degenerative disc disease such as nerve impingement that may contribute to symptoms. Fifth, blood tests need to be followed to assess for potential complications related to treatment such as side effects related to the stomach, kidney, or liver where early preclinical detection is critical.

Only this type of thorough and detailed assessment will allow proper identification and characterization of the polypain patient for purposes of individualized treatment as well as rendering prognosis. This type of assessment for a new patient with polypain may take several hours or more to complete. The typical 45-60 minute new patient assessment or 15 minute follow-up visit is simply not sufficient to cover the complexity and severity of the polyregional musculoskeletal pain issues and clinical components of polypain. After all, a new patient with just any one of the many clinical problems in polypain in isolation may take 45-60 minutes to be assessed. It is beyond reason or sense to expect the assessment of polypain with its polyregional musculoskeletal symptoms, sleep disruption, fatigue, functional impairment, psychological disturbances, cognitive impairments, and other associated clinical features could be performed in anywhere near that time.

Yet, such is the expectation of the current healthcare system. Healthcare administrators and insurers refuse to recognize the need for prolonged patient encounters even in the face of chronic widespread polyregional musculoskeletal pain. The healthcare system does not recognize the significant labor and time intensive cognitive effort that is reasonable and necessary to perform the required appropriate assessment that is mandatory to properly and adequately determine the diagnosis and characterization of the patient with chronic, widespread polyregional musculoskeletal pain such as fibromyalgia polypain. The health care system simply refuses to recognize the reality of chronic widespread musculoskeltal pain. Indeed, many health insurers have wrongly engaged in denial, deceit, and delay to reduce or avoid appropriate reimbursement for the care of chronic widespread musculoskeletal pain such as polypain to limit access to the individualized, specialized, and comprehensive healthcare services needed by patients with fibromyalgia polypain and by limiting access to appropriate medications through arbitrary formulary restrictions.

The only practitioners with the knowledge, skill, and training to assess and manage the polyregional musculoskeletal components of polypain are rheumatologists. This is contrary to current practice in which many patients with widespread musculoskeletal pain are often assessed and managed by pain specialist anesthesiologists, neurologists, orthopedic surgeons, and primary care physicians. Only rheumatologists can properly and adequately assess the polyregional musculoskeletal components of polypain. No one else. Unfortunately, many rheumatologists have no interest in the management of complicated, time-consuming, widespread musculoskeletal pain patients in their practice. Thus, it is crucial that the assessment and management of polypain be undertaken by a rheumatologist who understands that the source of pain is identifiable as arising from polyregional musculoskeletal sites, thoroughly comprehends how pain threshold modulates, and is committed the highly complex and time requiring challenges of polypain.

3. Polypain is a chronic disease – Treat by lysis, not by crisis.

The primary generalized osteoarthritis and spinal degenerative disc disease identified in polypain are chronic disease processes. Once the disease is present, it is always there. It does not necessarily have to be symptomatic, but even absent symptoms, established disease is established chronic disease. Indeed, there is a poor correlation between the biologic severity of osteoarthritis and spinal degenerative disc disease as measured against symptoms of pain and functional limitation across individuals. For instance, some individuals may have severe pain and limitation for what appears to be very mild osteoarthritis or degenerative disc disease on the basis of x-rays, CT scan, or MRI studies while others may have no symptoms in the face of severe radiographic joint damage changes.

However, in any one individual with symptoms, the symptomatic osteoarthritis and degenerative disc disease are due to the underlying established chronic disease processes regardless of the biologic and physiologic severity. Even in the face of intermittent symptoms that are modified by many factors including treatment and multiple factors associated with joint use and movement including extent and degree of usage, biomechanics, ergonomics and posture, it is crucial to recognize that such symptoms are being promoted and driven by a chronic, progressive disease process. Thus, treatment must not be limited to managing the symptom of the day. Treatment must not be based on the concept of a stubbed toe, a cut finger, or a sinus infection whereby the symptoms are managed acutely for a short period of time during which the body heals and eventually there is no residual health issue. Treatment of such self-limited, discrete episodes of illness is known as treatment by crisis, whereby, each event is a self-limited event requiring symptomatic intervention until it heals and goes way. To the contrary, the primary generalized osteoarthritis and spinal degenerative disc disease of polypain never go away, despite the variable intensity of clinical symptoms perceived. As such, treatment must focus on the chronic aspects of symptom management not only to control immediate symptoms but to reduce the progression of disease to control the long term evolution of symptoms. Further, the absence of symptoms is not the absence of disease. As such, even absent symptoms, treatment must also focus on the management of the underlying disease and disease processes to reverse the presence of all reversible elements of disease to prevent complications of the disease including the development of pain. This is known as treatment by lysis. Thus, effective treatment of polypain must be based on treatment by lysis, not crisis.

An obvious corollary to the chronic aspect of polypain is that once an individual has primary generalized osteoarthritis and degenerative disc disease, that person always has it. These chronic disease processes never go away. They are treatable. Reversible components can be managed. Symptoms can possibly be treated to the point where a patient might become asymptomatic and without functional limit. However, the underlying disease processes of polypain will persist in the background. Thus, chronic management involves a lifelong commitment to control the underlying primary generalized osteoarthritis and degenerative disc disease.

4. Polypain is progressive.

The primary generalized osteoarthritis and spinal degenerative disc disease as identified in polypain are not only chronic disease processes, but they are chronic and progressive disease processes. Additionally, the associated bursitis, tendinitis, and fasciitis of polypain are chronic and progressive if not effectively treated. Thus, treatment must also focus on the progressive aspects of these processes to reduce the progression of disease to control the long term evolution of symptoms. Once again, it is important to note that the absence of symptoms is not the absence of disease. As such, even absent symptoms, it is critical that treatment also focus on the management of the underlying disease and disease processes to reverse the presence of all reversible elements of disease to prevent complications of the disease including the development of pain.

5. Symptoms are not the same as disease.

The source of the pain drivers in polypain is primary generalized osteoarthritis predominantly involving the neck and back with associated degenerative disc disease and the variable combination of associated tendinitis, bursitis, and fasciitis. However, the perception of pain is dependent upon the relationship of the generated pain message to the pain threshold. Thus, despite the recognition that the primary generalized osteoarthritis and spinal degenerative disc disease of polypain are chronic and progressive disease processes, clinical symptoms such as pain do not correlate with other findings of biological disease severity. When osteoarthritis and degenerative disc disease initially manifest physiologically, there is a long period of time during which these processes are subclinical and without symptoms. As the disease process progresses, there may be evidence of osteoarthritis and degenerative disc disease by laboratory tests such as radiographic studies; yet again, without clinical symptoms or findings. This is depicted in Figure 6.1 above in which the recognized disease processes of polypain that generate pain message are below the individual's pain threshold, and thereby are not perceived by the individual as painful. This again demonstrates the important concept that the absence of symptoms is not the absence of disease. In those individuals who do develop pain symptoms, the pain generators due to the underlying primary generalized osteoarthritis, spinal degenerative disc disease, and associated tendinitis, bursitis, and fasciitis exceed the individual's pain threshold causing the perception of pain. However, this does not correlate with the biological severity of the osteoarthritis or degenerative disc disease. Therefore, clearly, symptoms are not the same as disease in polypain.

The two pain management principles of treating underlying disease first and treating pain thresholds independently by managing issues of pain processing have been addressed above. In addition to managing pain, controlling and reversing reversible components, and preventing progression of symptomatic established underlying primary generalized osteoarthritis with associated degenerative disc disease and the variable combination of associated tendinitis, bursitis, and fasciitis, it is equally important to identify sites of disease involvement that are not or never have been symptomatic. Treatment intervention at such involved but asymptomatic sites provides the ability to prevent progression of disease, reverse any reversible disease, and, most importantly, to prevent or limit the evolution of subclinical disease into painful disease.

6. Avoid chasing symptoms.

Polypain is a chronic, progressive disease. It is comprised of polyregional pain generated by underlying disease processes related to primary generalized osteoarthritis, degenerative disc disease, tendinitis, bursitis, fasciitis, and pain message processing abnormalities leading to reduced pain thresholds and referred pain with increased nociception. While the pattern of symptoms and disease may vary from individual to individual, the pattern of disease in any one individual tends to be consistent and reproducible. In other words, the mechanism of medication effect, extent and degree of joint usage, biomechanics, ergonomics, and posture that make symptoms better or worse in any particular region or site in any one individual varies within a limited range. How that individual trades off functional ability for pain tends to remain relatively consistent as well. What varies the most is the circumstance under which these reproducible events occur. The ability to recognize such common disease factors under different conditions and circumstances is the key to improving the feedback relationship of pain to function and ultimately stabilizing and reversing reversible disease. Thus, not only should we treat by lysis rather than crisis, but we must also to avoid chasing symptoms by failing to recognize or control external factors that drive or exacerbate musculoskeletal disease and drive or reduce pain thresholds. By getting ahead of symptoms, we are able to improve the relationship of pain stimulus to pain threshold, lessen perceived symptoms, and eventually allow the development of a therapeutic reserve/pain free gap whereby the extent and degree of joint usage, biomechanics, ergonomics, and posture do not generate sufficient pain message to be perceived as painful relative to the pain threshold as they would have prior to treatment intervention. This requires thorough, detailed, and vigilant rheumatologic follow-up to understand the impact of factors affecting symptoms and disease over time in order to maintain control of symptoms and disease. Failure to do such leads to ongoing but potentially treatable underlying disease activity and ongoing clinical symptoms punctuated by preventable exacerbations.

7. The polyregional musculoskeletal pain sources of polypain are all about the joints and their joint related structures.

The fundamental purpose of the human musculoskeletal system is for support. However, humans are not rigid or immobile like a tree. We are mobile and have purposeful mechanical interaction with our environment for survival and self-improvement. Thus, in addition to bones, we have joints that permit such mobility and movement. Of course, our joints would be of no use unless we had muscles to move them in various ways, ligaments to hold joints together and direct their movement, tendons to attach muscles to joint areas to permit motion, tendon sheaths in certain areas to provide smooth movement of tendons, bursa areas to reduce friction between tendons, and fascia combined with ligaments and bones to keep closely related joint structures aligned.

The joints themselves are highly specialized structures comprising different types, shapes, and sizes of joints depending on the site and need. The commonest joint type, found in most of the joint areas of the extremities and spine, is known as the diarthroidial joint in which two bones meet and are capped by cartilage known as hyaline cartilage and nourished and lubricated by a tissue known a synovial tissue. This is depicted in Figure 6.6.

A joint or a group of joints and the joint related structures exist for the sole purpose of movement of that joint area. Joint alignment, mobility, and motion subject joints to various forces at rest as well as movement

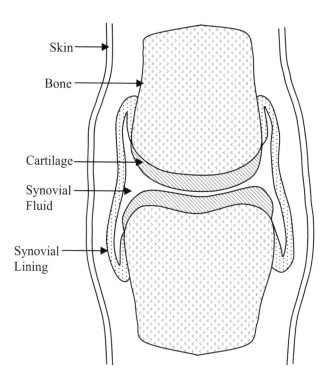

Figure 6.6: *The diarthroidial joint.*

related forces such as acceleration, deceleration, tension, compression loading, shear, torsion, and various combinations of these. Of course, in weight bearing joints, body weight is an additional loading force to consider. All of these elements are highly individualized given the number of joints an individual has, coupled with each individual's own inherited, genetically determined individual alignment of joints, degree of joint mobility, and factors and diseases affecting the health of the joint related structures and bone such as seen in osteoarthritis or other arthritic conditions. Further, all of this occurs against the background of highly individualized environmental interactions related to usage, biomechanics, ergonomics, and posture that have direct and specific effects on joint loading forces. Joints are meant to be moved and indeed depend on joint motion for joint cartilage health. And, therein lies the dilemma. It is the very movement and loading that the joints and periarticular structures were designed for that ultimately leads to the primary generalized osteoarthritis predominantly involving the neck and back with associated degenerative disc disease and the variable combination of associated tendinitis, bursitis, and fasciitis of polypain.

The symptoms of pain from the osteoarthritis and degenerative disc disease that occurs in polypain arises from multiple sites including stress on the bone adjacent to the joint, inflammation in the joint, stress and stretch on the joint capsule, stress and stretch on the joint ligaments and tendons, inflammation of the joint related periarticular structures, the joint related muscles with stretch or spasm, and torn meniscal cartilage. All these factors are affected by joint alignment, loading, and movement. Clearly, pain in polypain is intimately related to joint structure and alignment as well as joint and periarticular loading, usage, biomechanics, ergonomics, and posture. Furthermore, the evolution and progression of the underlying osteoarthritis and degenerative disc disease in polypain is similarly related to joint and spinal loading and usage, biomechanics, ergonomics, and posture. Therefore, treatment absolutely requires a thorough understanding how pain is generated at all affected joint, spine, and periarticular sites at a functional level related to the loading, structure, alignment, biomechanics, and ergonomics of these sites. Such information provides the opportunity for joint and site specific treatment related to improving alignment, posture, biomechanics, and ergonomic interactions through education, orthotics, appropriate neuromuscular re-education, appropriate toning and strengthening exercises, ergonomic training, and appropriate ergonomic accommodations and modifications.

Thus, a thorough assessment of the biomechanical state of the individual joint or joint regions and their interaction with the environment with regard to extent and degree of load bearing including weight related issues on weight bearing joints, usage, biomechanics, ergonomics, and posture is of paramount importance and this must continue on an ongoing basis. Only then can treatment be optimized to control site specific pain sources leading to generalized pain as well as underlying disease activity in order to optimize functional abilities.

8. Polypain is about multiple joints and sites that identify the polyregional pain.

As a corollary to the principle that polypain is about the joint and joint related structures, it is equally important to recognize that multiple or polyregional areas are involved in polypain at the same time. While virtually always involving the neck and/or low back, multiple other sites are involved simultaneously and often but not always in a symptomatic way. Thus, as stated above, treatment absolutely requires a thorough understanding of how pain is generated at all affected joint, spine, and periarticular sites at a functional level related to the loading, structure, alignment, biomechanics, and ergonomics of these sites. Such information provides the necessary information needed to provide joint and site specific treatment at all involved sites related to improving alignment, posture, biomechanics, and ergonomic interactions through education, orthotics, appropriate neuromuscular re-education, appropriate toning and strengthening exercises, ergonomic training, and appropriate ergonomic accommodations and modifications.

9. You can be better but not feel less pain or other symptoms: the role of functional activity and the Law of Unintended/Unrecognized Consequences.

A critical element of polypain relates to functional ability. After all, the ultimate major goal of any treatment plan for a chronic, painful musculoskeletal disease is to improve function. While frequently measured in research studies involving treatment interventions, it is virtually neglected in the clinical setting. In fact, in the usual clinical setting, essentially all treatment benefit is measured in terms of changes in the appreciation of pain devoid of context in terms of function, activities, and ergonomics.

However, as occurs in polypain, the perceived pain along with the under-lying joint and joint related structural alterations of primary generalized osteoarthritis, degenerative disc disease, fasciitis, bursitis, and tendinitis may lead to functional impairment of the specific areas involved as well as more generalized functional losses. This develops as a result of the im-pact of usage, biomechanics, ergonomics, and posture on the sources of pain in polypain. Increased pain will lead to reduced function in an effort to reduce symptoms and the patient will, as best as possible avoid activi-ties that trigger or worsen the osteoarthritis, bursitis, tendinitis, and fasciitis. This decrease in activity will result in lesser pain being driven by these sources of pain, thereby reducing the pain level, improving pain thresholds, and improving the relationship of pain to pain threshold. Fig-ure 5.9 in Chapter 5 depicts this change from Time A to Time B. There-fore, the polypain patient naturally trades pain reduction at the expense of functional activity when this is possible. This is depicted in Figure 6.7. Without determining the patient's functional activity, it would at least su-perficially appear that because the pain is improved, that the polypain process is indeed improved. However, the price of that perceived im-provement is reduced function. This exemplifies the Law of Unintended/Unrecognized Consequences in which a desired reduction in pain comes at the expense of reduced functional ability.

Conversely, as pain improves whether by avoidance or more specifi-cally by treatment, the natural tendency of the individual will be to in-crease the activity level. This will lead to increased usage and adverse biomechanics, ergonomics, and posture. This increased activity will cause an increase in joint and periarticular related symptoms and worsen the relationship of pain to pain threshold. This is depicted in Figure 5.9 in Chapter 5 as the change from Time B to Time C. When treatment is di-rected at managing the pain symptoms, functional activity increases with a lesser impact on pain for any given functional level. In essence, the indi-vidual can do more at any given level of pain and pain threshold as pain generation is reduced and/or pain thresholds are increased by treatment of pain. Therefore, we trade treatment benefit with reduction in pain for increased functional activity. This increased activity will in turn lead to increased pain. In fact, in the face of effective treatment, the benefit in controlling pain may be lost in exchange for increased functional activity. Thus, in the face of treatment, the benefit may not be in reported symp-

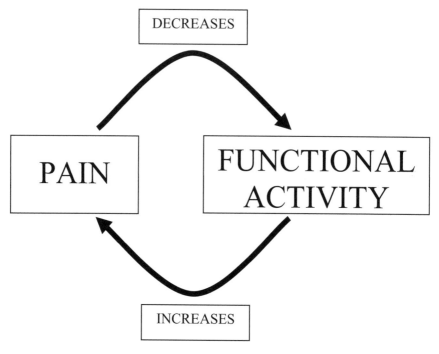

Figure 6.7: *Feedback loop relationship of pain to function in polypain.*

toms, but rather be found in changes in function. This exemplifies the Law of Unintended/Unrecognized Consequences in which improved functional ability comes at the expense of ongoing pain in the face of successful treatment of the pain. The correlation between pain and functional activity is that of a dynamic and ever changing feedback loop relationship as depicted in Figure 6.7. Therefore, a lack of reported pain symptoms does not equate with benefit from the therapeutic program and the ongoing presence of symptoms in the face of treatment does not equate with a lack of benefit.

Furthermore, today's pain is the worst pain, regardless of interval improvement by treatment. This occurs in part because of the relationship of pain to functional activity and the worsening of symptoms with increased functional activity as well as the issue of chronic pain memory as discussed in Chapter 5. The relative recent change in symptoms over time is what will be recalled as the time related recall of change in symptoms because patients with chronic pain are more biased to recall and recount more recent and more intense symptoms.

Therefore, it is absolutely vital that assessment in polypain always include a detailed functional activity assessment to avoid missing a therapeutically beneficial treatment.

10. Treat all manifestations of polypain starting with symptoms, then functional impairments, then reversible disease, and ultimately treat to prevent progression.

Polypain is a chronic, progressive disease comprised of polyregional pain generated by underlying disease processes related to: 1) primary generalized osteoarthritis, degenerative disc disease, tendinitis, bursitis, and fasciitis; 2) and pain message processing leading to reduced pain thresholds with tenderness and referred pain with increased nociception. It is highly susceptible to interaction with the environment with regard to extent and degree of usage, biomechanics, and ergonomics. Given the chronic, progressive nature of the underlying disease, the dynamic relationship of pain message to pain threshold, and the significant influence of the environment, it is absolutely critical that treatment be directed to all these components of polypain. Thus, treatment must account for and manage pain and pain threshold issues pharmacologically along with appropriate biomechanical and ergonomic accommodations and modifications regarding: the pain drivers related to primary generalized osteoarthritis, degenerative disc disease, tendinitis, bursitis, and fasciitis at all identified sites; and the altered pain thresholds with aberrant pain processing by first managing the pain drivers and then managing pain processing, sleep disruption and psychological disturbances; and the functional activity impairments.

11. Must do all of the above at the same time.

Further, all the interventions must be done concomitantly. Not in parts. Not one part to the exclusion of another. Not sequentially. Not as needed. But all together, accounting for all the identified processes and issues. This is another reason why treatments in fibromyalgia fail. Treating one component at a time does not work. It is absolutely mandatory to treat all aspects, components, and manifestations of polypain together. Targeting any one site, process, component, or manifestation simply leaves the other components to further manifest and progress. In essence, this leads to treating one area at the expense of another. Today's pain is the worst pain. Treatment is, thus of necessity, complex, comprehensive, and coordinated.

12. Cost and/or risk of treatment versus benefit: nothing is without risk and the issue of truly informed consent.

Nothing we do is without risk. Stepping into the shower entails a risk of slipping and falling. Driving a car entails a risk of accident. Eating entails a risk of choking, food poisoning, or potential allergic reaction to food. Day in and day out we are exposed to activities that impose risks or costs. We constantly make choices about the levels of risk we are willing to accept to achieve our activities. Often, this is done based on gut feeling or some innate knowledge on a subconscious level based on personal experience or observation without knowledge of formal research or statistics. Indeed, when we step into the car, we really do not give much thought about getting into a car accident, despite the real possibility that one could occur. In fact, in everyday life, we are willing to undertake risks without much obvious thought at all in order to benefit from the activities we wish to undertake.

On the other hand, when it comes to medical treatment, most patients are not as concerned about benefit to their condition, but rather more overwhelmingly concerned about risks and side effects with much lesser focus on possible benefits. Thus, in everyday life, we skew our decision making away from risk concerns to the benefits of our activities, but when it comes to medical treatment we skew our decision making away from benefits to frequently overwhelming and unsupported concerns regarding potential side effects or complications. This is especially true in the face of a chronic disease, such as polypain, when the treatment is expected to be prolonged. Yet, over-emphasis of risk aversion based on unfounded fears of complications or side effects to avoid otherwise beneficial treatment is in and of itself a risk factor for a poorer outcome and the avoidance of risk may in fact cause more harm than good.

It is important to reiterate that nothing is without risk; however, most everything is with some benefit. The question is: How much risk are we willing to undertake for what degree of benefit? The issue of truly informed decision making relates to how well we can define these risks and benefits using objective data and give them appropriate subjectively relevant due weight for the circumstance we find ourselves considering.

All treatment in medicine is provided with the understanding that there is a potential cost and/or potential risk in undertaking such therapy and that the benefit of treatment outweighs the potential cost or risk. The chronic, progressive nature of polypain lends itself to repeated such analyses both horizontally over the multiple components of polypain that require intervention and vertically over time of the chronic course of polypain. In addition, it is subject to repeated reevaluation relative to the severity of perceived pain which itself is highly variable as a result of any treatment already provided and the effects of usage, biomechanics, ergonomics, and posture.

A proper cost/risk-benefit analysis can only come from a comprehensive assessment as detailed earlier, addressing all the components of polypain. Further, the results of any cost/risk-benefit analysis in polypain management must also take into consideration the relative contribution of pain sources and the pain thresholds being driven by pain generators, sleep disruption, and psychological distress to the perceived pain in determining the allocation of treatment resources. Such analysis must also consider the distinction of symptoms and underlying disease processes and that the absence of symptoms is not the absence of disease. It must also consider the feedback relationship of pain and functional activity level to avoid failing to recognize unintended or unrecognized treatment benefit.

Similarly, it must not ascribe benefit to treatment that was generated by another mechanism such as the placebo effect, whereby the improvement noted was real, but not caused by the treatment given. Further, it must consider the chronic, progressive nature of the underlying disease processes generating pain in polypain and that all treatment must be directed toward treatment by lysis. In addition to the polypain related factors, the analysis must equally include treatment specific factors such as co-morbid medical conditions, other medications being taken, the development of prior complications related to treatment, the ability to comply with treatment, the convenience of undertaking treatment, the actual dollar cost of treatment, and the effect of past and current treatment. The recognition of all these relevant factors empowers the patient to be as informed as possible in providing consent to treatment.

13. The power of knowledge: informed decision making is therapeutic.

The understanding of the components of polypain and how they occur and vary within any one individual is crucial for the rheumatologist to
provide the most appropriate treatment plan. Even more important, however, is that the patient have as complete an understanding as possible of
how the symptoms develop and the factors that modulate them. Obviously, the more the patient understands, the more useful is the information available regarding the issues impacting the course of disease and
symptoms.

First, the effectiveness of any treatment program not only depends
on its appropriateness and anticipated effectiveness but also significantly
on the patient's ability and willingness to fully comply with the recommendations. This is especially true in patients with chronic musculoskeletal
diseases including those diagnosed with fibromyalgia. The ability and willingness to comply with recommendations correlates with the patient's
knowledge and understanding of how symptoms and disease develop and
what factors modulate them, how treatment is anticipated to interact with
and provide benefit to these processes, and at what cost or risk. Further,
the patient is more able to affect the environmental interactions that affect
polypain in both a positive and negative sense. This ability to directly and
effectively participate in one's own care is in and of itself is therapeutic.

Second, there is a further benefit from such knowledge and understanding that relates to knowledge unto itself. The very fact an individual
understands and knows things that can be done to affect how that person
feels has a direct effect on the processing of the pain information itself.
As reviewed earlier, the cognitive and psychological empowerment of such
knowledge provides input into the descending modulation pathway from
the brain to the dorsal horn whereby pain thresholds are elevated with a
reduction in the intensity of pain appreciated. This is the same effect as
occurs in the clinically beneficial placebo effect.

Thus, the provision of detailed knowledge to the patient empowers
the patient to actively participate in the management of polypain and is
itself a therapeutic tool that allows for the opportunity of truly informed
consent and decision making.

14. No matter how bad things are, things can always be better: but, reality dictates.

Indeed, everyone with polypain can be better. However, how much better one can get is balanced by what it takes to get better and at what cost for how much benefit. In this regard, reality dictates. Polypain occurs in the context of the individual and the life of the individual. While sharing common principles between individuals, it is ultimately the discrete and unique factors impacting the presence of joint and joint related disease that dictate management. These factors are related to genetic predisposition and to the individual's unique pattern of usage, adverse biomechanics, adverse ergonomics, and posture from moment to moment coupled with the individual's highly situation specific factors that affect psychological well-being and sleep. These are constantly subject to trade-offs and patients are faced with moment to moment, day to day, and long term decisions as to what the ideal balance is for their highly individual and specific circumstances.

15. The Principle of Diminishing Returns.

The Principle of Diminishing Returns is a term used in the study of economics to define the situation whereby increasing one input of production without increasing the others will lead to increased output but at a reduced rate or benefit. The same principle applies to many aspects of medicine and in particular to the management of polypain. It is also yet another reason why treatments for fibromyalgia fail. For instance, despite increasing intensities of intervention of a single line of treatment such as more potent analgesics or higher doses of medications or increased frequency of interventions such as physical therapy, most patients with chronic widespread pain and tenderness fail to receive significant added benefit. The polypain model readily explains why. The reasons include: 1) not recognizing or diagnosing all issues to treat; 2) failing to treat all issues; 3) failing to treat all issues at once; 4) failing to recognize unexpected or unintended treatment benefits. The importance of these has been discussed above in establishing an effective treatment program. The recognition of these factors should preclude them from creating diminishing benefits. However, even under ideal circumstances, the treatment of polypain is subject to the Principle of Diminishing Returns in relation to the fixed nature of underlying genetics, physical make-up, and established joint and joint related damage all of which are not subject to reversal in the current state of the art. Therefore, it must be again emphasized that treatment must maximize all areas of appropriate intervention thorough aggressive, intense, thorough assessment and management routines. At some point, however, optimal treatment will manage all treatable and reversible disease and there will be left irreversible damage changes for which there is no disease based treatment. At this stage, in those individuals whose pain generators could not be lowered sufficiently and/or whose pain thresholds could not be raised sufficiently, there is left only symptomatic treatment which may potentially become increasingly limited by reality driven cost/risk issues as treatment levels are intensified. Therefore, to achieve successful treatment, it is critical to treat early, treat all components, and treat aggressively to capture disease, reverse all reversible components, and prevent progression.

16. It's always about ability—not disability.

Fundamental treatment goals are not about limits. They may be constrained by reality and tempered by circumstance, but reality is nebulous and circumstance is evanescent as they yield to the next moment. Treatment must consistently focus on enabling the patient through symptom reduction and improved function. Indeed, the fundamental goals of treatment are always to eliminate symptoms, return function to normal levels, reverse reversible disease, and prevent progression.

The Polypain Treatment Framework

Based on the treatment principles enumerated above, the polypain model provides a framework for the treatment elements of polypain. The fundamental general treatment elements are first and foremost aligned with the need for proper, thorough, and comprehensive assessment on which to base treatment decisions. Only through such evaluation can the rheumatologist be sufficiently informed and knowledgeable as to be able to provide the needed patient education in order that the patient be able to fully participate in the management program and make truly informed decisions regarding treatment. Given that polypain is a chronic, progressive disease process, intensive follow-up with appropriate evaluation of progress and treatment effects is needed to provide optimal benefit from a properly designed treatment program.

Specific treatment starts with treating the sources of musculoskeletal pain. The polypain sources of pain are primary generalized osteoarthritis predominantly involving the neck and back with associated degenerative disc disease and the variable combination of associated tendinitis, bursitis, and fasciitis. It is crucial to identify these processes at all sites involved, whether symptomatic or not. Treatment is thus based on managing the underlying disease process as it affects each site. Initial treatment addresses the pain related symptoms at each of the affected sites. Subsequent, longer term therapy, deals with reversing reversible disease, prevention of progression of established osteoarthritis and degenerative disc disease, and preventing the development of osteoarthritis and degenerative disc disease as possible in unaffected sites.

The importance of treating the sources of pain first is paramount in view of the dual benefit to reducing pain generation as well as improving pain thresholds as described in the Polypain Model. As noted, the pain generators themselves, through their effect on pain processing at multiple levels, adversely reduce pain thresholds, sensitizing the patient to perceive more pain in a process whereby pain begets pain. Thus, the management of reduced pain thresholds from adverse pain processing generated by increased nociception first requires management of the pain sources. In addition, attention to sleep disruption issues is required to appropriately manage reduced pain thresholds by improving pain processing. Further, treatment of psychological disturbances related to stress, anxiety, depression, and psychosocial issues is critical to optimally improve pain message processing and treat reduced pain thresholds. These treatment elements are depicted in Figure 6.8.

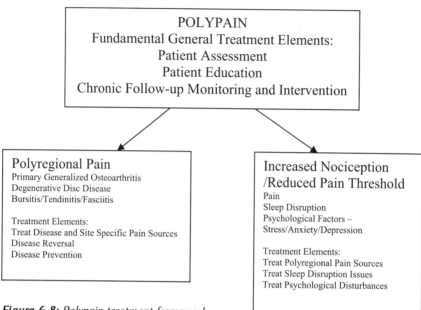

Figure 6.8: *Polypain treatment framework.*

Clinical Approach to Managing Polypain

A practical, clinical approach to managing the polypain treatment elements is summarized in Figure 6.9.

The approach to management again emphasizes the need for proper, thorough, and comprehensive assessment on which to base treatment decisions and the crucial importance of intensive follow-up with appropriate evaluation of progress to provide optimal benefit from a properly designed treatment program. Such comprehensive assessment provides the information necessary to devise an all-inclusive, in-depth, but individualized therapeutic protocol based on the distribution and degree of involvement of the polypain sites and components and the impact of this involvement on the individual. In essence, the assessment will determine the what, where, why, when, and which of treatment.

An appropriate treatment program will include as needed in some combination: pharmacologic intervention to control site specific symptoms, pain processing abnormalities, sleep disruption, and psychological disturbances; biomechanical and postural intervention through exercises, orthotics, neuromuscular re-education, and weight control; sleep hygiene management; ergonomic intervention through appropriate accommodation, modification, and sleep hygiene adjustments; and psychological support and counseling.

Furthermore, as polypain is a chronic disease process, intensive follow-up with appropriate evaluation of progress and monitoring treatment effects is needed to modify treatment based on: 1) issues specific to the treatment itself; 2) and treatment response regarding: a) osteoarthritis, degenerative disc disease, and periarticular disease; b) evolution of the biomechanical, postural, and ergonomic issues; c) evolution of sleep issues; d) and evolution of psychological issues. Treatment must be responsive to changes in these variables as well the Law of Unintended/Unrecognized Consequences in regard to unrecognized or unmeasured treatment benefit.

As polypain is a chronic and progressive process, treatment must not only focus on the control of the immediate symptoms, but also on reducing the progression of disease to control the long term evolution of symptoms and their consequences. Treatment must also be directed toward the management of the underlying primary generalized osteoarthritis and spinal degenerative disc disease processes at all sites, including asymptomatic areas, as the absence of symptoms is not the absence of disease. Over the long term, the goal of treatment is to manage all symptoms and functional impairments, to reverse the presence of all reversible elements of disease, to prevent progression, and to prevent the development of new complications of the disease including the development of new pain.

Fundamental Elements	Management Areas	Specific Interventions
General	Thorough, comprehensive assessment	
	Patient education	
	Close monitoring and follow-up	
Polyregional Pain		
	Medication	
		Anti-inflammatory medication
		Analgesic medication/Pain processing medication
	Biomechanics/Posture	
		Orthotics
		Neuromuscular re-education
		Muscle strengthening
		Range of motion exercises
		Weight loss
	Ergonomics	
		Education
		Accommodation
		Modification
	Injection – joint/bursa/tendon insertion/fascia	
	Surgery – rarely for irreversible refractory disease or nerve related complications	
Sleep		
	Biomechanics/Posture	
		Orthotics
		Neuromuscular re-education
		Range of motion exercises
		Weight loss
	Ergonomics	
		Sleep hygiene
		Accommodation
		Modification
	Medications	
		Sleep modifiers
		Sleep inducers
Psychological		
	Support	
	Counseling	
	Medication	

Figure 6.9: *Clinical approach to managing polypain.*

Part Four

The Fibromyalgia Polypain Wellness Core 9 Step Program

Chapter 7

Step 1: Successfully Using Medication to Treat Pain From Where It Starts In Your Body To Where It Ends In Your Brain

"...Thou has blest Thine earth, Thy rivers and Thy mountains with healing substances; they enable Thy creatures to alleviate their sufferings and to heal their illnesses..." —The Prayer of Maimonides

The fundamental principle of all polypain management is that the introduction of any specific treatment in the management of polypain be based upon a thorough cost/risk-benefit analysis. If there is no contraindication to the planned treatment, the selection of that treatment is based upon a benefit-risk analysis looking at such factors as pain severity and extent relative to pain thresholds, disease severity and extent, functional impairment, the outcome of prior treatments, co-morbid medical conditions, concomitant medications, complication risk, compliance, convenience, and cost. Reality dictates. Further, as polypain is a chronic disease process, intensive follow-up with appropriate and comprehensive evaluation of progress and monitoring treatment effects is needed to modify treatment based on: 1) treatment specific issues such as co-morbid medical conditions, concomitant medications, complications, compliance, convenience, and cost; 2) and treatment response issues related to the osteoarthritis, degenerative disc disease, and periarticular disease progression; evolution of biomechanical, postural, and ergonomic issues; evolution of sleep issues; and evolution of psychological issues. Treatment must be responsive to changes in these variables as well the Law of Unintended/ Unrecognized Consequences in regard to unrecognized or unmeasured treatment benefit.

Medication To Manage Polyregional Musculoskeletal Pain

Management of polypain requires treatment of both the sources of pain and the abnormalities of the pain message processing pathways as optimally as possible. This approach allows the targeting of treatment specifically based on correlating the clinical features to their physiologic processes. Thus, all treatment will be directed at: 1) managing polyregional pain from the underlying primary generalized osteoarthritis predominantly involving the neck and back with associated degenerative disc disease and the variable combination of associated tendinitis, bursitis, and fasciitis that are the sources of pain generation; 2) and improving pain thresholds through treatment of the pain signal processing pathways. Furthermore, in using medications to manage these two target components, it is crucial to recognize that a stepwise, combination approach is the most appropriate strategy to pursue.

Medication Target	Specific Sites
Pain Source	Primary generalized osteoarthritis, degenerative disc disease, tendinitis, bursitis and fasciitis
Pain Threshold/Nociception	Pain processing

Table 7.1: Fundamental pharmacotherapy principles of polypain management.

Treating Where Pain Comes From

Why Nonsteroidal Anti-inflammatory Drugs (NSAIDs) Work To Reduce Pain and How To Use Them

Treating the Source of Pain

The source of pain in polypain is polyregional musculoskeletal pain related to primary generalized osteoarthritis, degenerative disc disease, fasciitis, bursitis, and tendinitis. Pain from osteoarthritis derives from multiple sites including stress on the bone adjacent to the joint, inflammation in the joint, stress and stretch on the joint capsule, stress and stretch on the joint ligaments and tendons, inflammation of the joint related periarticular structures, the joint related muscles with stretch or spasm, and, where applicable, torn meniscal cartilage. Similar sources of pain are noted in degenerative disc disease. The pain from fasciitis, bursitis, and tendinitis is due to inflammation. Thus, the pain stimulus of polypain stimulates nociception directly as well as indirectly through the process of inflammation. Inflammation is identified locally at joint sites affected by osteoarthritis and by the presence of inflammatory markers at these sites as well as in the circulation.

Prostaglandins, thromboxanes, and leukotrienes are products of a metabolic pathway that comprise a group of inflammatory mediators that stimulate the production of pain, redness, local heat, swelling, as well as fever. They do these by modulating tissue specific cell function and regulation as well as inflammatory cell function and regulation. The synthesis of prostaglandins is controlled by an enzyme family known as cyclooxygenase (COX). There are two well known forms of this enzyme: COX-1 and COX-2. COX-1 is a regularly produced enzyme found in most tissues in the body. COX-2, on the other hand, is an enzyme found in a much more limited distribution in cells involved in inflammation including cells in joints and joint related structures and its production is stimulated by inflammation. Increased synthesis of prostaglandins occurs almost invariably in response to tissue injury of any kind including physical, chemical, thermal, or immunologic causes of injury and is seen to occur in osteoarthritis and other inflammatory musculoskeletal diseases.

Nonsteroidal anti-inflammatory drugs (NSAIDs) are a class of medi-

cations that inhibit the COX enzyme and reduce the production of prostaglandin pathway products. Specifically, they exhibit anti-inflamatory and
analgesic properties as well as being anti-pyretic (fever reducing). NSAIDs
have been shown to demonstrate other anti-inflammatory properties as
well.

The biologic basis for the use of NSAIDs in osteoarthritis, degenerative disc disease, fasciitis, bursitis, and tendinitis is clearly established
and supported by clinical studies. Studies also clearly demonstrate that as
a single therapy, NSAIDs are more effective than acetaminophen alone in
treating osteoarthritis related pain. Thus, the biologic basis for using
NSAIDs to treat the primary generalized osteoarthritis, degenerative disc
disease, bursitis, tendinitis, and fasciitis of polypain is well established
and clinically supported.

The first step in the management of polypain is the prescription of
an NSAID absent a contraindication based upon a thorough benefit-risk
analysis. If there is no contraindication to using an NSAID, the selection
of NSAID is based upon a benefit-risk analysis looking at such factors as
pain severity and extent relative to pain thresholds; disease severity and
extent; functional impairment; the outcome of prior treatments; co-morbid medical conditions; concomitant medications; complication risk; compliance; convenience; and cost. Reality dictates. Different NSAIDs have
variable potencies as some are more potent COX inhibitors than others
and some demonstrate more potency in some tissue sites compared to
others. Different NSAIDs have different rates of absorption and different
rates and mechanisms of metabolism. Even when controlling for all these
identifiable factors, all things being equal, two individuals may have vastly
different responses to the same NSAID. This may be related to the
individual's pharmacodynamics, the genetically and environmentally determined ability to respond to the physical and chemical structure of the
NSAID.

There are a number of NSAIDs currently available. They are available in a variety of formulations including tablets, capsules, oral solutions, topical solutions, intravenous solutions, and ophthalmic solutions.
They can be grouped into 2 large categories. The larger of these groups
include the nonselective COX inhibiting NSAIDs that inhibit both the
COX-1 and COX-2 enzymes to some degree, which varies from NSAID to

Group	NSAID
Non-selective COX inhibiting NSAID by chemical classification	
Carboxylic Acids	Acetylated salicylate: Aspirin (acetylsalicylic acid) Enteric coated aspirin Non-acetylated salicylates: Choline magnesium trisalicylate (Trilisate) Salsalate (Disalcid, Salflex, Monogesic) Difluorophenyl salicylate: Diflunisal (Dolobid)
Proprionic Acids	Ibuprofen (Motrin, Advil, Midol, Nuprin) Naproxen (Naproxyn, Napron-X) Naproxen Sodium (Anaprox, Aleve) Ketoprofen (Orudis) Oxaprozin (Daypro) Flurbiprofen (Ansaid) Fenoprofen (Nalfon)
Acetic Acids	Indomethacin (Indocin) Sulindac (Clinoril) Tolmetin (Tolectin) Diclofenac (Voltaren, Cataflam)
Oxicams	Piroxicam (Feldene) Meloxicam (Mobic)
Pyranocarboxylic Acid	Etodolac (Lodine)
Pyrrolizine Carboxylic Acid	Ketorolac (Toradol)
Naphthylalkanones	Nabumetone (Relafen)
Fenamates	Meclofenamate (Meclomen) Mefenamic Acid (Ponstel)
Selective COX-2 inhibiting NSAID	Celecoxib (Celebrex)
	Rofecoxib (Vioxx) – Withdrawn from market
	Valdecoxib (Bextra) – Withdrawn from market

Table 7.2: *Non-selective cyclooxygenase inhibiting NSAIDs by chemical class and selective COX-2 inhibiting NSAIDs.*

NSAID. The other group comprises the selective COX-2 inhibitors which have little effect on COX-1 inhibition. The non-selective NSAIDs can be further grouped according to their chemical class structure which in part determines the interaction of these medications with tissues as well as their metabolism which in turn determines their benefits and adverse effects. This is shown in Table 7.2.

When choosing an NSAID based on the above criteria, the lowest dose should be selected that is anticipated to meet the needs of treatment. However, under-treating the patient to reduce risk carries no benefit but only risk of complications from treatment as well as allowing progression of symptoms given that pain begets pain. Further, patience is required as it takes time to build up a steady state NSAID blood level and, once achieved, for the NSAID to optimally interact with the underlying inflammatory processes. Absent an adverse reaction or contraindication otherwise, an NSAID should be slowly titrated to the highest dose needed up to the maximal dose to obtain a maximal response or to absolutely rule out lack of efficacy if a lower dose does not produce a maximal response. In the face of an adverse reaction or lack of adequate response at the safest maximal dose, the NSAID under consideration should be discontinued and replaced with one of another chemical class absent any contraindication and the same process should be undertaken with the new NSAID. Typically, only one NSAID at a time should be used as there is no demonstrated benefit demonstrated when additively combining NSAIDs. Typical NSAIDs, their dosing frequency, doses, and relative costs are detailed in Table 7.3.

The benefits of NSAIDs in managing the components of polypain must be balanced by their potential adverse effects. Many, but not all, of the adverse effects of the NSAIDs are mediated by their primary mechanism of action, the inhibition of COX and the attendant inhibition of prostaglandin production. The major potential adverse effects related to NSAID use are gastrointestinal complications, renal (kidney) complications, hepatic (liver) problems, and cardiovascular adverse effects. Other potential adverse effects include skin reactions, hematological complications, respiratory difficulties, neurological side

NSAID	DOSING FREQUENCY	DAILY ORAL DOSING RANGE	RELATIVE COST
Salicylates			
Enteric Coated Aspirin	BID-QID	1800-4000 mg or more as titrated to serum salicylate level	Low
Choline Magnesium Trisalicylate	BID-QID	975-3600 mg	Very High
Salsalate	BID-QID	975-3600 mg	High
Short Half-Life NSAID			
Ibuprofen	TID-QID	1200-3600 mg	Low
Indomethacin	TID-QID	75-200 mg	Middle
Ketoprofen	TID-QID	75-300 mg	High
Tolmetin	TID-QID	600-2000 mg	Middle
Meclofenamate	TID-QID	150-400 mg	Very High
Fenoprofen calcium	TID-QID	900-2400 mg	High
Intermediate Half- Life NSAID			
Diclofenac	BID-QID	100-200 mg	Middle
Naproxen	BID-TID	500-1500 mg	Low
Naproxen Sodium	BID-TID	550-1650 mg	Low
Sulindac	BID	150-400 mg	Middle
Etodolac	BID-QID	400-1200 mg	High
Flurbiprofen	BID-QID	100-300 mg	High
Diflunisal	BID	500-1000 mg	Middle
Long Half-Life NSAID			
Nabumetone	QD-BID	1000-2000 mg	High
Oxaprozin	QD-BID	600-1800 mg	Middle
Piroxicam	QD	10-20 mg	Middle

Table 7.3: *Typical NSAIDs , their oral dosing frequency, daily oral doses, and relative costs. (QD = once daily. BID = twice daily. TID = three times daily. QID = four times daily.)*

effects, drug interactions, and allergic reactions.

Adverse gastrointestinal side effects include dyspepsia, gastric erosions, peptic ulcers, gastric perforation, and upper and lower gastrointestinal bleeding. Often, serious gastrointestinal complications develop without any warning symptoms. NSAID related gastrointestinal complications may be fatal. Risk factors for the development of NSAID associated ulcers include a past history of peptic ulcer, combining multiple NSAIDs at the same time, higher doses of NSAIDs, age greater than 65 years, concomitant use of glucocorticoids, and sicker individuals with multiple organ dysfunction. The selective COX-2 inhibitors demonstrate reduced upper gastrointestinal complications such as upper gastrointestinal blood loss and ulcers compared to non-selective NSAIDs. However, this protective effect was lost when celecoxib was used in higher than standard doses for almost one year.

The more frequent renal side effects include fluid retention, elevated potassium levels, and blunting the effect of diuretics. NSAIDs can produce impaired renal function, especially in individuals with pre-existing impairment of renal function or dehydrated individuals. Hepatic complications generally consist of mild drug related hepatitis with mildly abnormal elevations of liver function tests noted on blood work without any clinical symptoms or findings otherwise. This reverses upon discontinuation of the NSAID. Acute liver injury is very uncommon and liver failure is very rare.

Adverse cardiovascular side effects include hypertension, thromboembolic (clotting) complications, and hypertension. NSAIDs may cause the development of hypertension in non-hypertensive individuals, the elevation of blood pressure in patients with known hypertension, and the impairment of antihypertensive medications, especially those that block the renin-angiotensin-aldosterone system and beta blockers. An increased risk of coronary thromboembolic disease with attendant increased risk for myocardial infarction and sudden cardiac death as well as stroke has been more recently identified. NSAID related congestive heart failure has been reported as well as worsening of pre-existing congestive heart failure especially in those individuals with pre-existing heart disease.

Adverse reactions in the skin generally produce a variety of rashes that resolve upon discontinuation of the NSAID. Severe life-threatening rashes are rare. Adverse hematological complications include anemia, thrombocytopenia (reduced platelet count), and neutropenia (reduced neutrophil count). Bone marrow failure with aplastic anemia has been noted with indomethacin. NSAIDs that inhibit COX-I, but not the selective COX-2 inhibitors, interfere with blood clotting leading to an increased risk of bruising, bleeding, and more prolonged bleeding at sites of tissue damage or surgery. The effect on clotting is eventually reversed upon discontinuing the NSAID. Adverse side effects involving the respiratory tract are rare and include asthma and lung infiltrates. Neurological adverse effects include headache, psychosis, cognitive impairment, aseptic meningitis, tinnitus, and possibly central nervous system mediated dyspepsia. NSAIDs interact with many drugs increasing risks of potential toxicity or medical complications.

Despite the many potential adverse reactions, the first step in the management of polypain is the prescription of an NSAID absent a contraindication to using an NSAID based upon the thorough benefit-risk analysis discussed earlier. Awareness and vigilance are critical in monitoring patients for potential adverse effects of treatment and this is accomplished through intensive follow-up with appropriate and comprehensive evaluation of progress and monitoring of treatment risk.

Treating Pain Processing

Inflammation is a significant factor in the biological genesis of primary generalized osteoarthritis, degenerative disc disease, fasciitis, bursitis, and tendinitis. Prostaglandins are important mediators of this process. The presence of inflammation activates nociception and the appreciation of pain. In response to inflammation, especially driven by prostaglandins, as well as ensuing tissue damage, peripheral sensitization develops. The ongoing stimulation of nociception produces a state of central sensitization in the dorsal horn of the spinal cord. Initially, the central sensitization is caused by activation of the nerves carrying the pain message. This is followed in several hours by a delayed phase in which there is a large increase in the production of prostaglandins in the spinal cord itself which is driven both by the inflammation of primary generalized osteoarthritis, degenerative disc disease, fasciitis, bursitis, and tendinitis as well as unto itself independent of the pain. This further drives central sensitization. Thus, prostaglandins are not only important mediators in the genesis of primary generalized osteoarthritis, degenerative disc disease, fasciitis, bursitis, and tendinitis, but they are also important mediators of pain processing through nociception, primary peripheral sensitization, and subsequent central sensitization.

The benefit of NSAIDs in treating the inflammatory components of primary generalized osteoarthritis, degenerative disc disease, fasciitis, bursitis, and tendinitis is well established for reducing inflammation, treating the source of pain, and improving the reduced pain thresholds of primary peripheral sensitization. The presence of prostaglandin mediated central sensitization clearly identifies another site in the pain processing pathway where NSAIDs can act to reduce pain by improving reduced pain thresholds. Thus, NSAIDs not only treat the source of pain but also treat the abnormalities of pain processing that develop as a result of the primary generalized osteoarthritis, degenerative disc disease, fasciitis, bursitis, and tendinitis. This leads to a combined benefit of reducing pain message and improving pain thresholds, causing a significant improvement in the pain gap. Thus, there is less pain for any increased demand on the joints, tendons, bursae, and fasciae. Furthermore, there is an increased ability to carry out activities without obvious or significant flare of symptoms and there is a more rapid and greater ability to recover from an exacerbation.

Treating Where The Pain Goes

Clearly, managing the origin and sources of pain generation is a critical, crucial, and necessary component of managing polypain. However, through pain message processing, the pain generators lead to peripheral and central sensitization which in turn lead to pain amplification, pain magnification, wind-up or temporal summation, and referred pain through a process whereby pain begets pain and pain begets further inflammation. Thus, treatment must also address issues of pain processing unto itself. As noted, NSAIDs are the ideal first line treatment choice because they treat the underlying disease processes as well as manage crucial areas of abnormal pain processing. Therefore, the first medication step in the management of polypain is the prescription of an NSAID absent a contraindication based upon a thorough benefit-risk analysis. Reality dictates how this is done. Sometimes, the development of an optimal NSAID medication program in concert with optimal biomechanical and postural intervention through exercises, orthotics, neuromuscular re-education, and weight control; sleep hygiene management; ergonomic intervention through appropriate accommodation, modification, and sleep hygiene adjustments; and psychological support and counseling suffices to manage the pain processing component. Often, however, additional pharmacologic intervention is required to treat persistent, unresolved abnormalities of pain processing. These interventions do not specifically treat the underlying primary generalized osteoarthritis, degenerative disc disease, fasciitis, bursitis, and tendinitis, but address the abnormal pain processing and reduced pain thresholds these processes generate.

The next step is to add medications that reduce nociceptive pain processing and improve reduced pain thresholds. Absent a contraindication, the selection of such analgesics is based upon a benefit-risk analysis looking at such factors as pain severity and extent relative to pain thresholds, disease severity and extent, functional impairment, the outcome of prior treatments, co-morbid medical conditions, concomitant medications, complication risk, compliance, convenience, and cost. Reality dictates. Further, a critical polypain treatment principle is that it is necessary to treat all aspects of polypain and all components and manifestations together. Thus, at the same time medications are being introduced to manage the sources of pain and the pain threshold processing, concomitant treatment for the sleep disruption and psychological disturbances should be taking place, and this may also include the introduction of medications specifically to manage these issues. It is important to recognize that in addition to their intended primary benefit in managing sleep and psychological disturbances related to polypain, the medications used for sleep modification and psychological treatment also beneficially impact pain processing pathways and improve pain thresholds. Therefore, when considering which steps to take and what combinations to use in managing the pain processing component of polypain, it is crucial to identify the medications being used to manage psychological and sleep disturbances and to assess their role and contribution in the control of pain processing.

Table 7.4 lists medication classes that demonstrate potential analge-

Medication Class	Benefit in Comprehensive Polypain Treatment Program
NSAID	Yes
Acetaminophen	Yes
Opioids	Yes
Antidepressants	Yes
Sleep modifiers	Yes
Antiepileptic drugs	Yes (for Pregabalin)
Capsaicin Receptor Blockade	Yes
Local anesthetics	?
Antispasticity drugs	?
Others-NMDA (N-methyl-D-aspartate) antagonists, 5-HT3 (serotonin) antagonists, NK1(neurokinin-1) antagonists	?

Table 7.4: *Medication classes that potentially improve pain processing and reduce pain thresholds.*

sic benefit through improved pain processing and improved pain thresholds. Not all of these classes provide benefit in all circumstances. The likelihood of benefit relates directly to the presence of a complication of disease that is directly treated by the medication with parallel concomitant improvement in pain processing. In treating polypain, the medication classes of greatest benefit in treating pain message processing are NSAIDs, acetaminophen, opioids, antidepressants, sleep modifiers, the antiepileptic drug pregabalin, and capsaicin. The role of other antiepileptic drugs, local anaesthetics, antispasticity drugs, and other drugs have not been determined.

Medications used to manage pain processing increase pain thresholds and improve pain processing by reducing central sensitization which in turn leads to improved pain amplification, pain magnification, wind-up or temporal summation, and reduce referred pain through a process whereby less pain begets less pain and less pain begets reduced inflammation. By improving pain thresholds, the pain gap narrows or the pain free reserve deepens and not only is there less pain for any increased demand on the joints, tendons, bursae, and fasciae but there is an increased ability to carry out activities without obvious or significant flare of symptoms and there is a more rapid and greater ability to recover from an exacerbation.

Acetaminophen:
An Underestimated Yet Effective Medication

Acetaminophen is an antipyretic (fever reducing), non-narcotic analgesic. Its mechanism of action is not clearly understood. It is not considered to be an NSAID despite evidence suggesting it is considered to be a weak and/or indirect inhibitor of COX and attendant prostaglandin production including inhibiting a possible third form of COX found in the central nervous system. The biologic basis for the use of acetaminophen alone or in combination with NSAIDs in osteoarthritis is clearly established and supported by clinical studies. No such benefit for the use of acetaminophen alone for the management of degenerative disc disease, fasciitis, bursitis, and tendinitis has been established. This is not surprising. Acetaminophen is not considered to be anti-inflammatory and does not affect the source of pain. Its analgesic benefit appears to derive from improved pain processing.

In the management of polypain, if an optimal NSAID medication program in concert with optimal biomechanical and postural intervention through exercises, orthotics, neuromuscular re-education, and weight control; sleep hygiene management; ergonomic intervention through appropriate accommodation, modification, and sleep hygiene adjustments; and psychological support and counseling fail to adequately control the pain sources and pain processing and related pain thresholds, then the next step is to add acetaminophen. Absent a contraindication to using acetaminophen, the selection of acetaminophen is based upon a benefit-risk analysis looking at such factors as pain severity and extent relative to pain thresholds, disease severity and extent, functional impairment, the outcome of prior treatments, co-morbid medical conditions, concomitant medications, complication risk, compliance, convenience, and cost. Reality dictates.

As with the NSAIDs, the lowest dose of acetaminophen should be selected that is anticipated to meet the needs of treatment. However, under-treating the patient to reduce risk carries no benefit but only risk of complications from treatment as well as allowing progression of symptoms given that pain begets pain. Absent an adverse reaction or contraindication otherwise, acetaminophen should be slowly titrated to the highest dose needed up to the maximal dose to obtain a maximal response or to absolutely rule out lack of efficacy if a lower dose does not produce a maximal response.

Acetaminophen is generally well tolerated with a relative lack of side effects. However, it is toxic to the liver in doses exceeding 1g of acetaminophen per 10 kg of body weight or sometimes in lower doses. Therefore, it is recommended that the maximum dose of acetaminophen not exceed 4 g daily and that the maximal dose be reduced if there are concerns about the health or function of the liver. Caution must be exercised when taking other medications containing acetaminophen such as over-the-counter medications or combination analgesic medications as they may contain acetaminophen and may increase the total dose of acetaminophen if the required dose adjustments to not exceed the maximum daily dose are not undertaken.

Opioids: Overcoming the Addiction to Unfounded Fear

Opioids are a group of compounds that occur naturally or that can by synthesized. They combine with receptors to produce effects on the body similar to morphine. These receptors are distributed on cells in tissues throughout the body with a high concentration found within specific areas of the central nervous system including the spinal cord and particularly the brain. Opioids bind to one or more receptors identified as Mu, Delta, Kappa, and ORL_1. In the nervous system, opioids affect neurotransmitter release and subsequent nerve signal transmission. Activation of the opioid receptors induces a variety of responses, the most predominant one being that of analgesia, as seen in Table 7.5. They mimic the effects of endogenous natural neurotransmitters known as endorphins, enkephalins, and dynorphins.

The opioid receptive nerve cells in the spinal cord are found predominantly in the dorsal horn of the spinal cord where significant processing of pain takes place as reviewed in Chapter 6 and where opioid receptor stimulation reduces nociception and improves pain thresholds. Opioid responsive areas in the brain are found in the periaqueductal grey matter, rostroventral medulla, thalamus, hypothalamus, and amygdala. These are sites involved in the integration and processing of pain signals. The stimulation of opioid receptors in the periaqueductal grey matter and rostroventral medulla improves pain thresholds and reduces pain via increased activity of the descending pain modulation pathways that terminate in the dorsal horn.

While opioids improve pain processing and pain thresholds at the level of the dorsal horn and through descending pain modulation pathways from the brain, there is also evidence of enhanced effectiveness of opioids in the face of inflammation as seen in the primary generalized osteoarthritis, degenerative disc disease, fasciitis, bursitis, and tendinitis of polypain. This develops as a result of inflammation stimulating increased opioid responsiveness in the peripheral nerves involved in nociception in the inflamed tissue itself.

Thus, opioids improve pain processing and reduce pain thresholds by acting at the level of dorsal horn pain processing, pain processing in the brain via descending pain modulation, and, in the face of inflammation mediated nociception, opioids demonstrate enhanced effectiveness in reducing nocicption and improving pain thresholds at the site of inflammation itself by acting on the peripheral nerves.

In the management of polypain, if an optimal NSAID and acetaminophen medication program in concert with optimal biomechanical and postural intervention through exercises, orthotics, neuromuscular re-education and weight control; sleep hygiene management including medication; ergonomic intervention through appropriate accommodation, modification, and sleep hygiene adjustments; and psychological support including medication and counseling fail to adequately control the pain sources, pain processing, and related pain thresholds, then the next step is to add an opioid. Absent a contraindication to using an opioid, the selection of opioid is based upon a benefit-risk analysis looking at such factors as pain severity and extent relative to pain thresholds, disease severity and extent, functional impairment, the outcome of prior treatments, co-morbid medical conditions, concomitant medications, compli-

Receptor Type	Effects of Stimulating Receptor
Mu	Analgesia, respiratory depression, sedation, euphoria, physical dependence
Kappa	Analgesia, depression, sedation, respiratory depression
Delta	Analgesia, respiratory depression
ORL$_1$	Analgesia

Table 7.5: Opioid receptor stimulation effects.

cation risk, compliance, convenience, and cost. Reality dictates.

The analgesic potency of an opioid varies according to three major factors: which receptors it binds to, how potently it binds to the receptors, and dose limiting side effects. The first factor is the affinity of the opioid to bind to each particular opioid receptor. Opioids can bind to multiple receptors with different potencies for each receptor. However, the analgesic effects of opioids are predominantly controlled by binding to the Mu receptor. The second factor is whether the opioid purely stimulates the receptor (a pure agonist), weakly stimulates the receptor (a partial agonist), or stimulates one or more receptors and antagonizes another or more receptors (a mixed agonist-antagonist). Pure agonists such as morphine produce ongoing increasing analgesic benefit as the dose is progressively increased and the maximum dose is limited by side effects only. A partial agonist produces lesser analgesia than a pure agonist. The benefit of a mixed agonist-antagonist is limited by a ceiling effect whereby as the dose increases the benefit of the agonist component is increasingly impaired by the antagonist component, following the Law of Diminishing Returns. This ability to stimulate or antagonize analgesic receptors provides for a functional classification of opioids as shown in Table 7.6. The third factor relating to potency is the development of dose limiting side effects precluding potential additive benefit from higher dosing. Another way to look at opioids is to subjectively categorize the potency of opioids as weak or strong based on their observed clinical effects through clinical experience and such a categorization by the World Health Organization is shown in Table 7.6 as well. This breakdown into weak and strong potencies does not relate to the pharmacodynamics of the opioids nor their chemical properties or structures, but rather a perception of their effectiveness relative to side effects. While different opioids may have different levels of bioavailability, different pharmacokinetics, and different mechanisms and rates of metabolism, their doses can be titrated to provide equianalgesic benefit absent a side effect or dose limiting drug antagonism.

The biologic basis for the use of opioids in managing osteoarthritis related pain including temporomandibular joint disease and chronic low back pain is clearly established and supported by clinical studies, especially in addition to NSAIDs and acetaminophen. This is further supported

Characteristic	Opioid Name	World Health Organization Potency Description
Full Agonists		
	Morphine (Roxanol, MSIR, MS Contin)	Strong
	Fentanyl (Duragesic)	Strong
	Hydromorphone (Dilaudid)	Strong
	Codeine (Fiorinal, Fioricet, Tylenol with Codeine)	Weak
	Methadone (Dolophine)	Strong
	Tramadol (Ultram)	Weak
	Meperidine (Demerol)	Strong
	Oxycodone (Percodan, Percocet, Roxicet, Roxicodone, Tylox, Oxycontin)	Strong
	Hydrocodone (Vicodin, Norco)	Strong
Partial Agonists		
	Buprenorphine (Suboxone, Subutex)	Strong
	Butorphanol (Stadol)	
Agonists-antagonists		
	Pentazocine (Talwin)	Weak
	Nalbuphine (Nubain)	
	Nalorphine	

Table 7.6: *Functional classification of opioids.*

by clinical experience as seen by the inclusion of opioid treatment in the American College of Rheumatology guidelines for the medical management of hip and knee osteoarthritis. Thus, the biologic basis for using opiods to treat the nociception and pain message processing abnormalities of primary generalized osteoarthritis, degenerative disc disease, bursitis, tendinitis, and fasciitis of polypain is well established and clinically supported.

There are a number of opiods available. They are available in a variety of different formulations including tablet, liquid, sublingual, rectal, transdermal, parenteral, inhalational, intranasal, and intraspinal preparations. When choosing an opioid based on the above criteria, the lowest dose and least potent should be selected that is anticipated to meet the needs of treatment. Given that polypain is a chronic, progressive, and polyphasic disease process, consideration must be given to using longer acting opioids over the shorter acting ones. It is also very important to take note that many opioids are available in medications that combine them with acetaminophen or aspirin and extreme caution is required to monitor the dosing of these additional medications to avoid complications and overdosing. However, under-treating the patient to reduce risk carries no benefit but only risk of complications from treatment as well as allowing progression of symptoms given that pain begets pain. Further, patience is required as it takes time to build up a steady state opioid blood level, and once achieved, for the opioid to optimally interact with the underlying aberrant pain processing. Absent an adverse reaction or contraindication otherwise, an opioid should be slowly titrated to the highest dose needed up to the maximal dose to obtain a maximal response or to absolutely rule out lack of efficacy if a lower dose does not produce a maximal response. In the face of an adverse reaction that is not specifically dose related, the opioid under consideration should be discontinued.

In the face of a dose escalation adverse reaction and in the face of a positive but inadequate response, the dose should be reduced to the safest tolerated level at which a positive response is noted and, absent any contraindication, a second more potent opioid may be added and the same process should be undertaken to introduce and dose adjust the new opioid. If the combination is not sufficient to control symptoms, then consideration of discontinuing both and switching to a more potent opioid following the same process may be undertaken. However, in my experience, this is rarely indicated in polypain and usually suggests that other elements of the treatment program are not in place, other elements of the treatment program not being complied with as prescribed, an unidentified factor contributing to polypain has not been identified, or a new component contributing to polypain has developed.

Typical opioids, their dosing, doses, and weight for weight potencies relative to morphine are detailed in Table 7.7. Take note that the weight for weight potencies are related to the amount of medication needed to produce an analgesic effect equivalent to one unit of morphine and that all medications in the opioid class of drugs can produce similar levels of analgesia if tolerated at sufficient doses. It is important to note that these weight for weight potencies are approximations with variability between individuals as well as within an individual at different times depending on their metabolic state, comorbidities, and concomitant medications. Further, these comparative potencies may be dose dependent and vary according to the actual dose.

Tramadol is a unique, centrally acting analgesic in that it possesses a

Opioid	Relative Oral Dosing Potency Compared to Morphine	Duration of Action (hours)	Starting Dose
Codeine	0.1	3-6	30-60 mg every 4-6h
Tramadol	0.25	4-6	50-100 mg every 6h
Hydrocodone	0.5	2-4	5-10 mg every 3-4h
Oxycodone	1.5	2-4	5-10 mg every 3-4h
Morphine sulfate	1	3-6	15-30 mg every 4 h
Hydromorphone	5	4-5	2 mg every 4-6h
Levorphanol	5	4-6	2 mg every 6-8h
Methadone	10	8-12	2.5-5 mg every 3-4h
Sustained release morphine	1	NA	15-30 mg every 12-24h
Sustained release oxycodone	1.5	NA	10-20 mg every 12-24h
Transdermal fentanyl (skin patch – not oral)	150	72	25 micrograms/hour

Table 7.7: *Typical opioid potencies relative to morphine, duration of action and starting doses (h = hour, NA = not applicable).*

dual mechanism of action. It is a pure, but weak, agonist of the Mu receptor and improves pain thresholds by the opioid responsive pathways as described above. However, it also inhibits the reuptake of norepinephrine and serotonin, two neurotransmitters intricately involved in pain message processing at the level of the dorsal horn. This dual and possibly synergistic mechanism of action provides for enhanced effectiveness with lesser risk of opioid side effects. Thus, tramadol is a good early choice when the introduction of opioids is considered to manage polypain absent a contraindication to its use.

The benefits of opioids in managing the components of polypain must be balanced by their potential adverse effects. Many, but not all, of the adverse effects of the opioids are mediated by their primary mechanism of action through the stimulation of opioid receptors. The major potential adverse effects related to opioid use are related to the gastrointestinal tract, the nervous system, respiratory system, dermatologic system, genitourinary system, and cardiovascular system. Common adverse gastrointestinal effects include nausea through stimulation of the chemoreceptor trigger zone in the brain, vomiting, and constipation. Dry mouth, abdominal distension, and functional obstruction of the gastrointestinal tract may occur more rarely. Common neurological side effects include sedation, drowsiness, cognitive impairment, and pupil narrowing. Less commonly, mood changes, hallucinations, seizures, muscle twitching, or muscle rigidity may occur. In the respiratory system, opioids frequently promote cough suppression. In high enough doses they reduce the sensitivity of the brain respiratory center leading to respiratory depression. An asthma-like condition may develop occasionally. Dermatologic complications include occasional itchiness as well as hives, sweating, and flushing. Genitourinary tract complications include urinary retention. Sexual dysfunction can develop and in males reduced testosterone levels may occur with long term use. Cardiovascular complications include hypotension (lowered blood pressure) and bradycardia (slow heart rate). In very large doses, opioids have demonstrated a paradoxical hyperalgesia in association with other dose escalation side effects.

The use of narcotic class analgesics is shunned by the medical community primarily out of concern regarding addiction. Unfortunately, the term addiction is often and mistakenly used interchangeably with the terms dependency and tolerance.

Addiction is a state, psychological or physical, characterized by behavioral or other responses causing a compulsion to take the drug on a regular basis to experience its psychic effects or to avoid the discomfort of its absence. It is the abnormal, compulsive, and self-destructive use of the medication that significantly deviates from the medically recommended use and outside approved standards accompanied by drug seeking behavior due to psychological dependence. It is not a normal process. Characteristic features of addiction include: 1) a loss of control characterized by compulsive drug overuse even in the face of side effects, running out of medications early, frequent reports that medications or prescriptions are lost or stolen, requesting the medications from multiple physicians at the same time, using different pharmacies to fill prescriptions, altering prescriptions, obtaining street drugs, and unapproved use of other addictive drugs such as alcohol, sedatives, and hypnotics; 2) a compulsive preoccupation with drug use at the expense of other treatments and medical follow-up other than for refills of opioids and reports of no benefit from other medications or the presence of adverse reactions to other medications precluding their use; 3) and adverse physical, psychological, social, or financial harm including progression of symptoms, disease and functional decline, and being "high" or sedated with associated cognitive impairment. The process should not be confused with pseudo-addiction, which represents a drug seeking behavior to obtain relief of legitimately under-treated pain. The presence of pseudo-addiction usually suggests that other elements of the treatment program are not in place, not being complied with as prescribed, an unidentified factor contributing to polypain has not been identified, a new component contributing to polypain has developed, or there has been a change in metabolism or bioavailability of the existing medication routine.

Physical dependence is a normal physiologic effect of opioids as well as other medications such as steroid anti-inflammatory medications and blood pressure medications whereby the abrupt discontinuation of the medication results in symptoms of withdrawal. Physical dependence is a normal process. These types of medications can be withdrawn using an appropriate tapering program.

Tolerance is also a physiologic process whereby increasing doses of medication may be required to maintain the same biological effect. This often occurs with many different types of medications when they are first introduced. However, tolerance is not an ongoing process in the case of long term opioid treatment and increasing medication requirement is usually due to pseudo-addiction or, rarely, addiction. Tolerance is a normal process.

The evidence for the development of addiction in valid chronic pain syndromes as a consequence of treatment is unfounded, however. Only 0.5% of opioid treated chronic pain patients develop addiction. Notably, it has been suggested that the disease of addiction itself may affect about 10% of the population as a whole irrespective of other comorbidities and this 10% of addicted individuals would be represented in the chronic widespread musculoskeletal pain group as well, independent of any medically recommended treatment for their pain. Thus, through careful assessment and monitoring, the individuals at risk of addiction can be identified and managed accordingly whereas the likelihood of causing opioid addiction in the remainder is very small and opioids should not be avoided out of fear of creating addiction in those for whom opioid treatment is appropriate.

Despite the many potential adverse reactions, the addition of an opioid to an NSAID and acetaminophen in the management of polypain should be considered absent a contraindication to using an opioid based upon a thorough benefit-risk analysis as discussed earlier. Awareness and vigilance are critical in monitoring patients for potential adverse effects of treatment and this is accomplished through intensive follow-up with appropriate and comprehensive evaluation of progress and monitoring of treatment risk in terms of co-morbid medical conditions, concomitant medications, complications, compliance, convenience, cost, and treatment benefit.

Antidepressants Treat Pain Independent of Depression

Depression has been noted to occur two to four times more often in patients with chronic pain compared to individuals without chronic pain. When antidepressants were originally introduced to manage chronic pain, it was specifically done to treat the accompanying depression of chronic pain. During the course of this treatment, it was observed that there was an element of pain relief that was independent of the antidepressant effect. Subsequent studies have confirmed these distinct and separate mechanisms of pain modulation. Further, a recognizable benefit of antidepressants in reducing pain is that pain reduction may occur more rapidly and in lower doses than would be expected for an effect on depression. Additionally, and significantly, certain antidepressants have been shown to demonstrate analgesic benefit in non-depressed patients with chronic pain as well. The relationship, however, between the effect of these medications on mood and their effect on pain is complex and challenging to separate given the overlapping beneficial effects of antidepressants in treating coexisting depression in individuals with chronic pain.

In this section, we shall explore the role and use of antidepressant medications specifically for the purpose of impacting pain message processing either directly and primarily independent of psychological effect or impacting pain message processing secondarily through their benefit in treating psychological disturbances and sleep disruption. The use of these medications to manage the more specific psychological components and sleep issues of polypain are further discussed in the respective chapters devoted to these issues.

Antidepressant medications can be classified by their pharmacologic mechanism of action with regard to treating depression as noted in Table 7.8. In general they are classified as tricyclic antidepressants (TCA), selective serotonin reuptake inhibitors (SSRI), serotonin norepinephrine reuptake inhibitors (SNRI), reversible inhibitors of monoamine oxidase A (RIMA), norepinephrine specific reuptake inhibitors (NARI), and a miscellaneous group with various mechanisms of action. Despite the commonly shared antidepressant benefit, the multiple classes of antidepressants exhibit varied and different neurotransmitter mechanisms of action. However, in summary, all the antidepressants noted in Table 7.8 stimulate neurotransmitter pathways involving norepinephrine (NE) and/or serotonin (HT). The NE and HT neuronal pathways are involved in the integration and processing of pain signals. The neurons involved in these pathways originate in the brain in the rostroventral medulla and dorslateral pons and terminate in the dorsal horn where significant processing of pain takes place as reviewed in Chapter 6. Thus, antidepressant medications directly improve nociception and reduce pain via increased activity of the descending pain modulation pathways that terminate in the dorsal horn. This also leads to an improvement in pain processing in the dorsal horn of the spinal cord by reducing central sensitization. In addition, the antidepressants alter neurotransmission in other parts of the brain as part of their antidepressant effect and stimulation of these areas may result in the further stimulation of brain areas involved in pain processing resulting in further reduction in pain through descending pain modulation. Further, antidepressants may have beneficial effects not only on mood but also on the cognitive-behavioral aspects and disrupted sleep patterns related to pain.

The oldest and best known group of antidepressants is comprised of the tricyclic antidepressants. It is notable that the tricyclic antidepressants are also not only the most studied group, but they are also demonstrated to be the most effective of the antidepressants in managing pain thresholds and nociception. Placebo controlled trials have demonstrated superiority of the antidepressant medications that inhibit the reuptake of both norepinephrine and serotonin simultaneously, such as the tricyclic antidepressants, in the treatment chronic pain. However, the tricyclic antidepressants are considered to be "dirty drugs" in that they have multiple

Drug Class	Antidepressant Name	Neurotransmitter Effects
Tricyclic Antidepressants (TCA)	Amitriptyline (Elavil)	NE-reuptake inhibition
	Nortriptyline (Pamelor, Aventyl)	5-HT-reuptake inhibition
	Doxepin (Sinequan)	Possible NMDA antagonist
	Desipramine (Norpramin)	Possible sodium or calcium channel blocker
	Imipramine (Tofranil)	
	Clomipramine (Anafranil)	
	Trimipramine (Surmontil)	
SSRI Antidepressants	Fluoxetine (Prozac)	5-HT-reuptake inhibition
	Paroxetine (Paxil)	
	Citalopram (Celexa)	
	Fluvoxamine (Luvox)	
	Sertraline (Zoloft)	
	Escitalopram (Lexapro)	
SNRI Antidepressants	Venlafaxine (Effexor)	NE-reuptake inhibition
	Milnacipran (Savella, Ixel, Midalcipran)	5-HT-reuptake inhibition
	Duloxetine (Cymbalta)	
RIMA Antidepressants	Moclobemide (Manerix, Aurorix)	Reversible MAO-A inhibition
	Pirlindole	
NARI Antidepressants	Reboxetine (Edronax, Vestra)	NE-reuptake inhibition
Other antidepressants	Nefazodone (Serzone) Trazadone (Desyrel)	5-HT2 antagonist Weak NE-reuptake inhibition Weak 5-HT-reuptake inhibition
	Mirtazipine (Remeron)	Alpha-2 antagonist 5-HT2 antagonist 5-HT3 antagonist
	Bupropion (Wellbutrin)	Dopamine reuptake inhibition 5-HT-reuptake inhibition NE-reuptake inhibition
	Maprotiline (Ludiomil)	NE-reuptake inhibition

Table 7.8: *Antidepressant medication classes, specific antidepressants and their effect on neurotransmitters (NE = norepinephrine, 5-HT = serotonin, MAO = monoamine oxidase, NMDA = N-methyl-D-aspartate).*

other effects that may impact pain message transmission and processing. Such beneficial effects may include N-methyl-D-aspartate (NMDA) antagonism and blocking of sodium or calcium channels. Other antidepressants that inhibit the reuptake of both norepinephrine and serotonin, known as SNRI class or dual reuptake inhibitors, also appear to demonstrate favorable superiority in the treatment of chronic pain. SNRI antidepressants demonstrating improvement in symptoms of chronic pain include venlafaxine (Effexor) although a controlled trial using a lower average dose showed no benefit, duloxetine (Cymbalta), and milnacipran (Savella Ixel, Midalcipran).

The muscle relaxant cyclobenzaprine (Flexeril) has a chemical structure similar to the tricyclic antidepressants and demonstrates similar norepinephrine and serotonin reuptake inhibition neurochemistry despite not being classified as an antidepressant.

Unlike the tiered or serial addition approach to the use of NSAIDs, acetaminophen, and opioids, antidepressant medications should be introduced as early as possible as appropriately indicated in a parallel treatment track in concert with optimal biomechanical and postural intervention through exercises, orthotics, neuromuscular re-education and weight control; sleep hygiene management including medication; ergonomic intervention through appropriate accommodation, modification, and sleep hygiene adjustments; and psychological support including medication and counseling. The antidepressants are introduced either as an adjunct to specifically and directly treat issues related to pain processing independent of their effects on psychological issues and sleep or to primarily treat the associated psychological disturbances and/or sleep disturbances and with concomitant benefits in managing pain processing. Absent a contraindication to using an antidepressant, the selection of antidepressant is based upon a benefit-risk analysis looking at such factors as pain severity and extent relative to pain thresholds, disease severity and extent including severity and extent of psychological disturbances as well as severity and extent of sleep disturbances, functional impairment, the outcome of prior treatments, co-morbid medical conditions, concomitant medications, complication risk, compliance, convenience, and cost. As always, reality dictates.

The biologic basis for the use of antidepressant medications that particularly inhibit both NE-reuptake and 5-HT-reuptake in managing osteoarthritis related pain including chronic low back pain and widespread chronic musculoskeletal pain such as fibromyalgia is clearly established and supported by clinical studies. Thus, the biologic basis for using antidepressants to treat the nociception and pain message processing abnormalities of primary generalized osteoarthritis, degenerative disc disease, bursitis, tendinitis, and fasciitis of polypain is well established and clinically supported.

Like NSAIDs and opioids, antidepressants are available in more limited formulations including tablet, liquid, topical and parenteral preparations. When choosing an antidepressant based on the above criteria, the lowest dose and least potent should be selected that is anticipated to meet the needs of treatment. In the management of polypain, antidepressants are introduced for one or more of three components of polypain. They are used to directly affect nociception and pain processing, to treat depression, and to treat sleep disturbances. Thus, dosing of antidepressant medications is highly dependent on the purpose for which the antidepressant is being used. However, under-treating the patient to reduce risk carries no benefit but only risk of complications from treatment as well as allowing progression of symptoms given that pain begets pain. Further, patience is required as it takes time to build up a steady state antidepressant blood level and once achieved for the antidepressant to optimally interact with the underlying aberrant pain processing, and/or sleep disturbances, and/or depression. Absent an adverse reaction or contraindication otherwise, an antidepressant should be slowly titrated to the highest dose needed up to an appropriate maximal dose for the purpose it was introduced to obtain a maximal response or to absolutely rule out lack of efficacy if a lower dose does not produce a maximal response. In the face of an adverse reaction or lack of efficacy, the antidepressants may not be readily interchangeable with each other in regard to treating pain processing and thresholds due to their different neurotransmitter effects and the fact that there may be other treatment areas affected by the antidepressant medication such as psychological disturbances and sleep disturbances.

Treatment with antidepressants is further complicated by the fact that they are used in parallel with other treatment modalities that are being adjusted at the same time and treatment benefits as well as complications need to be assessed against the background of the treatment effects and complications of these other medications and any potential interactions between them. Further, in view of the selective benefit of tricyclic antidepressant medications in treating pain processing independent of depression and at lower doses than needed to treat depression, side effects seen at higher doses as needed to treat depression with tricyclic medications are thereby avoided. Thus, the use of tricyclic antidepressant medications to manage pain processing and/or sleep disturbances may be combined with safer and better tolerated medications to specifically treat depression.

The benefits of antidepressants in managing the components of polypain must be balanced by their potential adverse effects. Many, but not all, of the adverse effects of the antidepressants are mediated by their various neurotransmitter mechanisms of action.

The major potential adverse effects related to tricyclic antidepressant use are related to: the inhibition of the release the neurotransmitter acetylcholine producing anticholinergic side effects and these are dose related; their antihistamine effect related to blocking histamine receptors; their inhibition of adrenaline effect related to blocking alpha-1 adrenergic receptors; and effects on the cardiovascular system, the gastrointestinal tract, the nervous system, and the genitourinary system. As the required doses of tricyclic antidepressants to manage pain processing or sleep disruption are usually much lower than that needed to treat depression, dose related adverse effects are seen much less frequently and, when noted, are usually much less significant when used in these settings. When depression itself requires pharmacologic intervention, the higher doses of tricyclic antidepressants needed are rarely used today in favor of other relatively safer and better tolerated medications for that purpose. Typical anticholinergic side effects include milder and frequently self-limited side effects such as dry mouth, constipation, and blurred vision as well as more serious side effects such as dizziness, loss of consciousness, aggravation of narrow angle glaucoma, urinary retention, and paralytic ileus (paralyzed gut). Cardiovascular side effects include tachycardia (rapid heart rate), palpitations, arrhythmias, orthostatic hypotension (postural dizziness), cardiac conduction blocks, and cardiac ischemia or myocardial infraction. Other gastrointestinal side effects include nausea, vomiting, dyspepsia or gastrointestinal distress, anorexia, altered taste sensation, liver abnormalities, and of significant note given the concern of patients, weight gain. Nervous system side effects include sedation, a side effect that we take advantage of in helping concomitantly manage the sleep disturbance of polypain as discussed in Chapter 11. Other nervous system adverse effects include cognitive impairment, gait disturbances, tremor, insomnia, manic features, delirium, and abnormal sensations in the skin. Genitourinary adverse effects also include sexual dysfunction, loss of libido, ejaculatory dysfunction, and impotence.

The SSRI class of antidepressants do not produce effects on acetylcholine, histamine, and adrenaline receptors and are thus relatively unlikely to produce adverse effects related to these. They are also unlikely to cause weight gain and may, in fact, cause weight loss. The major potential adverse effects related to SSRI use are related to the gastrointestinal tract, nervous system, and genitourinary system. Gastrointestinal side effects include nausea, gastrointestinal distress, and diarrhea. Nervous system side effects include insomnia, agitation, anxiety, mania or psychosis, headache, and tremor. Genitourinary side effects include sexual dysfunction, loss of libido, and orgasmic impairment.

Despite the many potential adverse reactions, the addition of one or more antidepressants to an NSAID with or without acetaminophen/opioid in the management of polypain should be considered absent a contraindication to using an antidepressant based upon a thorough benefit-risk analysis as discussed earlier. Awareness and vigilance are critical in monitoring patients for potential adverse effects of treatment and this is accomplished through intensive follow-up with appropriate and comprehensive evaluation of progress and monitoring of treatment risk in terms of co-morbid medical conditions, concomitant medications, complications, compliance, convenience, cost, and treatment benefit.

Medications to Improve Sleep Improve Pain

The role of sleep modifiers in a comprehensive program to manage poylpain is explored in detail in Chapter 11.

Antiepileptic Medications to Manage Pain

Antiepileptic drugs comprise a diverse group of medications that ultimately affect seizure activity by inhibiting ion channel systems involved in nerve activation. In addition to their benefit in treating seizures, they have been found to beneficial in treating a variety of neuropathic pain syndromes in randomized controlled trials including trigeminal neuralgia, post-herpetic neuralgia, diabetic neuropathy, other peripheral neuropathies, spinal cord pain, and central post-stroke pain.

In this section we shall explore the role and use of antiepileptic medications specifically for the purpose of impacting pain message processing either directly and primarily or secondarily through their benefit in treating sleep disruption.

Antiepileptic medications can be classified by their pharmacologic mechanism of action with regard to treating seizures. In general, they are classified as: impacting gamma-aminobutyric acid (GABA) molecular targets; glutamate receptor antagonists; direct ion channel modulators; and $GABA_A$ calcium channel alpha-2-delta subunit modulators. As noted however, despite the initial molecular target, the antiepileptic drugs ultimately impact nerve conduction through ion channel system modulation as a final common pathway.

Pregabalin (Lyrica) is a GABA analogue similar to gabapentin (Neurontin). Pregabalin binds to the $GABA_A$ alpha-2-delta subunit of calcium ion channels of nerve cells. $GABA_A$ receptors are distributed throughout the spinal cord neurons including the dorsal horn where significant processing of pain takes place as reviewed in Chapter 6. The dorsal horn contains intercommunicating nerves or interneurons that modulate pain message. The interneurons that express GABA in the dorsal horn as a neurotransmitter are inhibitory and act to inhibit nociceptive pain pathway nerve signal transmission to improve pain thresholds. In addition, there are neuronal pathways originating in the brain that descend into the dorsal horn and express GABA as a neurotransmitter with attendant inhibitory effects on nerve signal transmission. In addition, pregabalin reduces the release of other neurotransmitters including glutamate, noradrenaline, and substance P. Thus, the antiepileptic medication pregabalin directly improves nociception and reduces pain via inhibition of nociceptive pain signal in the dorsal horn through local interneurons as well descending pain modulation pathways originating from the brain and terminating in the dorsal horn. This leads to an improvement in pain processing in the dorsal horn of the spinal cord leading to reduced central sensitization. Further, pregabalin alters neurotransmission in other parts of the brain to improve psychological well-being with a reduction in anxiety and stimulation of these areas may result in the further stimulation of brain areas involved in pain processing resulting in further reduction in pain through descending pain modulation. In addition, pregabalin may have beneficial effects not only on anxiety but also on the cognitive-behavioral aspects and disrupted sleep patterns related to pain.

A randomized controlled trial of pregabalin in fibromyalgia demonstrated improvements in pain, sleep, fatigue, and global symptom severity in higher doses. A second larger randomized placebo controlled trial to assess the benefit of pregabalin in patients with fibromyalgia showed that of 63% of patients who achieved significant reduction of pain, after 26 weeks of treatment, 32% of those patients lost the therapeutic response achieved at onset but significantly more patients sustained a defined improvement compared to placebo treatment. Thus, the biologic basis for the use of pregabalin in managing widespread chronic musculoskeletal pain such as fibromyalgia is clearly established and supported by clinical studies. The biologic basis for using pregabalin to treat the nociception and pain message processing abnormalities of primary generalized osteoarthritis, degenerative disc disease, bursitis, tendinitis, and fasciitis of polypain is, therefore, well established and clinically supported.

Pregabalin is available in the limited formulation of a tablet preparation. When choosing pregabalin, the lowest dose should be selected that is anticipated to meet the needs of treatment. In the management of polypain, antiepileptics are introduced to directly affect the nociception of polypain and, possibly, to additionally treat associated anxiety and sleep disturbances. However, under-treating the patient to reduce risk carries no benefit but only risk of complications from treatment as well as allowing progression of symptoms given that pain begets pain. Further, patience is required as it takes time to build up a steady state pregabalin blood level and, once achieved, for the pregabalin to optimally interact with the underlying aberrant pain processing. Absent an adverse reaction or contraindication otherwise, pregabalin should be slowly titrated to the highest dose needed up to an appropriate maximal dose for the purpose it was introduced to obtain a maximal response or to absolutely rule out lack of efficacy if a lower dose does not produce a maximal response.

In the face of an adverse reaction or lack of efficacy, the other antiepileptics are not identified to be readily interchangeable with pregabalin in regard to treating pain processing and thresholds in polypain including fibromyalgia, despite some possible interchangeability in defined neuropathic states, due to their different neurotransmitter effects. Treatment with pregabalin is further complicated by the fact that it is used in parallel with other treatment modalities that are being adjusted at the same time and treatment benefit as well as complications need to be assessed against the background of the treatment effects and complications of these other medications and any potential interactions between them.

The benefits of pregabalin in managing the components of polypain must be balanced by its potential adverse effects. Many, but not all, of the adverse effects of the antiepileptics are mediated by their various neurotransmitter mechanisms of action. The major potential adverse effects related to pregabalin in treating fibromyalgia include predominant neurological side effects such as dizziness seen in 23-49% of patients in a dose dependent manner, somnolence in 16-28%, headache, asthenia, euphoria, abnormal thinking, confusion, and incoordination. Other side effects include dry mouth in 7-13%, water retention, weight gain in 8-10%, and sinusitis. Studies in other populations have identified other adverse effects including neurological side effects such as blurry vision, double vision, neuropathy, tremor, speech disorder, anxiety, and sensory changes. Rare hematologic side effects include reduction in platelet count and bleeding risk. Muscle weakness, twitching, and muscle damage have been noted. A notable side effect at high doses is a drug induced "high" similar to diazepam 30 mg in a single dose.

Despite the many potential and significant adverse reactions, the addition of pregabalin to an NSAID, acetaminophen, opioid, and antidepresant in the management of polypain should be considered absent a contraindication to using an pregabalin based upon a thorough benefit-risk analysis as discussed earlier. Awareness and vigilance are critical in monitoring patients for potential adverse effects of treatment and this is accomplished through intensive follow-up with appropriate and comprehensive evaluation of progress and monitoring of treatment risk in terms of co-morbid medical conditions, concomitant medications, complications, compliance, convenience, and cost weighed against treatment benefit.

Pregabalin should be considered as part of the sequential and serial addition approach to medication management following the introduction of NSAIDs, acetaminophen, opioids, and antidepressant medications. It should be introduced as appropriately indicated in a parallel treatment track in concert with optimal biomechanical and postural intervention through exercises, orthotics, neuromuscular re-education and weight control; sleep hygiene management including medication; ergonomic intervention through appropriate accommodation, modification, and sleep hygiene adjustments; and psychological support including medication and counseling. Absent a contraindication to using pregabalin, the selection of pregabalin is based upon a benefit-risk analysis looking at such factors as pain severity and extent relative to pain thresholds, disease severity and extent including severity and extent of psychological disturbances as well as severity and extent of sleep disturbances, functional impairment, the outcome of prior treatments, co-morbid medical conditions, concomitant medications, complication risk, compliance, convenience, and cost. As always, reality dictates.

Topical Capsaicin: Useful But Challenging

Extracts of red pepper have been used to treat pain for centuries. The principal ingredient responsible for this benefit is capsaicin. Studies have demonstrated that capsaicin inhibits and depletes the neuropeptide substance P from unmyelinated small fiber nociceptive neurons that transit pain impulses generated by heat and inflammation. Substance P promotes neurogenic inflammation whereby the nociceptive pain response promotes further inflammatory swelling, redness, warmth, and stimulates inflammatory cells in a process where pain begets inflammation. Substance P also causes central sensitization by altering pain thresholds at the dorsal horn in a process whereby pain begets pain. Thus, capsaicin is beneficial in reducing both peripheral and central sensitization caused by inflammation. However, the beneficial aspect of capsaicin is coupled with a paradoxical, transient, initial response of burning pain at the site of application with concomitant peripheral and central sensitization with accompanying pain magnification and pain amplification. This is driven by stimulation of the vanilloid receptor for capsaicin-like compounds with the initial substance P release. It is subsequent to this initially painful response that the improvement in pain thresholds is noted.

Unlike the tiered or serial addition approach to the use of NSAIDs, acetaminophen, opioids, antiepileptic medication, and similar to the anti-depressant medications, capsaicin should be introduced as early as possible as appropriately indicated in a parallel treatment track in concert with optimal biomechanical and postural intervention through exercises, orthotics, neuromuscular re-education and weight control; sleep hygiene management including medication; ergonomic intervention through appropriate accommodation, modification, and sleep hygiene adjustments; and psychological support including medication and counseling. The capsaicin is introduced as an adjunct to specifically and directly treat issues related to pain processing. Absent a contraindication to using capsaicin, the selection of capsaicin is based upon a benefit-risk analysis looking at such factors as pain severity and extent relative to pain thresholds, disease severity and extent including severity and extent of psychological disturbances as well as severity and extent of sleep disturbances, functional impairment, the outcome of prior treatments, co-morbid medical conditions, concomitant medications, complication risk, compliance, convenience, and cost. As always, reality dictates.

The biologic basis for the use of capsaicin in managing osteoarthritis related pain is clearly established and supported by clinical studies. Thus, the biologic basis for using capsaicin to treat the nociception and pain message processing abnormalities of primary generalized osteoarthritis, degenerative disc disease, bursitis, tendinitis, and fasciitis of polypain is well established and clinically supported. Unfortunately, as it is available in topical formulation only, its use in the widespread pain of polypain is not possible. However, the application of capsaicin to local sites that are more exceptionally painful and/or inflamed than others can be of benefit.

Capsaicin is available in topical formulations of varying concentrations only, usually at less than 1% concentration. It is poorly absorbed orally, is highly irritating to the gastrointestinal tract, and is not available therapeutically as an oral medication. When choosing capsaicin based on the above criteria, the lowest concentration should be selected that is anticipated to meet the needs of treatment. Further, patience is required to deal with the paradoxical initial burning pain and to allow time for it to interact with the underlying aberrant pain processing. Absent an adverse reaction or contraindication otherwise, capsaicin should be slowly titrated to the highest concentration needed up to an appropriate maximal concentration for the purpose it was introduced to obtain a maximal response or to absolutely rule out lack of efficacy if a lower concentration does not produce a maximal response. In the face of an adverse reaction, the concentration should be lowered or capsaicin should be discontinued. In the face of a lack of efficacy at the highest tolerable concentration, capsaicin should be discontinued.

The benefits of capsaicin in managing the components of polypain must be balanced by its potential adverse effects. Generally, capsaicin is challenging to use because it is a topical agent and because it causes the paradoxical initial burning pain. This occurs not only at the sites of intended application, but also at any site it contacts including the finger used to apply it. Contact at sensitive sites such as eyes, mouth, nose, genital areas, and cuts or sores may be accompanied by transient but severe and even excruciating burning pain. It is aesthetically challenging and unpleasant to use.

Despite the many potential adverse reactions, the addition of capsaicin to an NSAID with/or without acetaminophen/opioid/antidepressant/ antiepileptic in the management of polypain should be considered absent a contraindication to using capsaicin based upon a thorough benefit-risk analysis as discussed earlier. Awareness and vigilance are critical in monitoring patients for potential adverse effects of treatment and this is accomplished through intensive follow-up with appropriate and comprehensive evaluation of progress and monitoring of treatment risk in terms of co-morbid medical conditions, concomitant medications, complications, compliance, convenience, cost, and treatment benefit.

Optimizing Pain Medications By Understanding Where Pain Comes From and Goes To

The use and role of medications in managing the components, contributors, and different levels of pain in the pathway of pain processing have been reviewed in detail above. This understanding and knowledge provides the ability to specifically target medications to different sites of the pain driver and pain messaging systems as seen in Table 7.9. The key elements in developing an optimal pain medication program in polypain are: 1) individualized treatment programs based on complete, comprehensive, in-depth, and individualized assessment; 2) cost/risk-benefit analysis that thoroughly considers pain severity and extent relative to pain thresholds, disease severity and extent, functional impairment, the outcome of prior treatments, co-morbid medical conditions, concomitant medications, complication risk, compliance, convenience, and cost; 3) reality dictates; 4) intensive follow-up; 5) and the Law of Unintended/Unrecognized Consequences in regard to unrecognized or unmeasured treatment benefit.

	Sites of Action of Different Classes of Pain Medication					
	NSAIDs	Acetaminophen	Opioids	Antidepressants	Pregabalin	Capsaicin
Pain Pathway Process						
Source of Inflammation	X					
Peripheral Sensitization	X		X			X
Transmission of pain signal in dorsal horn			X		X	
Central Sensitization	X	?X	X	X	X	X
Descending Pain Modulation		?X	X	X	X	
Psychological/Perception			X	X	X	

Table 7.9: *Sites of action in the pathway of pain processing of different classes of pain medications in the treatment of polypain.*

Chapter 8

Step 2: Why Biomechanics and Posture Affect Pain and How to Optimize Them

"I think I could, if I only knew how to begin. For, you see, so many out-of-the-way things had happened lately that Alice had begun to think that very few things indeed were really impossible."
—Lewis Carroll, *Alice's Adventures in Wonderland*

The successful therapy of fibromyalgia polypain requires the consistent treatment of both the sources of pain in polypain as well as the pain message processing pathways as optimally as possible. Treatment is, therefore, specifically based on correlating the clinical features to their physiologic processes. Thus, treatment will be directed at: 1) managing polyregional pain from the underlying primary generalized osteoarthritis predominantly involving the neck and back with associated degenerative disc disease and the variable combination of associated tendinitis, bursitis, and fasciitis that are the sources of pain generation; 2) and improving pain thresholds through treatment of the pain signal processing pathways. As such, it is important to take note that joints and joint related structures are not static components. They are dynamic elements continually subject to movement and loading. Ultimately, it is the cumulation of the ongoing moment to moment movement and loading that the joints and periarticular structures are designed for that leads to the symptomatic primary generalized osteoarthritis predominantly involving the neck and back with associated degenerative disc disease and the variable combination of associated tendinitis, bursitis, and fasciitis of polypain.

Therefore, adequate treatment of polypain requires a thorough understanding how pain is generated at all affected joint, spine, and periarticular sites at a functional level as related to the loading, structure, alignment, biomechanics, and ergonomics of these sites. Such information provides the opportunity for joint and site specific treatment related to improving alignment, posture, biomechanics, and ergonomic interactions
through education, orthotics, appropriate neuromuscular re-education,
appropriate toning and strengthening exercises, ergonomic training, and
appropriate ergonomic accommodations and modifications.

Medications alone are never enough. Failure to recognize and manage the biomechanical and postural needs of a patient with polypain will
not only lead to a biomechanical purgatory, but will virtually guarantee,
inadequate, if not significantly failed, treatment. Further, an appropriate
biomechanics and posture treatment program incorporating orthotics,
neuromuscular re-education, muscle strengthening, range of motion exercises, and appropriate weight loss allows for lesser medication intervention. Additionally, such interventions are a better and more natural substitute for medications. Most importantly, they provide treatment elements
that medications simply can not. Such intervention also allows the opportunity to not only physically impact the immediate osteoarthritis process
symptomatically but also to slow its progression especially in terms of
potential joint damage and deformity.

An appropriate biomechanics and posture treatment program incorporating orthotics, neuromuscular re-education, muscle strengthening,
range of motion exercises, and appropriate weight loss improves pain at
the source and reduces the pain intensity and severity. This leads to improved pain processing by reducing peripheral and central sensitization
which in turn leads to improved pain amplification, pain magnification,
wind-up or temporal summation, and reduces referred pain through a
process whereby less pain begets less pain and less pain begets reduced
inflammation. By improving pain source intensity and severity, the pain
gap narrows or the pain free reserve deepens and not only is there less
pain for any increased demand on the joints, tendons, bursae, and fasciae,
but there is an increased ability to carry out activities without obvious or
significant flare of symptoms, and there is a more rapid and greater ability
to recover from an exacerbation. Further, unlike medications that treat

inflammation and pain processing, the management of biomechanics and posture provides the opportunity to directly treat the musculoskeletal structures involved in polypain and improve joint, spine, and periarticular loading, structure, alignment, and ergonomics to help reduce the progression of osteoarthritis and degenerative disc disease.

Improving Pain, Biomechanics, and Posture with Orthotic Supports

The goal of optimizing joint, spine, and periarticular loading, structure, alignment, and ergonomics is accomplished through the incorporation of orthotics, neuromuscular re-education, muscle strengthening, range of motion exercises, and appropriate weight loss. The selection of which strategies to use depends on the specific joint or periarticular sites or structures that are involved. In certain areas of the body, treatment of the posture and alignment issues can be accomplished by muscle strengthening or range of motion exercises. In other areas, muscle strengthening cannot compensate for ongoing abnormal joint loading and alignment and range of motion exercises simply load the joint region further without improving joint biomechanics. It is for these joint regions that orthotics are most appropriate. Orthotics are specially designed physical devices used to align and/or support joints and joint related structures. They are used in situations when the body's ability to maintain neutral positioning and support at rest or optimal alignment with use is impaired.

Supporting the Neck to Reduce Pain

The cervical spine joint region, the neck, exemplifies the circumstance whereby muscle strengthening and range of motion exercises have no significant benefit and may in fact be detrimental. The neck is one of the most mobilized joint areas in our bodies. The discs, joints, ligaments, tendons, and periarticular structures of the cervical spine are designed pre-eminently for movement in addition to supporting the head. During our waking hours, our necks are virtually never resting. The neck is constantly in motion adjusting to support the head and responds to the sensory inputs surrounding us that require the use of our special senses such as vision, hearing, smell, touch, and taste. The head is a major window of sensory information about the world around us and, as such, the neck is mobilized to position the head to obtain such information. The head and neck are in constant motion to optimize such sensory input. In order to accommodate this sensory input, we sacrifice, either consciously or without any innate awareness, neutral positioning or optimal biomechanics of neck motion. Even when sleeping, ideal neck posture and positioning are poorly understood or sacrificed. In the symptomatic individual, the impact of certain neck positions and activities is self-evident. In the asymptomatic individual, the cost of such abnormal alignment and support is not appreciated until symptoms related to the cervical spine such as pain and/or neurological symptoms in the neck, and/or head, and/or upper chest, and/or arms and hands develop, or headaches surface.

In patients with fibromyalgia polypain, the sources of pain are primary generalized osteoarthritis predominantly involving the neck and back with associated degenerative disc disease and the variable combination of associated tendinitis, bursitis, and fasciitis. Specifically, 97% of individuals report pain related to the cervical spine due to osteoarthritis and degenerative disc disease and 100% of individuals have objective findings of cervical spine pain.

The loading of the cervical spine related joints and discs is affected by everyday activities such as sitting at a desk while working or reading, sitting to drive, sitting on a couch to read or watch television, walking and looking around, housework, physical labor, exercise, hobbies, and recreational activities. In this electronic age of information and video screens, our attention is frequently placed upon video screens and monitors such as computer monitors and television screens creating constant visual tracking with attendant neck movement. Neck movement is invariably accompanied by abnormal posture and ergonomics related to seating position and video screen placement, inappropriate seating and desk arrangement relative to desk and chair height and arrangement, and other inappropriate ergonomics in the home, work, car, and recreational settings.

Such inappropriate posture, ergonomics, and biomechanics not only lead to adverse and excess loading of the cervical spine joints, discs, and periarticular structures unto themselves at rest, but also lead to amplified negative consequences related to motions of the cervical spine all of which, in total, lead to increased symptoms and progression of the underlying osteoarthritis and degenerative disc disease of the cervical spine.

It is really straightforward to see once you know what to look for. As you read this book, take a momentary break and consciously check out your body position and specifically your neck. The least likely position you are in at this moment is a neutral one whereby you are sitting upright with this book held at eye level with virtually no neck flexion and absolutely no neck side tilt. Indeed, if you are sitting at a desk, you are likely bent forward with your neck significantly flexed forward looking at the book on the desk. Your head is likely fairly closely buried into the book and your head is likely leaning into one of your hands as you support your head by leaning on an elbow. If you are sitting on a couch or sofa, you are most likely sprawled out and leaning to one side with your neck bent forward and to the side. If you are lying and reading the book, you are most likely lying chest down and severely hyperextending your neck. Unless you have been educated and trained in ergonomics, biomechanics, and posture, it is natural to adopt these poor positions. It is likely detrimental to all individuals, but unquestionably detrimental to those who have polypain.

Cervical spine muscle strengthening and range of motion exercises lead to additional abnormal joint loading and alignment with worsened pain in the presence of such pervasive and unrecognized adverse cervical spine ergonomics, biomechanics, and posture in polypain. Appropriate orthotic support providing optimal cervical spine positioning and alignment at rest overcomes the detrimental consequences of these other modalities. Due to the lack of an existing appropriate orthotic for the cervical spine, I developed a self-adjusting cervical collar to provide the needed support and optimal positioning to the neck. The Smart Support Neck Collar is a fiber-filled cervical collar that provides cushioned support to the head and neck while at the same time placing the head and neck in a relatively neutral position at rest and preventing significant neck movement that would increase loading on the joints and discs of the cervical spine.

The consistent use of the Smart Support Neck Collar provides longer term neuromuscular re-education and allows the body to better learn and understand more neutral positioning and lesser loading movements of the cervical spine. This neuromuscular re-education is accomplished by improved tone and coordination of the head and neck muscles and a concomitant improved sense of appropriate loading and alignment for the situations the cervical spine is exposed to through feedback mechanisms to the spinal cord and brain. This process allows the cervical spine to be better prepared for anticipated demands.

Thus, the Smart Support Neck Collar is therapeutic and improves cervical posture and biomechanics to reduce symptoms. It also helps to reduce progression of osteoarthritis and degenerative disc disease in the cervical spine through neuromuscular re-education and the trained maintenance of improved posture and biomechanics even absent the collar in the long term.

The Smart Support Neck Collar should be used in circumstances in which cervical spine symptoms are exacerbated to minimize loading and maintain as neutral a cervical position as possible. It is especially helpful when doing desk work or computer work as seen in figure 8.1. In addition to the improved neck mechanics, the collar provides feedback in terms of pressure or discomfort when the neck is not in reasonable alignment. This function of the collar as a feedback tool motivates the user to change the arrangement of the work area or computer set-up including adjusting the chair and desk height and the relative arrangement of the desk and chair as well as the location and layout of desk work and accessories such as keyboard, mouse, monitor, and telephone until neck symptoms are optimized. It is also very helpful when sitting or sprawled on the couch watching television. Some of my patients even wear the Smart Support Neck Collar when driving due the excess loading of the cervical spine from the neck motion related to driving. However, this should only be cautiously done by users familiar with the restriction of motion imposed by the collar as limited neck motion may be a risk factor for an accident. If uncertain as to the safety of the neck collar when driving, common sense obviously dictates to not wear it under that circumstance.

Approximately one third of the day is spent recumbent and sleeping. While not thought of typically as a time to be concerned about neck related problems, lying down creates positions in which abnormal loading and posturing of the cervical spine readily develops. This is particularly important in individuals with polypain. The amount of support the head and neck require greatly depends on the position of the head, neck, and body relative to the pillow. As seen in Figure 8.2, the distance between the neck and the mattress is generally much greater when side lying compared to when lying on the back. Side lying is greatly complicated by the shoulder in that it not only increases the distance of the head and neck from the mattress, but it also causes the shoulder girdle to push up into the lower neck region at the same time gravity is pulling the head down. This adds further to the excess loading from this side bending force in the side lying position.

   This discrepancy of positions and forces from the back compared to side lying positions clearly demonstrates that a single regular pillow cannot provide optimal support in both positions. Complicating the issue is that, in general, individuals do not stay in one position during sleep and turn from side to side, back to side, or end up in some combination position in between. Depending on the pillow arrangement at the start of sleep, ultimately as sleep progresses, the pillow support will either become inadequate or excessive and lead to abnormal positioning and ex-

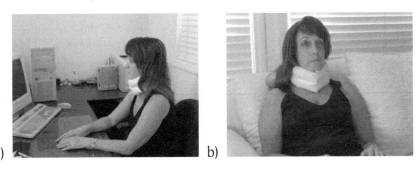

Figure 8.1: *Smart Support Neck Collar use: a) at a desk; b) sitting on sofa.*

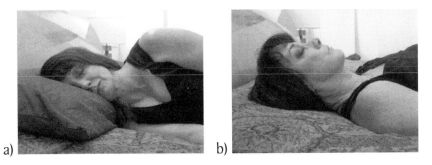

Figure 8.2: *Distance of neck to mattress when: a) side lying; b) back lying.*

cess loading of the cervical joints, discs, and periarticular structures leading to increased neck related pain and headache. This abnormal positioning and loading is further exacerbated by individuals who lie in a prone or face down position. As seen in Figure 8.3, prone lying leads to torquing, twisting, side bending, and hyperextension forces on the cervical spine with attendant excess joint and disc loading. Add all this to the fact that the head and neck are abnormally positioned and loaded for long portions of a 6-8 hour or longer sleep interval and it is easy to see the incredible cumulative abnormal posturing and excessive joint, disc, and periarticular structure loading the cervical spine undergoes during sleep.

To manage the challenges of appropriate cervical spine posturing during sleep, I developed a dynamic neck support pillow that adjusts the amount and height of support to accommodate the demands of different side and back lying positions. The Smart Support Pillow is a neck support pillow system that provides neck support at a lower height when lying on the back to accommodate the shallower distance needed to support the head and neck in this position. It automatically adjusts to provide increased head and neck support to help maintain relatively neutral head and neck alignment when turning to the side. This is shown in Figure 8.4. In addition, the construction of the Smart Support Pillow precludes prone lying, a position which is to be avoided at all costs because of the associated torquing, twisting, side bending, and hyperextension forces on the cervical spine. As sleep positions change through the night, the Smart Support Pillow will adjust to provide more optimal alignment and support of the head and neck automatically.

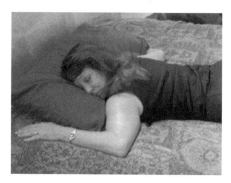

Figure 8.3: *Head and neck position with prone lying.*

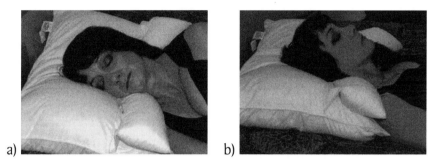

Figure 8.4: Smart Support Pillow support when: a) side lying; b) back lying.

Supporting the Feet to Reduce Pain

Patients with fibromyalgia polypain frequently have foot problems. Subjective pain in the feet is reported by 40% of patients and objective osteoarthritis findings are noted in 58% of patients. Loss of the arches in the feet is noted in 95% of patients. Deformities of the toes are present in 86%. Plantar fasciitis is identified in 27% of patients. The sources of pain in the feet are related to the primary generalized osteoarthritis in the feet with associated deformities combined with loss of natural and needed intrinsic arch supports.

The joints of the feet and joint related foot structures are subject to loading with weight bearing even without movement of the joints. They are also subject to joint loading related to movement as any other joint or joint area, especially repetitive loading with walking, and are further subject to the impact loading of body weight against gravity with the force of approximately four times body weight being transmitted to the foot with walking. These forces are not only loading, but they are significantly deforming as well. Any abnormality affecting the integrity of the joints or joint related support structures in the feet such as osteoarthritis and related deformities and/or weaknesses of the arch structure in the feet will be greatly magnified by the weight bearing and walking loads imposed upon the feet. Thus, pain arising from osteoarthritis and related foot deformities and/or loss of arches will be greatly magnified by the repetitive and excessive loading of the feet and joint damage and foot deformity will progress.

The need for appropriate support and cushioning of the foot with weight bearing and walking is clear and obvious to those with foot pain problems, especially in the context of polypain. Due to a complete absence of orthotics that address the heel and both metatarsal and longitudinal arch problems that are complicit in the evolution of the foot problems identified in fibromyalgia polypain, I developed a fully user adjustable arch support system insole that could readily accommodate the entire array of foot problems in patients with polypain. The Universole Arch Support System for regular shoes and regular use, and the Winsole Arch Support System for sport shoes and heavy duty applications are customizable and readily adjustable insoles that provide for individually adjustable amounts of support as needed to the metatarsal areas, the instep areas, and the heels to return the feet to the more natural alignment needed to sustain appropriate load bearing. The Universole or Winsole provides cushioning and support to treat the symptoms of any musculoskeletal foot problem in virtually any footwear.

Through its cushioning, energy return, support, and alignment features, the Universole or Winsole improves foot biomechanics with weight bearing or walking and reduces loading and deforming forces on the joints

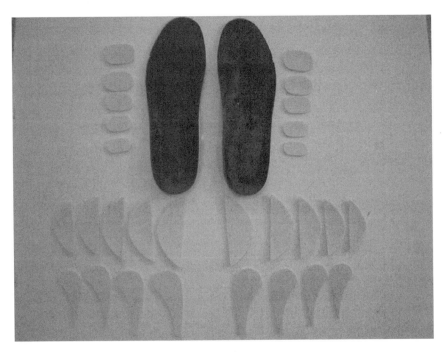

Figure 8.5: The Universole and Winsole Arch Support Systems.

of the feet and joint related foot structures. The heel cushion features provide the ability to not only help reduce pressure from complications such as plantar fasciitis but also provide for the ability to compensate for leg length discrepancies, as seen in 48% of patients with polypain, that cause unbalanced loading of the low back and lower extremities. These features not only improve alignment and treat the symptoms of pain, but they also improve the risk of ongoing deformity and damage to the joints of the foot and joint related foot structures.

Of course, the use of the Universole or Winsole Arch Support System should always be coupled with the wearing of appropriate footwear. In consideration of this, it is particularly important to be attentive to several areas of shoe design.

First, the heel should be as low as possible to provide as flat a support surface as possible to keep the foot parallel to the ground. The higher the heel relative to the forefoot, the greater the loading of the forefoot when standing and walking. This leads to the increased likelihood of forefoot pain. This also causes increased exposure to deforming forces that lead to loss of the metatarsal arch and deformities of the forefoot and toes adding to the progression of the local osteoarthritis. Avoid high heels.

Second, the front of the shoe where the toes reside, the toe box, should be wide enough and rounded enough to accommodate the toes not only at rest, but also standing and walking. The typical foot deformities seen in fibromyalgia polypain are similar to deformities seen in many foot conditions. The forefoot in particular is subject to loss of the metatarsal arch with attendant widening of the forefoot and the development of alignment deformities of the toes including hammer toes, claw toes, and side bending of the toes. These deformities are further exaggerated by weight bearing and walking. Thus, the forefoot and toes ultimately require more space in the toe box area of the shoe. Many individuals compensate for the forefoot problem by purchasing footwear in larger sizes. This is wrong to do, as the larger the size, the longer and wider the shoe, the looser the fit, and the greater the likelihood of inadequate support in other areas of the shoe. In other words, the shoe will be too loose and ill-fitting.

Third, the back of the shoe, known as the heel counter, should be sufficiently rigid and supportive prevent movement of the hindfoot in the shoe itself when walking and to minimize hindfoot alignment issues such as pronation that occurs in the flat foot deformity seen in 33% of patients with polypain. This is a challenge when buying footwear given the concomitant need for a wide forefoot and a more narrow heel.

Generally, a decent sport shoe such as a cross trainer shoe, walking, or running shoe with a readily removable insole to allow replacement with the Universole or Winsole Arch Support System works best to accomplish these needs. The shoe must be the correct length for the foot and must be of the correct width to accommodate the changes in foot anatomy and alignment already present. It should have sufficient depth inside to allow the placement of the Universole or Winsole. It should fit comfortably, should not be loose, and should not move relative to the foot with walking. In other words, the shoe should also fit snugly enough such that the foot, the Universole or Winsole, and shoe should move as a single unit when walking.

Improving Pain, Biomechanics, and Posture Through Strengthening and Toning

While all of the recommended exercises in the Polypain Wellness Core Program can be done by almost all individuals with polypain, there may be certain individuals who for other health reasons should avoid some or all of the recommended exercises. Always check with your doctor to make sure there is no reason why you should not do these exercises or if other accommodations or modifications are required. None of the exercises should ever cause more pain than you already have. If there is an increase in your symptoms, it is likely you have not followed all the recommendations and instructions correctly. In any case, if there is any increase in symptoms that cannot be eliminated by making any needed corrections to the exercise, immediately discontinue the exercise and contact your doctor. Do not continue any exercise that causes an increase in your symptoms. Having said all this however, virtually everyone, with rare exception should be able to perform and benefit from the Polypain Wellness Core exercise program for muscle strengthening and toning.

Muscle strengthening and toning are crucial components in the management of polypain. The ability to maintain neutral joint or joint region positioning and support at rest or optimal alignment with use is highly dependent on the balance of muscular, gravitational, and/or other forces acting on that region. Muscle weakness or loss of tone leads to abnormal alignment of the joint region. This abnormal alignment predisposes to abnormal joint loading at rest which in turn is magnified by use and loading of the joint area. Thus, muscle strengthening and toning are valuable in some joint areas where orthotics are not physically reasonable or cannot compensate for ongoing abnormal joint loading and alignment, and range of motion exercises simply load the joint region further without improving joint biomechanics. Joint regions that benefit from muscle strengthening and toning are those in which improved joint alignment and mechanics occurs without significantly abnormal or excess loading or biomechanical strain to the joint area while performing the exercises.

Reducing Low Back Pain Through Strengthening and Toning

The lumbar or lumbosacral spine joint region, more commonly referred to as the low back, is a typical area that greatly benefits from muscle strengthening, toning, and neuromuscular re-education. The discs, joints, tendons, ligaments, and periarticular structures of the lumbosacral spine are designed mostly for support in addition to mobility. Throughout the day, the low back is subjected to tremendous loading forces even during relatively simple activities such as sitting or standing. The low back undergoes enhanced loading demands with activities such as walking, bending, and sometimes coughing or sneezing. And while the low back is least demanded upon lying on the back with hips and knees flexed, it undergoes increased loading as one turns and adopts other positions while sleeping. The loading of the low back is further exacerbated by postures and positions that deviate from a neutral alignment that would otherwise minimize the impact of such activity. Just like the neck region, in the symptomatic individual, the impact of certain low back positions and activities is self-evident. In the asymptomatic individual, the cost of such abnormal alignment and support is not appreciated until symptoms related to the lumbosacral spine such as pain and/or neurological symptoms in the low back, and/or buttocks, and/or hip areas, and/or legs and feet surface.

In patients with fibromyalgia polypain, 97% of individuals have pain related to the lumbar spine due to osteoarthritis and degenerative disc disease. The loading and alignment of the lumbar spine related joints and discs is affected by everyday activities such as sitting at a desk while working or reading, sitting and driving, sitting on a couch to read or watch television, walking, bending, lifting, coughing, sneezing, housework, physical labor, exercise, hobbies, and recreational activities. We find ourselves frequently in front of video screens and monitors such as computer monitors and television screens in a variety of seating postures.

Such lumbosacral positions and movement are invariably accompanied by abnormal posture, adverse ergonomics, and excessive loading forces related to seating position and video screen placement, inappropriate seating and desk arrangement relative to desk and chair height and arrangement, and other inappropriate ergonomics in the home, work, car, and recreational settings. In addition to the normal loading demands upon the low back, inappropriate posture, ergonomics, and biomechanics lead to inappropriate and excess loading of the lumbar joints, discs, and periarticular structures and amplify the normally expected loading forces from motions of the lumbar spine. These, in total, lead to increased symptoms and progression of the underlying osteoarthritis and degenerative disc disease of the lumbar spine.

In patients with fibromyalgia polypain, the low back symptoms are driven by osteoarthritis and degenerative disc disease which are directly affected by loading, alignment, biomechanics, and ergonomics. In addition to the moment to moment loading and alignment issues affecting the lumbar spine of patients with polypain, there are notable biomechanical features of fibromyalgia polypain that frequently impact the lumbar osteoarthritis and degenerative disc disease. These include: I) hypermobility of the lumbar spine; 2) thoracic rotoscoliosis with unbalanced alignment and loading of the lumbar spine; 3) leg length discrepancy with unbalanced alignment and loading; 4) lumbosacral hyperextension; 5) iliotibial band tightness; 6) and trochanteric bursitis. Thus, there is a clear need for optimal lumbar spine alignment and support to reduce and eliminate the obviously abnormal loading, alignment, biomechanics, and ergonomics affecting the lumbar spine in polypain.

Strength, stability, and alignment of the lumbar spine is controlled mainly by the power and tone of the abdominal muscles and through their actions on aligning the pelvis and sacrum to neutral position relative to the lower lumbar spine and hips. Improved abdominal muscle strength and tone reduces and helps eliminate lumbar hyperextension, stabilizes hypermobility, and helps improve unbalanced alignment due to rotoscoliosis and/or leg length discrepancy. Thus, the most crucial component in managing the low back related symptoms of fibromyalgia polypain, and indeed another lynchpin of polypain treatment, is abdominal muscle strengthening. Think of the abdominal muscles as Nature's back support corset and abdominal muscle strengthening exercises as a means of tightening the corset to improve back support.

Through regular abdominal strengthening, the abdominal muscles develop improved tone. Through regular abdominal muscle strengthening, the abdominal muscles also develop a better sense of appropriate loading and alignment for the situations the low back is exposed to through feedback mechanisms to the spinal cord and brain. This process, known as neuromuscular re-education, allows the lumbar spine to be better prepared for anticipated demands.

It is important to note that virtually all exercise programs recommended for treating degenerative and mechanical low back problems, at their core, are fundamentally abdominal muscle strengthening, toning, and neuromuscular re-education programs. However, most low back exercise programs are either too complex to allow compliant self-management, provide insufficient or impractical strengthening, or include deleterious exercises that exacerbate the pain and alignment issues.

In addition to improving lumbar spine biomechanics, posture, and loading, the maintenance of normal abdominal muscle strength and tone is vital to sustaining balance, coordinating movements of the trunk, and providing sufficient strength and coordination to perform activities such as bending, lifting, carrying, kneeling, squatting, and getting up from and down into a chair or bed. The abdominal muscles are one of the most important muscle groups in your body.

In managing polypain, it has been my experience that the singular and most effective exercise program to provide the needed abdominal muscle strengthening, toning, and neuromuscular education to improve low back and related symptoms is a graded, self-managed, medically supervised, sit-up based, abdominal strengthening exercise program coupled with a self-managed daytime pelvic tilt program.

Sit-up Based Abdominal Strengthening Program
SETTING UP FOR THE SIT-UP BASED ABDOMINAL STRENGTHENING PROGRAM

To successfully accomplish the sit-up based abdominal strength-ening exercise program, proper set-up is critical. It is necessary to find a location in your house where there is a piece of furniture such as a sofa or dresser where you can comfortably and securely slip your feet and shoes under to anchor your feet flat to the floor and not allow movement of your feet when performing this exercise. It is important that the item of furniture be secure and not move or shift at all when performing the exercise. If no such location exists, you can purchase a T-bar type foot support that can be attached to the bottom of a door to anchor the feet and shoes. If using a T-bar, it may be necessary to adjust or modify it to allow it to anchor your feet and shoes firmly with your feet flat on the floor. It is also important when using a T-bar that the door remain securely closed without movement when performing the exercise. Another alternative is to have another person hold your

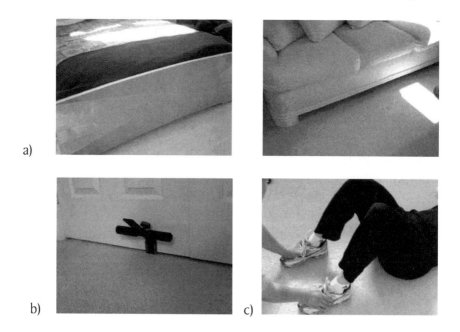

Figure 8.6: a) *Possible locations for abdominal strengthening exercises; b) alternative T-bar set-up; c) sit-up with another person anchoring your feet firmly.*

feet down flat in place of using furniture or a T-bar (Figure 8.6).

This exercise should only be done on the carpeted floor or on an exercise mat placed on the floor. It should never be done in bed, unless instructed by a medical professional, as the mattress compresses when doing the exercise and destabilizes your low back, placing you at risk of increased back symptoms. You must always wear a supportive sport shoe. There should be enough space in front of the foot support for you to lie flat on your back with your hips and knees bent in a flexed position (see Figure 8.7). Your knees should be flexed approximately 90 degrees. Your feet should be flat on the floor. Your feet should apart from each other approximately 6-10 inches. To protect and support your head and neck, you should place one or more fairly full pillows, with or without cushions depending on the grade of sit-up being performed, under your head and neck including the Smart Support Pillow and you should wear the Smart Support Neck Collar to stabilize the head and neck as you perform the exercise.

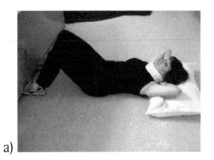
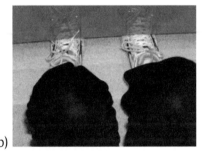

Figure 8.7: *a) Position and posture for abdominal strengthening exercises; b) foot spacing for abdominal strengthening exercises.*

PERFORMING THE SIT-UP BASED ABDOMINAL STRENGTHENING EXERCISE PROGRAM

1) **Grade of sit-up**—The grade of the sit-up is determined by the degree of elevation of the upper back, head, and neck relative to the floor. The higher the elevation, the easier the sit-up, however, the less intense the sit-up. When starting out, it is appropriate to start at an incline of about 30 degrees, about 1/3 of the way up. This is accomplished by using pillows and a seat cushion from a couch as shown in figure 8.8.

As abdominal muscle strength and tone improves, the incline is gradually reduced to allow you to lie flat with one or more full pillows to support your head and neck as shown in Figure 8.7a.

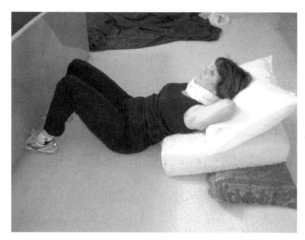

Figure 8.8: *Alignment and incline for sit-up based abdominal strengthening exercise program when first starting the program.*

2) Pelvic tilt—To perform the sit-up based abdominal strengthening exercise program correctly and safely, it is necessary to initially perform a pelvic tilt to reduce any residual lumbar hyperextension as shown in Figure 8.9a. This hyperextension is readily recognized by sliding your hand under your low back. The space between the floor and your low back represents the residual lumbar hyperextension we wish to eliminate. To do this, it is necessary to tighten the abdominal muscles and push the low back straight into the floor without lifting your buttocks off the floor. This produces a gentle roll of your pelvis on your hips and straightens and flattens the low back. Try this with your hand under your low back and you will feel the low back putting increased pressure on your hand as the pelvic tilt eliminates the space under your low back as seen in Figure 8.9b. This pelvic tilt should be done before each sit-up.

3) Stage of sit-up—The placement of your arms determines the stage of the sit-up. Stage I is the least demanding stage. For a Stage I sit-up, your arms are placed straight in front of you (Figure 8.10a). This is the

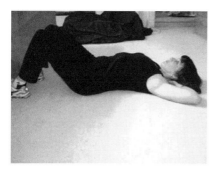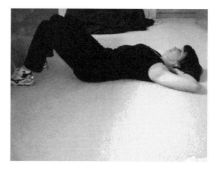

Figure 8.9: *a) Lumbar hyperextension and the space under your low back; b) successful pelvic tilting eliminates that space.*

stage to start with when starting any grade of sit-up as described above. Once you are proficient at Stage 1, you can increase the intensity to Stage 2 by folding your arms across your lower chest and upper abdomen as shown in Figure 8.10b. Once Stage 2 exercises are readily done, you can move on to Stage 3 sit-ups which are performed with your arms crossed in front of your chest with fingertips on your shoulders as depicted in Figure 8.10c. Success at Stage 3, will allow you to move on to Stage 4 with your arms raised, elbows bent, and fingers gently touching the outside of your neck as seen in Figure 8.10d. Finally, when Stage 4 sit-ups are performed with ease, you can move on to Stage 5 sit-ups, with your arms raised, elbows bent, and placing both hands behind your head, gently touching your head but not pulling on it or putting significant pressure on it. This is shown in Figure 8.10e.

4) **Once you have established the grade and stage** of sit-up, you are ready to perform the exercise.

5) **The sit-up starts with a pelvic tilt.**

6) **Contract your abdominal muscles** and start to pull straight up. It is necessary to avoid bending your neck or throwing yourself forward. All the work comes from the abdominal muscles. Your head, neck, and back should be straight and in neutral alignment throughout the entire sit-up. A good way to make sure this happens is to keep your eyes focused toward the ceiling and to imagine that a steel rod runs from the

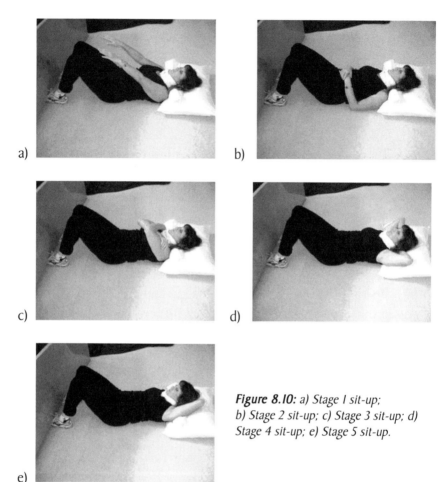

a)

b)

c)

d)

e)

Figure 8.10: a) Stage 1 sit-up;
b) Stage 2 sit-up; c) Stage 3 sit-up; d)
Stage 4 sit-up; e) Stage 5 sit-up.

top of your head down through your spine to the low back preventing
the bending of your head or any part of your spine. In other words, your
head, neck, and spine are locked straight. The only motion should be
your pelvis rotating on your hips and, in essence, you should be like a
door hinge with the bending taking place exclusively at the pelvis-hip
area only.

7) **Slowly, but steadily,** raise yourself as far as you can go which should
generally be about $^2/_3$ to $^3/_4$ of the way up. There should be gentle resistance and pressure against the top of the feet from whatever you have
selected to anchor your feet, however, at no time should your feet raise
off the floor during the getting up and going down phases.

8) Once you are up all the way, **stop and breathe**. Ensure that you head, neck, and back are straight and that your low back remains in a pelvic tilt. Then you can start to go back down. It is critical to maintain your abdominal muscle pull on the way down. You must go down as slowly as you came up. Going down is as critical a part of the exercise as coming up. Thus, it is done in a controlled, slow manner. Do not drop or plop down.

9) Once you have gently landed back on your pillow you can **catch your breathe** and let your abdominal muscles relax until you are ready for the next sit-up.

10) **There is no rush to do the sit-ups.** The key is to do them correctly. When starting out, it is okay to rest for a minute between sit-ups. Once you get stronger and more proficient, the rest time will decrease.

11) **Do 10 sit-ups every day.** Whether you are starting out or highly proficient, you should do 10 sit-ups every single day. As the purpose of the exercise is to improve abdominal muscle strength, tone, and neuromuscular coordination, the importance of consistency and compliance cannot be overemphasized. However, it is not necessary to increase the number of repetitions beyond 10 per day to accomplish these goals. Thus, the sit-up based abdominal strengthening exercise program is highly efficient and straightforward once you have mastered the basics.

12) While challenging, **abdominal strengthening exercises should never produce pain in the low back**. If you develop pain, it is likely you are not performing the exercise correctly. If pain recurs after reviewing how you are performing the sit-ups, then immediately discontinue them and consult your doctor.

Daytime Pelvic Tilt Program

The daytime pelvic tilt program is an extension of the sit-up based abdominal strengthening exercise program. In essence, pelvic tilts performed through the day provide the same benefits as the sit-up based abdominal strengthening exercise program in terms of strengthening and toning, albeit at a lower intensity. However, given that pelvic tilts can be performed in any position, in any situation including at rest such as sitting or lying as well as with activities such as standing or walking, they provide the opportunity to enhance neuromuscular education and coordination by training the abdominal muscles under specific conditions of loading and stress. Pelvic tilts are basically vertical sit-ups.

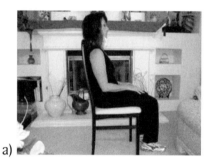

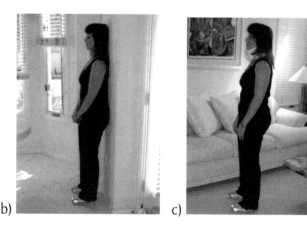

Figure 8.11: *a) Pelvic tilts when sitting; b) pelvic tilts when standing against a wall; c) pelvic tilts when standing.*

See the discussion above as to the performance of pelvic tilts as part of the sit-up based abdominal strengthening exercise program. That same pelvic motion and tightening of the abdominal muscles accomplishes the pelvic tilt in any position. For instance, when sitting in a chair, slide into the chair to rest your back against the chair back. Just as you did with the sit-up based abdominal strengthening exercise, slide your hand under the low back in the space between the low back and the chair back. The space between the chair and your low back represents the residual lumbar hyperextension we wish to eliminate. Now, tighten the abdominal muscles and push the low back straight into the chair back without sliding forward or lifting your buttocks. This produces a gentle roll of your pelvis on your hips and straightens and flattens the low back. You will feel the low back putting increased pressure on your hand as the pelvic tilt eliminates the space under your low back as seen in Figure 8.11a. You can do the same thing when you are standing by leaning into a wall with your heels about 4-6 inches out from the wall as depicted in Figure 8.11b. Tighten the abdominal muscles and push the low back straight into the wall without sliding forward or lifting your buttocks. This produces a gentle roll of your pelvis on your hips and straightens and flattens the low back. You will feel the low back putting increased pressure on your hand as the pelvic tilt eliminates the space under your low back. Indeed, the pelvic tilt can be accomplished while standing without a wall, as seen in Figure 8.11c, by placing your palms onto your abdominal muscles and tightening the abdominal muscles against the resistance of your hands. This produces a gentle roll of your pelvis on your hips and straightens and flattens the low back. Ultimately, you should be able perform the pelvic tilt in a vertical position without the need for other supports.

In addition to performing pelvic tilts for the sit-up based abdominal strengthening exercise, they should be done throughout the day under conditions of prolonged sitting, standing, or walking independent of symptoms in the low back. They should always be done if activities through the day start to exacerbate symptoms related to the low back or even if there is the development of a fatiguing sensation in the low back. Generally, 5-10 properly done pelvic tilts help relieve increasing low back symptoms. Pelvic tilts can be repeated as many times through the day as appropriate and as needed. Thus, the daytime pelvic tilt exercise program is another critical treatment component of polypain.

Reducing Knee Pain Through Strengthening and Toning

The knee joint is another typical area that greatly benefits from muscle strengthening, toning, and neuromuscular re-education. The knee joint compartments, tendons, ligaments, and periarticular structures of the knee are designed for support and mobility. Throughout the day, the knees are subjected to loading forces at rest such as when lying or sitting. With use, even when not bearing weight, they undergo additional forces such as acceleration, deceleration, tension, compression loading, shear, torsion, or some combination of these. These forces are further magnified by the additional loading force of body weight resisted against gravity with weight bearing activities such as standing, walking, kneeling, or squatting. The alignment of the knee, comprising the alignment of the upper leg on the lower leg, and the alignment of the kneecap, coupled with the strength of the muscles moving the knee all play a crucial role in the distribution of forces in the knee joint. These, in turn, are major determinants in the evolution and progression of osteoarthritis in the knee.

In patients with fibromyalgia polypain, subjective knee osteoarthritis symptoms are reported by 63% of patients. Objective findings in polypain identify patellofemoral osteoarthritis in 73%. The loading and alignment of the knee is affected by the activities as noted. While the knee is inherently designed to undergo a certain degree of loading, the underlying osteoarthritis predisposition in polypain increases the risk of osteoarthritis symptoms and the development of joint damage and deformity. In addition to the normal loading demands upon the knee joint, inappropriate posture, ergonomics, and biomechanics lead to inappropriate and excess loading of the knee joints and periarticular structures and amplify the normally expected loading forces motions of the knees. These in total lead to increased symptoms and progression of the underlying osteoarthritis of the knee.

In patients with fibromyalgia polypain, the knee symptoms are driven by osteoarthritis which is directly affected by loading, alignment, biomechanics, and ergonomics. In addition to the moment to moment loading and alignment issues affecting the knee joints of patients with polypain, there are notable biomechanical features of polypain that impact the knee osteoarthritis such as angular deformities of the knees. In addition the pes anserine bursa, a knee related periarticular structure, may become inflamed. Thus, there is a clearly identified need for optimal knee alignment and support to reduce and eliminate the abnormal loading, alignment, biomechanics, and ergonomics affecting the knee joints in polypain.

Strength, stability, and alignment of the knee are controlled by a careful interplay of joint structure and muscles supporting and moving the knee joint as well as the ligaments and capsule that hold the joint together. The predominant involvement of the patellofemoral joint and pes anserine bursa in polypain identifies abnormal alignment and support issues in the quadriceps muscle mechanism. Improved quadriceps muscle strength and tone reduces and helps eliminate patella tracking abnormalities, stabilizes hypermobility, and helps improve abnormal alignment. Thus, the most crucial component in managing the knee related symptoms of polypain, and indeed a further key component of polypain treatment, is quadriceps muscle strengthening. Through regular quadriceps strengthening, the quadriceps muscles develop improved tone. Through regular quadriceps muscle strengthening, the quadriceps muscles also develop a better sense of appropriate loading and alignment for the situations the knees are exposed to through feedback mechanisms to the spinal cord and brain. This neuromuscular re-education, allows the knee joints to be better prepared for anticipated demands.

It is important to note that virtually all exercise programs recommended for treating degenerative and mechanical knee problems, at their core, are fundamentally quadriceps muscle strengthening, toning, and neuromuscular re-education programs. However, most knee exercise programs, just like low back programs, are either too complex to allow compliant self-management, provide insufficient or impractical strengthening, or include deleterious exercises that exacerbate the pain and alignment issues.

In managing polypain, it has been my experience that the singular and most effective exercise program to provide the needed quadriceps muscle strengthening, toning, and neuromuscular education to improve knee related symptoms is a self-managed, graded, medically supervised, isometric resisted quadriceps strengthening exercise program.

Isometric Resisted Quadriceps Strengthening Exercises

SETTING UP FOR ISOMETRIC RESISTED QUADRICEPS STRENGTHENING EXERCISES

As with the sit-up based abdominal strengthening exercise program, proper set-up is critical for the isometric resisted quadriceps strengthening exercise. This exercise should be done on a carpeted floor or on an exercise mat placed on the floor. However, unlike the sit-up based abdominal strengthening exercise program, it can be done in bed if there is a firm supportive mattress. The head, neck, and back should be elevated to an incline of about 30 degrees, about 1/3 of the way up. This can be readily accomplished by using pillows and a seat cushion from a couch to provide an incline with a straight back as shown in Figure 8.12a. This exercise is always done semi-recumbent from this incline. It is never done when lying flat. The top pillow should be the Smart Support Pillow to stabilize the head and neck as you perform the exercise.

PERFORMING ISOMETRIC RESISTED QUADRICEPS STRENGTHENING EXERCISES

1) Slowly and carefully lift the right leg only at the hip, keeping the knee completely straight, and lift until the heel of the right foot is about one foot off the surface or at the level of the big toe of the other foot. This is depicted in Figure 8.12b.

2) Once the straight leg is up at about the one foot level, hold it there and tighten the muscles over the top of the right leg and gently bend your right foot and toes toward your head as shown in Figure 8.12b.

3) Now hold this right leg in this position for a 5 second count, then gently put the leg straight down.

4) Repeat this cycle for a total of 10 repetitions.

5) Following the same procedure, repeat the same cycle for the left leg for a total of 10 repetitions.

6) Do 10 repetitions of the isometric quadriceps strengthening exercise

on both sides every day. Whether you are starting out or highly proficient, you should do 10 repetitions on each side every single day. As
the purpose of the exercise is to improve quadriceps muscle strength,
tone, and neuromuscular coordination, the importance of consistency
and compliance cannot be overemphasized. However, it is not necessary to increase the number of repetitions beyond 10 per day per side
to accomplish these goals. Thus, the isometric quadriceps strengthening exercise program is also highly efficient and straightforward once
you have mastered the basics.

7) Isometric quadriceps strengthening exercises should never produce
pain in the low back or knees. If you develop pain, it is likely you are not
performing the exercise correctly. If pain recurs after reviewing how
you are performing the isometric quadriceps strengthening, then immediately discontinue them and consult your doctor.

8) The intensity of the isometric quadriceps strengthening exercise can be
increased by performing the exercise against added resistance by adding weight to the ankles. However, this should only be done under
supervision of your doctor when appropriate.

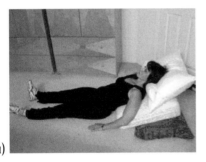 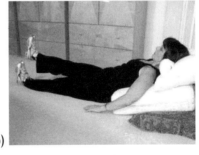

a)   b)

Figure 8.12: a) Position and posture for isometric quadriceps strengthening at
maximal elevation; b) tightening the muscles on the top of your leg and gently
bending the ankle and toes toward your head.

Improving Pain, Biomechanics, and Posture Through Range of Motion Exercises

Range of motion exercise programs are another strategy utilized to treat abnormal joint alignment and loading at rest and with use. The ability to maintain neutral joint or joint region positioning and support at rest or optimal alignment with use is highly dependent on the balance of muscular, gravitational, and/or other forces acting on that region. Muscle weakness or loss of tone leads to abnormal alignment of the joint region. This abnormal alignment predisposes to abnormal joint loading at rest which in turn is magnified by use and loading of the joint area. Range of motion exercises are valuable in some joint areas where orthotics are not physically reasonable or cannot compensate for ongoing abnormal joint loading and alignment and muscle strengthening exercises simply load or mal-align the joint region further without improving joint biomechanics. Range of motion exercises can be performed passively by moving the joint or joint region through a range by relaxing the muscles of the joint and using an external support or person to move the joint. Or, they can be self-performed actively by using the muscles of the joint to move the joint through its range. Joint regions that benefit from range of motion exercises are those in which improved joint alignment and mechanics occurs without significantly abnormal or excess loading or biomechanical strain to the joint area while performing the exercises.

Reducing Shoulder Pain Through Range of Motion Exercises

The shoulder joint and shoulder joint region is a classic site that benefits from range of motion exercises and the attendant neuromuscular re-education they provide. The shoulder joint and other shoulder related joint structures, tendons, ligaments, bursae, and capsule of the shoulder are designed for freedom of movement of the upper extremity. To achieve such a high degree of mobility, the innate structure of the shoulder sacrifices stability. This leaves the shoulder highly dependent on the capsule, ligaments, and muscles for support and alignment. Throughout the day, the shoulders are subjected to loading forces even at rest as the shoulder region muscles work to optimize stable alignment. With use, the shoulders undergo additional forces such as acceleration, deceleration, tension, compression loading, shear, torsion, or some combination of these.

These forces are further magnified by the additional forces of loading when the arms and hands are pushing, pulling, lifting, or carrying. The alignment of the shoulder comprising the alignment of the upper arm to the shoulder socket coupled with the tone of the muscles moving the shoulder all play a crucial role in the distribution of forces in the shoulder joint. These in turn are major determinants in the evolution and progression of bursitis, tendinitis, and capsulitis of the shoulder and osteoarthritis in the joints associated with the shoulder.

In patients with fibromyalgia polypain, subjective distinct shoulder symptoms are reported by 26% of patients. Objective findings in polypain identify the presence of subacromial bursitis and/or supraspinatus tendinitis in 21%. While the shoulder is inherently designed to undergo a wide range of movement, this is accompanied by an inherent instability of the joint to allow this freedom of range and, in the context of polypain, increases the risk of shoulder joint related symptoms and the development of joint damage and deformity. In addition to the normal loading demands upon the shoulder joint, inappropriate posture, ergonomics, and biomechanics lead to inappropriate and excess loading of the shoulder joint and shoulder related joint structures, tendons, ligaments, bursae, and capsule and amplify the normally expected loading forces through motions of the shoulders. These, in total, lead to increased symptoms and progression of the underlying osteoarthritis of the shoulder related joints and shoulder tendon, bursa, and capsule inflammation.

The mobility, strength, stability, and alignment of the shoulder joint region is controlled by a careful interplay of joint structure, the muscles supporting and moving the shoulder joint and shoulder related joints, the ligaments and capsule that hold the joint together, and the bursae protecting these structures. The predominant involvement of the shoulder tendons and bursae in fibromyalgia polypain identifies abnormal alignment and support issues in the shoulder joint region or shoulder girdle alignment mechanism. Improved shoulder muscle tone and coordination reduces and helps eliminate impingement abnormalities, stabilizes hypermobility, and helps improve abnormal alignment. Thus, the most crucial component in managing the shoulder related symptoms of polypain, and a further key component of fibromyalgia polypain treatment, is shoulder range of motion exercises. Through regular shoulder range of motion exercises, the shoulder muscles develop improved tone and a better sense of appropriate loading and alignment for the situations the shoulders are exposed to through feedback mechanisms to the spinal cord and brain. This neuromuscular re-education, allows the shoulder joint region to be better prepared for anticipated demands.

It is important to note that virtually all exercise programs recommended for treating shoulder joint region problems, at their core, are fundamentally shoulder range of motion toning and neuromuscular re-education programs. However, most shoulder exercise programs, just like low back and knee programs, are either too complex to allow compliant self-management, provide insufficient or impractical routines, or include deleterious exercises that exacerbate the pain and alignment issues.

In managing polypain, it has been my experience that the singular and most effective exercise program to provide the needed shoulder toning and neuromuscular education to improve shoulder joint region related symptoms is a self-managed, graded, medically supervised, active shoulder range of motion exercise program.

Shoulder Range of Motion Exercises
WALL CLIMBING

1) To set up for the wall climbing exercise, first find a wall without anything mounted on it.

2) Stand sideways to the wall at a distance such the when you raise your arm sideways, your fingertips will just touch the wall. This is depicted in Figure 8.13a.

3) Do a pelvic tilt and align your spine in a neutral position as reviewed earlier.

4) Gently and slowly use your fingers to climb the wall as you raise your shoulders. At the same time, side step in toward the wall with your feet. Do not lean into the wall or bend your body. By side stepping, you will keep your body straight and keep your spine aligned in a neutral position. See Figure 8.13b.

5) Continue climbing the wall and side stepping until your arm and hand are as elevated as possible by the support of the wall and you cannot side step any further without leaning your body or pushing your hip into the wall. Your body should remain in a vertically neutral position at the end of the wall climb. In most instances, your foot will be close to, but not touching, the wall and no other body part other than the forearm and hand will be in contact with the wall. See Figure 8.13c.

6) Once the arm is maximally raised, you will reverse the process and side step away from the wall gently and slowly using your fingers to climb down back to the starting position. Do not drop your arm.

7) Repeat this procedure for a total of 10 repetitions on the side you started with, then turn around to the other side and repeat the process for 10 repetitions.

8) Do 10 repetitions of the wall climb shoulder range of motion exercise on both sides every day. Whether you are starting out or highly profi-

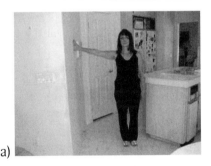

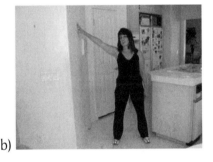

a)   b)

Figure 8.13: *Wall climbing exercise: a) initial stance for wall climbing; b) body position with wall climbing; c) body position with arm fully raised with wall climbing exercise.*

c)

cient, you should do 10 repetitions on each side every single day. As the purpose of the exercise is to improve shoulder joint region tone and neuromuscular coordination, the importance of consistency and compliance cannot be overemphasized. However, it is not necessary to increase the number of repetitions beyond 10 per day per side to accomplish these goals. Thus, the wall climb shoulder range of motion exercise program is also highly efficient and straightforward once you have mastered the basics.

9) If initially the shoulder does not seem to come up all the way, it may be there is a loss of range. This loss of range will usually improve as you continue to perform the exercise consistently over time.

10) There should be no new or additional shoulder pain when doing this exercise.

Arms Over Head

1) To set up for the arms over head exercise, you will need a yard/meter stick, or wooden dowel, or broom/mop handle of similar length. Taking the stick with you, seat yourself comfortably in a chair sitting upright and not sitting into the chair back.

2) Do a pelvic tilt and align your spine in a neutral position as reviewed earlier.

3) Facing forward, hold the stick in both hands in a palm down direction with both arms straight out resting on your knees. See Figure 8.14a.

4) Gently and slowly raise the stick with both arms evenly. If you have a painful shoulder, use the good side to help raise the painful side without adding to the underlying pain.

5) Raise both arms evenly, as far as they will go over your head. See Figure 8.14b and 8.14c. Maintain the pelvic tilt throughout the arm movement.

6) Once the arms and stick are maximally raised, you will reverse the process and gently and slowly lower your arms and stick until the stick is resting at your knees.

7) Repeat this procedure for a total of 10 repetitions.

8) Do 10 repetitions of the arms over head shoulder range of motion exercise with both arms every day. Whether you are starting out or highly proficient, you should do 10 repetitions every single day. As the purpose of the exercise is to improve shoulder joint region tone and neuromuscular coordination, the importance of consistency and compliance cannot be overemphasized. However, it is not necessary to increase the number of repetitions beyond 10 per day to accomplish these goals. Thus, the arms over head shoulder range of motion exercise program is also highly efficient and straightforward once you have mastered the basics.

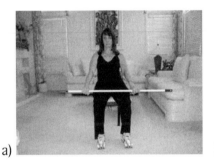
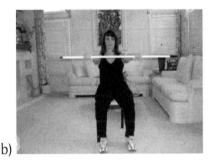
a) b)

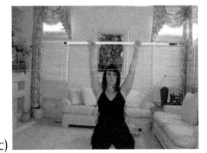
c)

Figure 8.14: *Arms over head exercise: a) initial seating position; b) arm, stick, and body position midway through raising the arms; c) arm, stick, and body position with arms fully raised.*

9) If initially one or both of the shoulders do not seem to come up all the way, it may be there is a loss of range. This loss of range will usually improve as you continue to perform the exercise consistently over time.

10) There should be no new or additional shoulder pain when doing this exercise.

TOWELING

1) To set up for the toweling exercise, you will need the same stick you used for the arm over head exercise. The toweling exercise is done standing.

2) Do a pelvic tilt and align your spine in a neutral position as reviewed earlier.

3) With the stick in your right hand, bring your right arm up and behind you so that the stick is behind your back and your right hand is near the top of your head. Bring your left arm and hand to your low back, upper buttock area and grasp the lower end of the stick. This is shown in Figure 8.15a.

4) Gently and slowly move your arms such that the stick creates a circular motion on your back. The benefit of the exercise is in moving the shoulder to create the circular motion similar to when toweling your back. Hence, the name "toweling" exercise. There is no benefit to the shoulder if there is only an up and down motion, as you are simply bending the elbows without ranging the shoulders. Complete the motion to make one full circle. See Figure 8.15b.

5) Repeat this procedure for a total of 10 circles.

6) Then release the stick and bring it in front of you and hold it in your left hand. Holding the stick in your left arm and hand, bring your left arm up and behind you so that the stick is behind your back and your left hand is near the top of your head. Bring your right arm and hand to your low back, upper buttock area and grasp the lower end of the stick. This is shown in Figure 8.15c.

7) Gently and slowly move your arms such that the stick creates a circular motion on your back, just as you did earlier. You will find the circles will automatically move in the opposite direction to the ones you had done in the reverse arm position. Repeat this for a total of 10 circles.

8) Do 10 repetitions of the toweling shoulder range of motion exercise in both positions every day. Whether you are starting out or highly proficient, you should do 10 repetitions in both positions every single day. As the purpose of the exercise is to improve shoulder joint region tone and neuromuscular coordination, the importance of consistency and compliance cannot be overemphasized. However, it is not necessary to increase the number of repetitions beyond 10 per day per position to accomplish these goals. Thus, the toweling shoulder range of motion exercise program is also highly efficient and straightforward once you have mastered the basics.

9) If initially the circles are difficult to make or seem very small, it may be there is a loss of range. This loss of range will usually improve as you continue to perform the exercise consistently over time. The circles

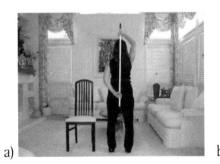

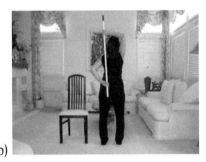

a)   b)

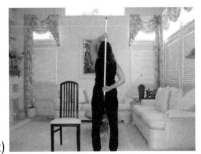

c)

Figure 8.15: *Toweling shoulder range of motion exercise: a) position of stick with right arm up and left arm down; b) circular motion of exercise; c) position of stick with left arm up and right arm down.*

are usually smaller than the space between your shoulder blades, even under ideal circumstances.

10) There should be no new or additional shoulder pain when doing this exercise.

Walking More While Reducing Pain: An Integrated Daily Walking Program

In terms of biomechanics and posture, one of the most challenging activities we undertake on a regular basis is walking. Walking demands optimal alignment, posture, biomechanics, and ergonomics of the toes, feet, ankles, knees, hips, low back, mid back, and neck. It requires the seamless coordination of joint movement and function to accomplish mobility efficiently and without pain or damage to the musculoskeletal structures. In patients with polypain, the presence of primary generalized osteoarthritis predominantly involving the neck and back with associated degenerative disc disease and the variable combination of osteoarthritis and associated tendinitis, bursitis, and fasciitis involving the toes, feet, knees, hips, low back, and neck may impair the fundamental mechanics of walking and limit the amount of weight bearing and walking that can be sustained. Of greater concern in polypain is that weight bearing and walking load the neck, low back and discs, hips, knees, feet, and toes and even more so in the face of abnormal joint structure and alignment. This promotes the evolution and progression of the underlying osteoarthritis and degenerative disc disease and the variable combination of associated tendinitis, bursitis, and fasciitis related to joint and spinal loading and usage, biomechanics, ergonomics, and posture. Thus, patients with polypain have multiple joint, joint region, and periarticular sites that are negatively impacted by the seemingly simple act of walking and the underlying primary generalized osteoarthritis predominantly involving the neck and back with associated degenerative disc disease and the variable combination of associated tendinitis, bursitis, and fasciitis greatly impact the biomechanics and ergonomics of walking leading to abnormal patterns of gait and limitations in ambulatory ability.

Managing polypain with appropriate medications and an appropriate biomechanics and posture treatment program incorporating orthotics, neuromuscular re-education, muscle strengthening, range of motion exercises, and appropriate weight loss not only reduces the pain intensity and severity but improves functional capability such as walking. In addition to specifically managing the individual joints and joint regions involved, the coordination of function of these multiple and separate regions to accomplish functional tasks such as walking requires retraining and re-educating the process under the treated conditions of these individual sites. This level of neuromuscular re-education is achieved through an integrated daily walking program promoting improved alignment, posture, biomechanics, and ergonomic interactions.

It is important to note that the integrated daily walking program is an exercise program that is distinct and separate from the regular and daily walking undertaken to accomplish activities such as walking to and from the car, shopping, and walking around the house or around the office. The integrated daily walking program should be done at a time set aside specifically for this activity as part of the Biomechanics and Posture portion of the Polypain Wellness Core. In so doing, you maximize the opportunity to be attentive to and respond to the biomechanical and ergonomic requirements of the walking program.

Fundamentals of the Integrated Daily Walking Program

While this integrated daily walking program can be done by virtually all individuals with polypain, there may be certain individuals who for other health reasons should avoid this walking program. Always check with your doctor to make sure that there is no reason why you should not do this walking program or if other than the recommended accommodations or modifications are required. This walking program should never cause more pain than you already have. If there is an increase in your symptoms, it is likely you have not followed all the recommendations and instructions correctly. In any case, if there is any increase in symptoms that cannot be eliminated by making any needed accommodations or modifications to the exercise, immediately discontinue the exercise and contact your doctor. Do not continue the walking program if there is an increase in your symptoms or you develop any new symptoms including new pain or breathing difficulties. Having said all this however, virtually everyone, with rare exception, should be able to perform and benefit from the Polypain Wellness Core Integrated Daily Walking Program.

1) In the presence of polypain, the most important fundamental step in initiating a walking program is the proper identification of all the joints, joint regions, and periarticular sites that are involved in your specific circumstances. This is necessary to ensure that site specific treatment, especially in terms of medications, posture, biomechanics, and ergonomics, is undertaken appropriately prior to starting a walking program. It is also necessary to ensure that there is no contraindication to a walking program such as involvement of joint sites or regions that may worsen by walking or the presence of other comorbid conditions such as cardiovascular or respiratory contraindications to a walking program.

2) You must have the Smart Support Neck Collar and be comfortable with its use. You must have the Universole or Winsole Arch Support System appropriately set up and in place in a good pair of running, cross trainer, or sport walking shoes. You must be adept at performing daily abdominal muscle strengthening and toning exercises and isometric resisted quadriceps strengthening exercises. You must be able to perform pelvic tilts correctly on demand. Most importantly, you must be able to perform vertical pelvic tilts when standing and walking, correctly, on demand.

3) In preparing for the walk, you must do the abdominal strengthening exercise and isometric resisted quadriceps strengthening exercise portions of the Polypain Wellness Core Program before walking.

4) You must wear the Smart Neck Support Collar. You must wear the sport shoes with the Universole or Winsole Arch Support System.

5) This walking program requires you to be knowledgeable and vigilant about your posture and biomechanics. Thus, walking outdoors is preferable to walking on a treadmill as you can control the rate and pace including stopping and starting in response to your abilities and the biomechanical and ergonomic demands of walking. Treadmill walking is much more challenging and demanding as the treadmill forces you to keep a certain pace regardless of symptoms or need for change in biomechanics and posture. Treadmill walking should only be undertaken by individuals experienced in the requirements of outdoor walking and under the supervision of your doctor.

6) This is a walking program. Therefore, walk comfortably and don't run.

7) When starting this program, you should walk at a comfortable regular walking pace, which, depending on your symptoms and health status, is usually about 1-1½ miles per hour.

8) As you walk, incorporate pelvic tilts intermittently and do pelvic tilts if you feel any symptoms in your low back, buttocks, or legs such as a sense of fatigue, increased pain, or new pain. This is depicted in Figure 8.16. If pelvic tilts performed while walking do not alleviate such symptoms, find a nearby wall and do the pelvic tilt routine as described in the section on pelvic tilts. These should be sufficient to control any increase in symptoms and permit you to complete the walk. Any new or persistent symptoms should be reported to your doctor and the walk should be discontinued pending resolution. You must be constantly vigilant to your body position and needed adjustments to maintain neutral posture and biomechanics.

9) In general, when starting this program, you should endeavor to walk 15 minutes daily. As the walking becomes easier, you can increase the walk by 5 minute increments. Generally, the increments should occur every several weeks barring any complications. The goal is to gradually increase the walking time while maintaining the initial pace of 1-1½ miles per hour. Depending on time availability, most individuals eventually manage to get in 30-60 minutes of walking. Once the walking program is established at this time interval without difficulty, then the pace can be slowly increased

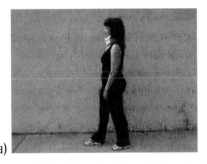 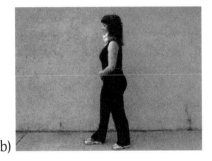

a) b)

Figure 8.16: *Pelvic tilt while walking: a) without hands bracing abdominal muscles; b) with hands bracing abdominal muscles.*

adding one-tenth to two-tenths miles per hour every several weeks barring any complications. Eventually, the walking pace can be increased to 3 miles per hour. Speeds greater than 3 miles per hour generally are brisk walking, jogging, or running speeds and are not part of the fundamental walking program but may be undertaken under the care and advice of your doctor as appropriate.

This Integrated Daily Walking Program improves the coordinated action of the joints, discs, muscles, ligaments, tendons, bursae, and fasciae involved in walking through neuromuscular re-education, strengthening, and toning. This also allows the opportunity to not only physically impact the immediate osteoarthritis process symptomatically but also to slow its progression especially in terms of potential joint damage and deformity. This also leads to improved pain message processing. Thus, by improving pain source intensity and severity, the pain gap narrows or the pain free reserve deepens and not only is there less pain for any increased demand on the joints, tendons, bursae, and fasciae but there is an increased ability to walk without obvious or significant flare of symptoms and there is a more rapid and greater ability to recover from an exacerbation related to walking. Further, the Integrated Daily Walking Program provides the opportunity to directly treat the musculoskeletal structures involved in polypain and improve joint, spine, and periarticular loading, structure, alignment, and ergonomics to help reduce the progression of osteoarthritis and degenerative disc disease that would develop absent these interventions.

In addition to the musculoskeletal benefit, the Integrated Daily Walking Program provides the other identified benefits of regular physical exercise. Such benefits of regular physical exercise include aerobic conditioning, improved weight control with increased calorie burn, psychological well-being with reduction in depression and stress, improved bone density and reduction in risk of osteoporosis, reduction in blood pressure and reduced risk of developing hypertension, reduced risk of developing diabetes and improved diabetic control in those affected, improved cognitive and physical functioning in the elderly, reduction of risk of developing stroke, reduction in risk of dying from heart disease, reduction in risk from developing colon cancer, and reduction in risk of dying prematurely.

Improved weight control with concomitant weight reduction leads to reduced load on the low back and weight bearing joints leading to improvement in the pain and biomechanics of fibromyalgia polypain. Similarly, walking related improvement in depression and stress improves pain processing in polypain with increased pain thresholds. Thus, in addition to the beneficial impact to each of these individual components of polypain, the interaction of these components identifies additional synergistic benefits of the Integrated Daily Walking Program.

Why Current Exercise Programs and Physical Therapy For Fibromyalgia Fail

In the face of musculoskeletal pain, many individuals undertake self-directed exercise programs in the belief that moving their joints is of benefit. Many physicians refer patients to physical therapy for the same reason. While specifically targeted and controlled intervention with orthotics, neuromuscular re-education, muscle strengthening, range of motion exercises, and weight loss are critical modalities of treatment for fibromyalgia polypain, the introduction of self-directed exercises including pool exercises or undirected physical therapy invariably causes a worsening of polypain symptoms. Patients with polypain usually get worse when undertaking self-directed programs specifically due to a complete lack of knowledge or understanding about the polyregional nature of the disease and the biomechanical and ergonomic demands on unrecognized joint or joint regions or due to misunderstood mechanisms or sources of pain. Such endeavors eventually cause the involved areas to worsen. Swimming programs and aquatic therapy programs are the worst culprits in this regard. Despite the notion that the buoyancy of water helps reduce joint pressure, the movement induced by water waves, the body's resistance to that movement, and exercises performed against the drag resistance of water load the upper and lower extremity joints as well as the neck and low back excessively and exacerbate the underlying osteoarthritis, degenerative disc disease, and the associated tendinitis, bursitis, and fasciitis of polypain. Any exercises other than those recommended in this book should not be undertaken without a comprehensive evaluation of the effect of such exercise on the targeted area and the other areas involved in the polypain process.

Chapter 9

Step 3: The Real Facts About Weight Management, Pain, and What To Do

"According to statistics, everyone who eats, dies."—Jeff Sarkozi, M.D.

The importance of weight management in the treatment of fibromyalgia polypain relates to the association of overweight and obesity in the development and evolution of symptoms associated with osteoarthritis, tendinitis, bursitis, and fasciitis in the low back, hips, knees, ankles, feet, as well as the hands. While many factors influence an individual's weight independent of the presence of fibromyalgia polypain, clearly, the presence of chronic widespread pain and musculoskeletal impairments from primary generalized osteoarthritis, degenerative disc disease, tendinitis, bursitis, and fasciitis may lead to reduced physical activity predisposing to weight gain, overweight, and obesity. Other components of fibromyalgia polypain may contribute as well. Effective treatment of fibromyalgia polypain should be expected to decrease these activity limitations and reduce any related weight gain. However, overweight and obesity due to factors not related to fibromyalgia polypain also adversely impact fibromyalgia polypain and require independent management to reduce their burden to the pain.

How Overweight And Obesity Contribute To Pain

The primary mechanism by which overweight and obesity impact osteoarthritis results directly from weight related increased loading of the spine, weight bearing joints, and periarticular structures. Yet clearly, other factors also play a role especially given the association of hand osteoarthritis to overweight and obesity. These include metabolic factors correlated with obesity such as abnormalities of lipid and glucose metabolism and obesity associated inflammation.

Weight bearing and walking demand optimal alignment, posture, biomechanics, and ergonomics of the toes, feet, ankles, knees, hips, low back, mid back, and neck to accommodate the normally expected loading of the joints and joint related structures. In patients with polypain, the presence of primary generalized osteoarthritis predominantly involving the low back with associated degenerative disc disease and the variable combination of associated tendinitis, bursitis, and fasciitis involving the toes, feet, knees, hips, and low back may impair the fundamental mechanics of weight bearing and walking through abnormal joint structure and alignment and may limit the amount of weight bearing and walking that can be sustained. The impact of loading the low back and discs, hips, knees, feet, and toes through weight bearing and walking is magnified in the face of such abnormal joint structure and alignment. Excess weight adds to this burden and further promotes the evolution and progression of the underlying osteoarthritis, degenerative disc disease, and the variable combination of associated tendinitis, bursitis, and fasciitis related to joint and spinal loading and usage, biomechanics, ergonomics, and posture in the low back, weight bearing joints, and joint related structures. Thus, overweight and obese patients with polypain have multiple joint, joint region, and periarticular sites that are additionally impacted by excess weight, especially when weight bearing and walking.

Distorted Perceptions Of Overweight and Obesity

The issue of overweight and obesity receives considerable attention in our society. From mainstream media, to public and private healthcare agencies and groups, to the commercial sector promoting weight loss treatments and programs, there is an ongoing barrage of information regarding a purported burgeoning epidemic of fat and gluttony. The general message is that we are becoming alarmingly fat, that this is occurring rapidly in front of our very eyes, and that we are doomed because of it. Indeed, one group of medical experts has postulated that gains in life expectancy seen in the past thousand years will level off, or worse, will reverse solely because of obesity. Such dire warnings, based on hypotheses and assumptions, serve only to fuel fear and panic rather than inform a confused public whose common sense is being manipulated. The situation is further complicated by the fact that population risk studies are much removed from the clinical setting of determining risks for any one individual patient.

There is an important additional force adding to the exaggerated perception of massive obesity overtaking society. It is found in the contradictory cultural view of the ideal body image. Despite some increase in weight in the population of the United States over the decades as discussed below, the ideal female image of today is thinner and weighs less than her counterpart of decades ago as seen in the weights of Miss America contestants, Playboy models, and other models and actresses. These factors have led to the current circumstance in which virtually everyone wrongly believes they are too fat and that their mission in life is to be as thin and light as they were when they were twenty or, worse yet, the thinnest person they could think of. Such cognitive distortions persist despite the real fact that the majority of the population is not obese as we will see further on. On the other hand, there is a minority group of individuals who have true obesity at age twenty onward, in whom fat and weight critically exceed that of their peers, and for whom many real health concerns emerge.

What Is Obesity?

Conceptually, the definition of obesity is straightforward. It is a condition of excess body fat. The controversial points in this understanding are what is meant by "excess" and what is meant by "condition". These terms mean different things depending on the era and circumstance and are driven by social, cosmetic, medical, and personal bias. From a health standpoint, given that weight is a continuous measure, that we all weigh something, and we all have some body fat, the question is: At what point is body fat excessive enough to be considered an unhealthful state making it a medical condition? From a clinical standpoint, the degree of body fat is expressed as the Body Mass Index, the BMI. The BMI is a measurement of weight relative to height. Importantly, the BMI correlates with total body fat content. Specifically, the BMI is defined as body weight in kilograms divided by the height in meters squared as shown in Figure 9.1. If measuring weight in pounds and height in inches, a correction factor can be multiplied in to derive the BMI.

BMI = WEIGHT in Kilograms ÷ (HEIGHT in Meters)²

BMI = [WEIGHT in Pounds ÷ (HEIGHT in Inches)²] x 703

Figure 9.1: Calculation of BMI.

Based on risk stratification, the National Institute of Health has classified overweight as a BMI greater than 25 and obesity as a BMI greater than 30. Note that overweight and obesity are not the same category. Overweight people are not obese. I repeat, overweight people are not obese people and are not necessarily over-fat people. Obese individuals are, on the other hand, by definition, excessively fat from a health standpoint. It is also important to not get lost in the rhetoric of overweight and obesity and fail to recognize that there are many individuals whose weight is quite normal and others who are downright relatively too light. Normal or healthy weight is classified as a BMI of 18.5-24.9 and underweight as a BMI of less than 18.5. This is depicted in Table 9.1.

	Obesity Class	BMI (kg/m²)
Underweight		Less than or equal to 18.5
Normal/Healthy Weight		18.5 – 24.9
Overweight		25 – 29.9
Obesity	I	30 – 34.9
	II	35 – 39.9
Extreme Obesity	III	Greater than or equal to 40

Table 9.1: Classification of overweight and obesity by BMI. (Adapted from National Institute of Health, National Heart, Lung and Blood Institute. Clinical Guidelines on the Identification, Evaluation and Treatment of Overweight and Obesity in Adults: The Evidence Report. Washington, D.C.: NIH Publication No.: 98-4083; 1998)

The weights at which an individual falls into the normal/healthy weight category, overweight category, and obese category are displayed in Table 9.2. A five foot three inch woman is not considered to be even overweight until she weighs 141 pounds and a five foot ten inch man is not overweight until he reaches 174 pounds. The same five foot three inch woman is not considered obese until she weighs 169 pounds and the five foot ten inch man is considered to obese at a weight of 209 pounds.

Height in Inches	Normal/Healthy Weight (in pounds) BMI 18.5-24.9	Overweight (in pounds) BMI 25-29.9	Obesity (in pounds) BMI 30 or greater
58	88-119	119-143	Over 143
59	91-123	124-148	Over 148
60	95-127	128-153	Over 153
61	98-132	132-158	Over 158
62	101-136	136-163	Over 164
63	104-140	141-168	Over 169
64	108-145	145-174	Over 174
65	111-149	150-179	Over 180
66	114-153	155-185	Over 185
67	118-159	159-191	Over 192
68	121-163	164-196	Over 197
69	125-168	170-202	Over 203
70	129-173	174-208	Over 209
71	132-178	179-214	Over 215
72	136-183	184-220	Over 221
73	140-188	189-226	Over 227
74	144-194	194-232	Over 233
75	148-199	200-239	Over 240
76	152-204	205-245	Over 246

Table 9.2: *Weight in pounds based on Body Mass Index and height in inches.*

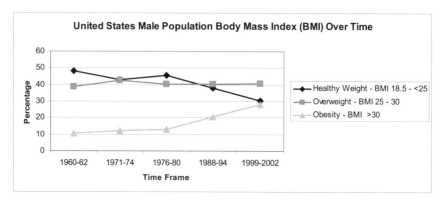

Figure 9.2: *The age-adjusted prevalence of BMI independent of age, race, and ethnicity for men age 20-74 years over time. (Data from National Center for Health Statistics. Health, United States, 2005 with Chartbook on Trends in the Health of Americans. Maryland: U.S. Government Printing Office; 2005)*

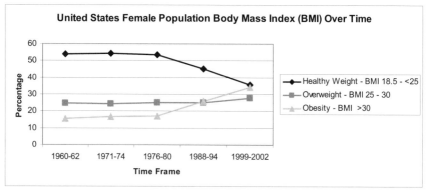

Figure 9.3: *The age-adjusted prevalence of BMI independent of age, race, and ethnicity for women age 20-74 years over time. (Data from National Center for Health Statistics. Health, United States, 2005 with Chartbook on Trends in the Health of Americans. Maryland: U.S. Government Printing Office; 2005)*

Why Do We Gain Weight?

In exploring the question as to why obesity develops, we must consider the issue of obesity from two perspectives. The first is the issue of societal weight shift. The second issue is about the factors that contribute to weight gain in any one individual.

Everybody Is Gaining Weight

Population studies based on national health and nutrition surveys since 1960 performed by the National Center for Health Statistics have gathered data on the age-adjusted prevalence of BMI independent of age, race, and ethnicity for individuals age 20-74 years. The results are depicted in Figures 9.2 and 9.3 for men and women respectively.

These data clearly show that until the 1976-80 time frame, the prevalence of the healthy weight, overweight, and obese BMI groups was relatively stable with a very slight reduction in the prevalence of healthy weight individuals and a very slight concomitant increase in the obese group. Between the 1976-80 through 1999-2002 time frames, there was a marked decline in the absolute prevalence of healthy weight individuals measuring 15.2% less men and 18.1% less women. At the same time, there was an absolute 15.3% increase in the prevalence of obesity in men and 16.9% in women.

The relative increase in obesity is an impressive number with a 120% relative increase in the prevalence of obesity in males and a 99% increase in females or about a doubling in the relative presence of obesity. These relative numbers are used to promote the concept of an epidemic of obesity. The real magnitude of change, though, is a 15.3% increase in the prevalence of obesity in men and 16.9% in women.

However, the prevalence of individuals classified as overweight has remained essentially unchanged as seen by the relatively straight line for this group in both the male and female graphs. What this tells us is that there has not been a sudden explosion of obesity at all, but rather there has been a gradual increasing shift of the overall weight of everybody to cause 15% of men and 17% of women who were at the high end of healthy weight in 1976-80 to gain enough weight to enter the lower levels of the BMI category of overweight by 1999-2002. Similarly, the same weight gain in the overweight group caused the same percentage of individuals in the lower levels of overweight BMI to shift to the higher BMI levels in the same overweight category, the higher levels of overweight BMI individuals to shift into the lower levels of obese BMI, and, ultimately, lower levels of obese BMI individuals to shift into the higher levels of obese BMI. In other words, it appears that everybody in the United States population gained some weight and increased their BMI category accordingly.

The magnitude of such weight gain can be gleaned from data from health surveys from the National Center for Health Statistics. The actual measured mean weight gain for men age 20-74 from the latter time period of 1976-80 through 1999-2002 is 17.2 pounds resulting in a 10% increase in weight. The mean weight gain for women age 20-74 is 18.9 pounds resulting in a 13% increase in weight over that time period. This increase in the weight of the general adult population has been gradual, not sudden. Thus, the issue of the epidemic of obesity is not an epidemic in the true sense of the concept but, rather, is really a gradual, but nonetheless real, shift in weight with gain in mean weight of the population in the order of about 17 to 19 pounds over the past two to three decades. While clearly of significant health concern, it is important to keep a perspective on these absolute numbers with regard to the measured weight shift as the experts and media have many believing everybody is becoming obscenely obese and distorting perspectives by implying this is occurring at an alarmingly rapid rate.

Expect to Gain Weight After Your Twenties

Another important consideration in the understanding of weight issues is the effect of age on weight. It is surprising and disappointing to many of my patients that they gain weight as they get older. This occurs despite their knowledge that other friends and family in their age group invariably have also gained weight. The fact is that everybody naturally gains weight in their early to mid-adult life. Anthropometric reference data collected between 1988-1994 for the National Health and Nutrition Examination Survey (NHANES) regarding weight as measured in pounds in men and women over 20 years of age is depicted in Figure 9.4. The data clearly show that there is weight gain in both men and women that starts in their twenties and peaks in their fifties. Subsequently, weight naturally declines returning closer to their weight in their twenties. The peak weight gain from the age twenties to the fifties is 17.1 pounds in men and 22 pounds in women representing an overall 10% gain in body weight in men and 16% gain in body weight in women. Of course, this natural cycling of weight gain is added to the up-shift of weights over the past two-three decades putting individuals at increased risk of increasing weight sufficiently to fall into the obese category for a period of time. Nonetheless, weight gain of about 10-20% from one's twenties to one's fifties is normal, natural, and expected.

Socio-environmental Contributors

Sociological factors affecting weight patterns in society are simply the summation of specific factors that otherwise impact each individual's weight but affect large numbers of the population-at-large in the same time frame generally by virtue of public heath policy, social attitude, or commonly shared environmental events. As noted, the more significant shift in incremental weight gain began its onset in the 1976-80 time frame as seen in Figures 9.2 and 9.3. A significant public health campaign was underway in the same time frame encouraging discontinuation of smok-

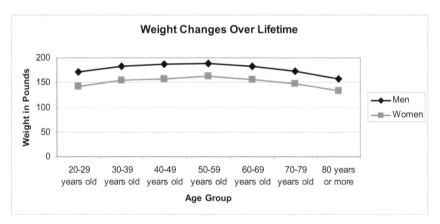

Figure 9.4: *Mean weight of men and women over lifetime as measured in pounds between 1988 to 1994 spanning a lifetime. (Data from National Health and Nutrition Examination Survey. Anthropometric reference data, United States, 1988-1994. Center for Disease Control, National Center for Health Statistics. 3 June 2006 <www.cdc.gov/nchs/about/major/nhanes/Anthropometric%20Measures.htm>)*

ing. This was coupled with changing societal attitudes toward smoking in recognition of the negative health consequences attributed to smoking. Indeed, a significant reduction in smoking took place between 1965 to 1990 with a reduction of current smokers from 41.9% to 25.3% as seen in Figure 9.5. This was followed by an ongoing but slower rate of decline from 25.3% in 1990 to 21.5% in 2003.

The significance of cigarette smoking lies in the well documented phenomenon of weight gain in smokers who quit. Within 10 years of smoking cessation, the mean weight gain of smokers who quit, beyond time related weight gain in ongoing smokers, is 9.7 pounds for men and 11 pounds for women. However, weight gains of greater than 28 pounds have been reported in 10% of men and 13% of women who have quit smoking. It has been estimated that cessation of smoking has contributed to about 25% of the prevalence of overweight/obesity in men and 16% of the prevalence of overweight/obesity in women. Thus, a portion of the so-called epidemic of obesity is actually a by-product of social engineering in the area of smoking cessation for which the benefit-cost/risk analysis was not fully comprehended. Indeed, this is another example of the Law of Unintended, but in this case bad, Consequences. Clearly, smokers who quit smoking

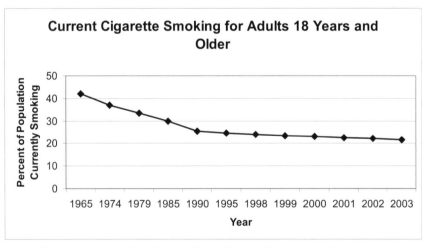

Figure 9.5: *Prevalence of smoking in the adult United States population age 18 years and older. (Data from National Center for Health Statistics. Health, United States, 2005 with Chartbook on Trends in the Health of Americans. Maryland: U.S. Government Printing Office; 2005)*

improve their health and survival from quitting smoking. However, they get fatter and often sufficiently fat to become obese. Coupled with their improved smoking cessation survival, they survive longer in their overweight and obese state. They then get to suffer the health consequences and increased mortality related to obesity. Thus, in regard to the public health issue of smoking cessation, we traded off the morbidity and mortality of smoking for the morbidity and mortality of obesity which has now become the new focus of public health intervention. In the realm of public health and social engineering, when it comes to free will choice behaviors, social scientists and the public must very wisely be careful what they wish for.

Another factor contributing to the weight gain of our population is the increasing sedentary nature of our culture by virtue of labor saving machines, computers, and video screens. After controlling for exercise, age, diet, and smoking status, a large study found that each two hour increase in television watching was correlated with a 23 percent increase in obesity. In contrast, in communities in which physical activity and walking are a way of life, individuals weigh less on average than comparison groups and there is a reduced prevalence of obesity. It has been suggested that reduced energy expenditure is a more significant contributor to obesity than increased food intake and reduced activity accounts for almost all the weight gain in the population. In a 10 year study of weight change, it was noted that recreational activity correlated inversely with weight. In other words the less activity performed, the heavier the weight. The tradeoff for reduced physical demands at work and leisure especially coupled with the highly sedentary increase in video screen time is the reduction in calorie expenditure which, absent a reduction of caloric intake, results in weight gain. Again, note the Law of Unintended Consequences.

Finally, the ready availability of cheap food through efficient agriculture, food processing, and food delivery has led to an overall increased consumption of calories with women eating 300 calories per day more in the year 2000 than compared to 1971 and men about 200 calories more. This increased caloric intake coupled with reduced activity contributes significantly as well to the increase in weight and increased prevalence of obesity in the past two to three decades. Once again, note the Law of Unintended Consequences.

It is likely that, as these socio-environmental factors come into balance, the population weight shift will also come into balance, albeit at a higher set point in the given circumstances. There is no substantiation for the concern that there will be an endless pattern of weight increase in the population.

Individual Factors:
Those We Control and Those We Don't

Factors that influence weight in any one particular individual can be categorized into 2 groups. The first group is composed of the genetic factors we inherit that comprise our fundamental biological make up. The second group are the socio-environmental factors that affect us not only individually, but as noted above, can cause population shifts in weight when large numbers of individuals are impacted at the same time.

Hereditary genetic factors comprise the genetic components that relate to obesity and include obesity or weight control genes, sex, and race. Evidence supporting the genetic role of obesity is found in data showing that BMI is correlated amongst first degree relatives. Further support comes from twin studies correlating BMI between twins with the stronger association amongst identical twins even if twins were raised apart in distinctly separate environments. The BMI of adopted children correlates with the BMI of their biological parents and not their adoptive parents.

There are genetic rodent models of obesity identifying specific genes that cause obesity such the Agouti gene and the leptin gene. The relevance of these genes and their products is yet to be determined in humans and in and of themselves do not account for obesity in most obese individuals. In addition, there are rare metabolic diseases in humans with specific gene abnormalities in which obesity is a component of the disease complex. In terms of common everyday obesity, it is clear that genetic factors contribute to the variation in weight and fat distribution between individuals and the contribution of genetics to weight and fat distribution has been estimated to be about 50% with a range of between 25% to 70%. In other words, about half the contribution to an individual's weight is inherited and predetermined. Individuals inherit half their risk of overweight and obesity. The bottom line is: If you want to know why you are as fat (or as thin) as you are, or how fat you are going to be, look at the old family photos. If one's relatives are overweight or obese, it should come as no surprise that an individual might be overweight or obese. It is a tough challenge to overcome genetics, however, genetics only determine where the set point for weight is to be. Genetics yields a predetermined, potential target weight. Where an individual's actual weight ends up, however, is also controlled by socio-environmental factors that control the other 50% contribution to weight, for good or for worse.

Clearly, the socio-environmental factors discussed above are impacts that develop at the level of each individual. The consequences of smoking and smoking cessation, fitness and activity level, caloric intake, body image, and age related factors are vital contributors to the weight status of any one individual. Amongst adult women, pregnancy is another important factor contributing to weight gain. In addition to the expected weight gain related to pregnancy itself, there is the issue of weight retained following delivery. One study reported that 41.6% of women reported retaining 9 or more pounds of their pregnancy weight with 33.8% reporting retaining 14 or more pounds. Following a first pregnancy, women retain 4.4-6.6 pounds of their pregnancy weight. In a group followed for 10 years, sustained weight gain from one live birth was 3.7 pounds and for 3 live births during that period, retained weight was 4.9 pounds.

Another important contribution to weight gain amongst individuals under medical care is medication associated weight gain. In general, drugs that cause non-water related weight gain fall into six categories: psychoactive medications; anticonvulsant drugs; diabetes therapy; serotonin/histamine antagonists; beta blockers; and hormonal interventions. Typical medications known to produce weight gain are listed in Table 9.3.

While not often addressed, sleep deprivation also appears to possibly contribute to weight gain through increased hunger and appetite.

What Are The Consequences of Obesity?

The health risks of overweight and obesity are risks. Not absolute guarantees. They are risks of disease, disease complications, and mortality that are linked to increased weight. Thus, overweight and obesity correlate with adverse health outcomes but the strength of the correlation varies directly with the degree of excess weight above normal weight and more specifically with the abdominal obesity as determined by the amount of fat around the waist. As depicted in Table 9.4, compared to normal

Category	Class	Medications
Psychoactive		
	Antipsychotic	Thioridazine, clozapine, olanzipine, sertindole, risperidone, quetiapine
	Antidepressant	Tricyclic antidepressants: Amitryptiline, nortriptyline, imipramine, doxepin; Selective serotonin reuptake inhibitors: paroxitene; Other: mirtazapine
	Lithium	Lithium carbonate
Anticonvulsant		Gabapentin, valproate, carbamazepine
Diabetes Therapy		Insulin, sulfonylureas, metiglinide, thiazolidenediones
Serotonin/Histamine Antagonist		Cyproheptadine, pizotifen
Beta Blocker		Propanolol, atenolol, metoprolol
Steroid Hormones		Glucocorticoids; Progestins: megestrol acetate, medroxyprogesterone acetate

Table 9.3: *Medications known to cause weight gain.*

weight individuals, the disease risk for type II diabetes mellitus, hypertension, and cardiovascular disease is increased in overweight individuals and the risk continually increases as weight increases. The presence of excess abdominal fat as defined as a waist circumference greater than 35 inches in women and 40 inches in men increases the risk of these complications, particularly in those who are in the overweight or class I obesity group.

While clearly increased weight above normal identifies an increased risk of medical complications compared to normal or underweight individuals, even individuals with normal weight or underweight carry a degree of risk for the same diseases. Weight is simply one factor amongst many other genetic and environmental influences that contribute to the development

	Obesity Class	BMI (kg/m^2)	Disease Risk	
			Waist Circumference ≤ 40 inches (Men) ≤ 35 inches (Women)	Waist Circumference > 40 inches (Men) > 35 inches (Women)
Underweight		Less than or equal to 18.5	Baseline	Baseline/↑
Normal/Healthy Weight		18.5 – 24.9	Baseline	Baseline/↑
Overweight		25 – 29.9	↑	↑↑
Obesity	I	30 – 34.9	↑↑	↑↑↑
	II	35 – 39.9	↑↑↑	↑↑↑
Extreme Obesity	III	Greater than or equal to 40	↑↑↑↑	↑↑↑↑

Table 9.4: Classification of weight status according to BMI and waist circumference with associated disease risks of type II diabetes mellitus, hypertension, and cardiovascular disease. (Adapted from National Institute of Health, National Heart, Lung and Blood Institute. Clinical Guidelines on the Identification, Evaluation and Treatment of Overweight and Obesity in Adults: The Evidence Report. Washington, D.C.: NIH Publication No.: 98-4083; 1998)

and progression of these complications. Indeed, there is ongoing debate as to whether these increased risks are solely attributable to obesity and fat or the accompanying lack of physical activity and fitness – the fat versus fitness debate. It is also notable that there are obviously many overweight, obese, and even some extremely obese individuals without such health complications.

Diseases and disorders correlated with overweight and/or obesity include lipid disorders; type II diabetes mellitus; hypertension; ischemic heart disease; congestive heart failure; stroke; osteoarthritis; cancers of the colon, breast in post-menopausal women, prostate, uterus, and gall-bladder; respiratory disorders and sleep apnea; gallstone disease; and psychological disturbances such as depression. Another complication of obesity that is frequently overlooked is the social impact of obesity. Individuals who appear fat to other people are viewed as less sincere, less friendly, meaner, and more obnoxious. Obese women earn less money than their non-obese counterparts and are less likely to be married. Indeed, when a non-obese job applicant is made up to appear 30 pounds

Age Group	BMI				
	<18.5 (Underweight)	18.5 to <25 (Normal weight)	25 to <30 (Overweight)	30 to <35 (Class I Obesity)	35 and over (Class II/III obesity combined)
25-59 years	1.38 (greater risk)	1	0.83 (lesser risk)	1.2 (greater risk)	1.83 (greater risk)
60-69 years	2.3 (greater risk)	1	0.95 (lesser risk)	1.13 (greater risk)	1.63 (greater risk)
70 years and over	1.69 (greater risk)	1	0.91 (lesser risk)	1.03 (greater risk)	1.17 (greater risk)

Table 9.5: *Relative risk of mortality at BMI categories of underweight, normal weight, overweight, class I obesity, and class II/III obesity in 3 age groups. Values are relative risk compared to normal weight individuals and values less than 1 indicate reduced risk of mortality and values greater than one indicate increased risk of mortality with the risk increasing as the value increases. (Data from Flegal KM, Graubard BI, Williamson DF et al. Excess deaths associated with underweight, overweight, and obesity. JAMA 2005; 293: 1861-1867)*

heavier and applies for the same job, the overweight appearing individual is less likely to be hired. Such negative attitudes toward obesity evolve into discrimination not only in the employment sphere but also in college acceptance and rental housing.

While the risk of health complications associated with excess weight correlates with increasing BMI and abdominal fat, the risk of mortality related to obesity is much less clear and significantly more controversial. Combined mortality data obtained from the National Health and Nutrition Examination Survey (NHANES) I, II, and III stratified according to BMI for age groups 25-59 years, 60-69 years, and 70 years and over provides the relative risk of mortality compared to the normal weight group that served as the reference point. The results are detailed in Table 9.5 and demonstrated graphically in Figure 9.6.

The results of this data reveal, contrary to common belief and implication in the media and community, that being overweight, but not specifically obese, carries no increased risk of dying from the excess weight and indeed appears to be associated with a reduced risk of mortality.

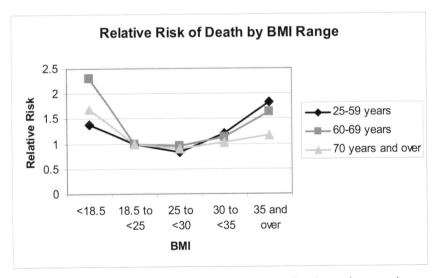

Figure 9.6: *Relative risk of mortality at BMI categories of underweight, normal weight, overweight, class I obesity and class II/III obesity (see Table 9.5 for category descriptions and risk meanings) in 3 age groups. (Data from Flegal KM, Graubard BI, Williamson DF et al. Excess deaths associated with underweight, overweight, and obesity. JAMA 2005; 293: 1861-1867)*

Class I obesity, BMI 30-35, carries only a slight relative increase risk of mortality if one is under 70 years of age, but no increased added risk if one is older. Overall, significantly increased relative risks for dying in any age group occur if an individual is underweight with a BMI less than 18.5 or significantly overweight with a BMI of 35 or greater. This results in the U shaped curves seen in Figure 9.6. The data also reveals another important relationship with regard to age and weight. In essence, the older the individual, the lesser the impact of obesity on mortality. Indeed, this makes perfect sense given the natural, normal, and expected weight gain seen from one's twenties to fifties. After all, why would the body naturally accumulate some weight and fat from one's twenties to one's fifties if it was going to kill that person? Conversely, being underweight carries increased mortality risk in the older age groups compared to the youngest age group of 25-59 years. Similar results have been obtained in numerous studies. What this means from a mortality perspective is that individuals should keep their weight down when they are young and allow it to climb naturally but not excessively with age. Being underweight in old age is a bad sign and being obese in one's youth is just plain bad.

Another important issue raised by the data presented relates to the significance of weight gain after age 20. After all, it is normal and natural to gain weight from one's twenties to one's fifties. Clearly, the relative risk of health complications such as diabetes, hypertension, and cardiovascular disease increases with increasing weight even in those in the normal weight BMI category. Thus, any age related increase in weight would be expected to add to that relative risk. Indeed, this is confirmed in a large study of women in which weight gain of 5-7.9 kg after age 18 mildly increased the risk of coronary heart disease compared to a weight gain of 5 kg or less and the relative risk increased with further increases in weight correlating with increased BMIs. Further, even within the normal weight BMI category, weight gain over 5 kg was associated with increased cardiovascular risk. This is consistent with the association of increased risk of cardiovascular disease with increasing BMI values even in the normal weight BMI category as described above for the general population.

Thus, there is consistent and strong evidence regarding increased relative risk compared to normal weight individuals of health complications such as diabetes, hypertension, and cardiovascular disease and increased mortality in individuals who are obese, as defined by a BMI of 30 or greater, especially when there is increased abdominal and waist area fat accumulation, and especially if under age 70. However, the data presented above with regard to a lesser, but nonetheless increased, relative risk of medical complications in overweight but otherwise not obese individuals falling in the BMI categories between 25 to less than 30 seems paradoxical given that there is no associated increase in mortality from being overweight but not obese. This is likely explained by the lesser severity and prevalence of these disease complications in the overweight only group, the availability of treatments for these complications if they occur, the responsiveness of milder disease to simpler treatments, and the better responsiveness of milder disease to the available treatments.

Weight Reduction Has Benefits

Clearly, the rationale for weight loss lies in increased relative health risks associated with overweight and/or obesity and increased relative mortality risks associated with obesity. Relative risks, however, are not absolute risks. As such, each person must be assessed individually in order to determine his or her absolute risk or actual presence of health complications related to overweight and obesity. There are many individuals who are overweight and fewer in the obesity categories who do not have sufficient individual absolute risk factors to justify weight loss. If, in fact, an evaluation determines significant individual absolute risks of obesity related complications or the actual presence of obesity related complications, then it is reasonable to ask: What benefit would there be to losing weight?

There is clear evidence that weight loss is associated with: 1) a reduction in blood pressure and/or a reduction in the need for antihypertensive medication in overweight and obese patients; 2) improved blood glucose with and without the presence of diabetes in overweight and obese patients; 3) and improvement in triglyceride levels and HDL cholesterol levels in obese individuals. There is a report of reduced mortality from obesity related cancers and diabetes in overweight women with obesity related health complications. However, despite improvement in related risk factors, there is no conclusive data that any weight loss intervention improves morbidity and mortality from cardiovascular disease.

More specifically, with regard to polypain, the risk of knee osteoarthritis is reduced by over 50% in women who reduce their weight by 2 BMI units or approximately 5.1 kg over the preceding 10 years. This benefit is noted in individuals with baseline BMI in the normal weight, overweight, and obese categories. Further studies have identified the benefits of weight loss in managing osteoarthritis especially combined with a biomechanics and posture exercise program to promote aerobic conditioning and strengthening. Weight reduction leads to associated improvement in knee biomechanics with each pound of weight loss translating into a fourfold equivalent reduction of knee loading forces. Weight reduction similarly reduces loading of the lumbar spine. In addition, the presence of increased abdominal girth due to fat accumulation leads to abnormal lumbar biomechanics by causing a forward shift in the body's center of gravity, thereby exacerbating lumbar hyperextension. Lumbar hyperextension is present in 88% of patients with polypain and contributes to the low back pain reported by 97% of patients. Weight loss with reduction in abdominal fat leads to improved lumbar loading and biomechanics with attendant reduction in low back related symptoms.

Dieting Works for Most

Anybody and everybody can lose weight. Weight loss develops when caloric expenditure exceeds caloric intake. It's that simple. If individuals burn more calories than they take in, they will lose weight. Weight loss requires reduced caloric intake and/or increased caloric expenditure relative to baseline needs. Similarly, weight gain occurs in the face of increased caloric intake and/or decreased caloric expenditure relative to baseline needs. The baseline caloric needs of the body are determined in part by genetics and in part by the functional demands of the body in response to the environment such as food intake, activity level, body temperature regulation, and metabolic needs. When weight is steady, the total calories eaten in a day represents the total calories expended. This daily caloric requirement set point is basically like a thermostat, that I will refer to as a caloristat. No matter what one's weight is, the caloristat sets the required number of calories the body determines it needs. The caloristat is independent of weight and the same caloric set point requirement can exist in underweight, normal weight, overweight, and obese individuals. No matter where the caloristat set point, however, if intake is reduced below the set point of the caloristat with stable activity levels and/or total caloric expenditure is increased above the set point of the caloristat with stable intake, weight loss will occur. Similarly, if intake is increased above the set point of the caloristat with stable activity levels and/or total caloric expenditure is decreased below the set point of the caloristat with stable intake, weight gain will ensue.

While anybody can lose weight, sustaining weight loss is the greater challenge. This is due in part to the fact that the caloristat is responsive to changes in circumstances and conditions in order to adapt and protect the body from food induced weight gain and diet induced weight loss. In the face of maintaining a weight loss of 10 percent or more of body weight, there is a corresponding reduction in the set point of the caloristat leading to an average 6 kcal/kg/day reduction in the body's energy expenditure in non-obese individuals and 8 kcal/kg/day reduction in the body's energy expenditure in obese individuals. In the face of weight loss, the body reduces the number of calories it expends in order to counter the weight loss. Thus, it is harder to lose the next pound than it was the last and it becomes increasingly difficult to sustain any particular weight loss as the body works to return weight to its stable, pre-weight loss baseline. Similarly, weight gain of 10% is associated with an increase in energy expenditure to counter the increase in weight. In essence, the caloristat adjusts to maintain established, stable weight in the face of weight loss, as well as weight gain, as shown in Figure 9.7. Therefore, the Law of Diminishing Returns is an important factor in limiting the degree of sustained weight loss possible in typical diet induced weight loss.

The other significant issue with regard to maintenance of weight loss is recidivism and regaining the lost weight. Most individuals who lose weight in weight loss programs simply do not maintain the weight loss. While anybody can lose weight with any reduced calorie diet in which calories out exceed calories in, such weight loss is not sustained and individuals regain 30-35% of the lost weight within one year even with added behavioral therapy. Furthermore, 50% or more regain their lost weight by 5 years.

The difficulties in achieving and maintaining weight loss lead to the yo-yo phenomenon whereby an attempt to diet leads to actual inadequate weight loss due to lack of knowledge and understanding of how to lose weight or perceived inadequate weight loss with unfulfilled expectations. Even in the face of real weight loss, either circumstance leads to abandonment of the diet attempt with subsequent regain of the weight that was actually lost. Anybody can lose weight. To reiterate: Anybody can lose weight. The real challenge is to keep it off.

The ability to initiate and maintain any diet requires a complete understanding of caloric intake and expenditure. The issue of dietary intervention for weight loss is further complicated by the fact that normal weight individuals underreport what they eat by 10-30 percent and this underreporting increases to 30 percent or more in overweight individuals. This clearly affects how well an individual can participate in any dietary program.

While diet programs include interventions such as reduced fat, reduced carbohydrate, or combining different foods or eating patterns, there is little evidence that any diet program provides benefit independent of caloric reduction. In other words, the ability to lose weight requires reducing caloric intake below the calories expended.

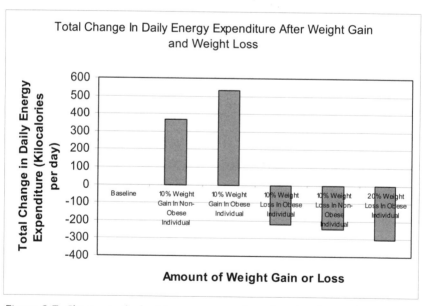

Figure 9.7: *Changes in the body's energy expenditure from baseline with 10% weight gain and weight loss of 10% and 20%. (Data from Leibel RL, Rosenbaum M, Hirsch J. Changes in energy expenditure resulting from altered body weight. N Engl J Med 1995; 332: 621-628. Erratum in: N Engl J Med 1995; 333: 399)*

Physical Activity and Exercise Intervention Helps

Weight loss occurs when caloric expenditure exceeds caloric intake. Reducing calories through reduced dietary intake clearly promotes this balance in favor of weight loss. Similarly, increasing caloric expenditure through increased physical activity and exercise that increases calories burned over baseline activity levels favors weight loss. Physical activity correlates inversely with weight. All things being equal, the lesser the activity, the greater the weight. The benefits of exercise are many and include reduced risks of: dying prematurely; dying from heart disease; developing a stroke; developing diabetes; developing high blood pressure; developing colon cancer; and developing osteoporosis. Exercise reduces depression and anxiety and promotes psychological well-being. It improves strength, mobility, and reduces the risk of falling. As a treatment without specific diet intervention, the introduction of exercise causes weight loss and reduction in body fat that varies with the intensity of exercise. On the other hand, when an exercise program is added to a calorie restricted diet, there appears to be little added benefit to the amount of weight loss independent of the diet. This is explained by the fact that burning calories by exercise is much more difficult than simply not taking them in. Indeed walking 1¾ miles in 35 minutes or running 1½ miles in 15 minutes burns only about 150 kilocalories. That's the equivalent of about one chocolate chip cookie!

While the effect of exercise in promoting weight reduction is small, exercise is important in helping maintain dietary weight loss and helps prevent weight regain noted with diets. Any benefit from exercise to promote weight loss is complicated by the observation that obese individuals overestimate their physical activity levels just as they underestimate their caloric intake resulting in an impaired ability to introduce and maintain an appropriate exercise program.

The potential risks of exercise are predominantly related to musculoskeletal injuries. This is especially of concern in individuals with polypain with symptoms and underlying disease related to primary generalized osteoarthritis predominantly involving the neck and low back with associated degenerative disc disease and the variable combination of associated tendinitis, bursitis, and fasciitis. Other potential risks include cardiac arrhythmia, acute myocardial infarction, and exercise related asthma.

Medication and Surgical Treatments of Obesity Are Associated With Significant Complications

The role of medications in managing obesity above and beyond diet and exercise is very small. The added benefit in weight loss is less than 5 kg at one year. While improved glucose metabolism, lipid levels, and blood pressure may be noted with pharmacotherapy, there is no evidence of improved survival. These medications have significant side effects. They are not replacements for diet and exercise. Medications to treat obesity might be considered in a very limited group of obese individuals who have failed adequate diet and exercise intervention and who have significant complications related to the obesity.

Surgical treatment of obesity should only be considered in extremely obese individuals with BMI of 40 or greater who have failed diet and exercise intervention with or without medication intervention and who have significant obesity related health complications.

Weight Issues in Fibromyalgia Polypain

Individuals with fibromyalgia polypain undergo the same weight issues and weight concerns as all individuals do. In addition, the weight of individuals with polypain is further potentially affected by the impact of: 1) polyregional pain from the underlying primary generalized osteoarthritis predominantly involving the neck and back with associated degenerative disc disease and the variable combination of associated tendinitis, bursitis, and fasciitis; 2) reduced pain thresholds; 3) sleep disturbances; 4) psychological disturbances; 5) and treatment of polypain and its components. Just like any weight gain, the weight gain that occurs in polypain is a result of eating more calories than expended; expending fewer calories due to functional impairments from polypain that limit activity; or changes in appetite, energy expenditure, or caloric requirements driven by medications and other treatment interventions. In fibromyalgia polypain, 42% note a weight gain averaging 22.8 pounds. Thus, issues related to weight gain and weight management are of significant concern in individuals with polypain.

How To Manage Weight In Fibromyalgia Polypain To Reduce Pain And Improve Health

1) Since 1976-80, there has been a gradual increase in the weight of the population of an average of 17-19 pounds, with an average 10% increase in weight in men and 13% average increase in weight in women. This is not an epidemic, but rather a gradual weight shift.

2) Factors impacting weight include genetics, smoking and smoking cessation, fitness and activity level, caloric intake, body image, age related factors, pregnancy, medications, and sleep.

3) As genetics contribute to about 50% of your weight and fat, look at your old family photos to know why you are as fat or thin as you are and learn how fat or thin you will be.

4) Being fat isn't the same as "I'm not as thin or light as I used to be". It is normal, natural, and expected that you will gain weight starting from your twenties into your fifties. The average weight gain for men is 17.1 pounds in men and 22 pounds in women representing an overall 10% gain in body weight in men and 16% gain in body weight in women. It is normal and natural. The goal is to start at the lowest point of normal weight BMI that you can when you are in your twenties to prepare for this natural weight gain and to avoid falling into the obese category as you naturally gain weight.

5) Health related complications correlated with overweight and/or obesity include: lipid disorders; type II diabetes mellitus; hypertension; ischemic heart disease; congestive heart failure; stroke; osteoarthritis; cancers of the breast, prostate, colon, uterus and gallbladder; respiratory disorders and sleep apnea; gallstone disease; psychological disturbances such as depression; and the negative social impact of obesity.

6) There appears to be an increased risk of mortality from being underweight as well as being obese. Being normal weight or overweight only does not appear to decrease survival. You should keep your weight

down when you are young as obesity is a greater risk when you are younger compared to when you are older. Allow weight to climb naturally, but not excessively, with age. Being underweight in old age is a bad sign just as being obese when you are young is bad.

7) Weight loss is associated with: a reduction in blood pressure and/or a reduction in the need for antihypertensive medication in overweight and obese patients; improved blood glucose in overweight and obese patients; improved triglyceride levels and HDL cholesterol levels in obese individuals; and reduced mortality from obesity related cancers and diabetes in overweight women with obesity related health complications. There is no conclusive data that any weight loss intervention improves morbidity and mortality from cardiovascular disease.

8) Osteoarthritis, tendinitis, bursitis, and fasciitis in the low back, hips, knees, ankles and feet, as well as the hands are associated with overweight and obesity. Weight loss benefits osteoarthritis especially combined with a biomechanics and posture exercise program to promote aerobic conditioning and strengthening even if weight is in the normal range.

9) The Rule of Thirds Polypain Weight Loss Program

The management of polypain with appropriate medications and an appropriate biomechanics and posture treatment program incorporating orthotics, neuromuscular re-education, muscle strengthening, and range of motion exercises should always include an appropriate weight loss program in overweight and obese individuals to optimally promote improved alignment, posture, biomechanics, and ergonomic interactions.

While the Rule of Thirds Polypain Weight Loss Program can be done by almost all individuals with polypain, there may be certain individuals who for other health reasons should avoid this weight loss program or should undertake a different weight loss program. Always check with your doctor to make sure there is no reason why you should not do this program or if a different weight loss program is required.

One of the significant problems with weight loss programs is that they are deprivational. Deprivational diets are doomed to fail. When people are forced to eat foods they don't like or eat in a pattern that does not fit their lifestyle, they will not maintain such a diet even when the stakes are their physical well being or appearance. People who are not underweight or losing weight because of health reasons take pleasure in eating in addition to the obvious survival benefit of food. Unless the issue is survival eating, people will avoid deprivational diets or, if in fact they undertake such a diet, will eventually fail to maintain it. The issue is compounded by the fact that weight loss is accompanied by the Law of Diminishing Returns and that expectations of weight loss far exceed reality.

The Rule of Thirds Polypain Weight Loss Program overcomes these limitations. Basically, if your weight is steady and not climbing, you continue to eat your usual food in your usual way taking your usual portions onto your plate. However, rather than eating the entire portion on your plate, you leave 1/3 behind. And, that's it.

It is estimated that 22-27 kcal/kg of energy is needed to maintain each kilogram of body weight daily in a normal adult plus or minus about 20 percent with higher requirements in males. In an average 80 kg (176 pound) individual, the daily metabolic calorie requirement is about 2000-2400 kcal. If weight is steady, then intake also equals 2000-2400 kcal. Using the Rule of Thirds, intake can be reduced by nearly 600-800 kcal per day and more practically will result in a reduction of about 500 kcal per day in the give and take of things. This will result in a reduced caloric intake of about 3500 kcal per week. This translates into a weight loss of about 1 pound per week at least initially.

The Rule of Thirds Polypain Weight Loss Program, when introduced to manage weight for polypain independent of other obesity related health issues, should result in a weight loss of 5-10% of initial weight. At a rate of 0.5-1.0 pound of weight loss weekly, this may take 4-8 months to achieve. However, reality dictates. The caloristat will reset at a lower level as weight loss progresses, making weight loss more difficult due to a reduction in the basal metabolic rate induced by the weight loss. Nonetheless, the Rule of Thirds Polypain Weight Loss Program provides such an initial reduction in caloric intake, that even as the caloristat resets lower, there should be an ongoing balance in favor of weight loss.

It is my experience that patients with polypain who cannot lose weight using the Rule of Thirds Polypain Weight Loss Program are not successful in any other non-medication weight loss program in the long term.

10) In view of the sleep disturbances identified in polypain, liquids, caffeine, chocolate, and dietary or pharmacologic stimulants should be avoided at least 4 hours before bedtime.

11) Complementing the Rule of Thirds Polypain Weight Loss Program is the Polypain Wellness Core Biomechanics and Posture exercise program as well as the Integrated Daily Walking Program. These exercises promote weight loss and, more importantly, help sustain the weight loss attained by the Rule of Thirds Polypain Weight Loss Program. An average 70 kg individual, walking at a rate of 1½ miles per hour (40 minute /mile), a very slow casual walk, will burn about 60 kcal in 30 minutes of walking. At a more standard walking rate of 3 miles per hour (20 minute/mile), walking for 60 minutes will burn about 250 kcal. The contribution of the Polypain Wellness Core Biomechanics and Posture exercise program and Integrated Daily Walking Program is significant to the Polypain Weight Loss Program.

12) Some medications used in the management of polypain may promote some weight gain. Such weight gain is generally small, consisting of several pounds. However, the benefit of these medications in managing inflammation, pain, sleep, and psychological disturbances outweigh the concerns regarding the minor weight gain. Furthermore, the Rule of Thirds Polypain Weight Loss coupled with the Polypain Wellness Core Biomechanics and Posture exercise program and Integrated Daily Walking Program is effective in managing any medication related weight gain. Indeed, the benefit of these medications in reducing symptoms and improving function provide for the ability to increase activity levels and exercise, thereby allowing increased calorie usage with corresponding benefit to weight control.

Chapter 10

Step 4: Ergonomics: Understanding How Pain Interacts With The World At Large and What To Do About It

"Carpe diem" ("Seize the day")—Anon

Ergonomics relates to the analysis of the physical interaction of individuals with their surrounding environment to permit a safe, healthy, comfortable, and productive process. Joints and joint related structures are meant for purposeful use. They are not static structures but, rather, dynamic elements continually subject to voluntary, task oriented positioning, movement, and loading. Through posture, the joints and joint related structures are subjected to loading forces at rest such as when lying or sitting. With use they undergo additional loading forces depending on the activity required and through a combination of loading and positioning with use undergo additional forces such as acceleration, deceleration, tension, compression loading, shear, torsion, or some combination of these. These forces are further magnified by the additional loading force of body weight or added loads resisted against gravity, especially with weight bearing activities such as standing, walking, kneeling, or squatting. The alignment of the joints and joint regions relative to the load and expected movements coupled with the strength of the muscles moving these joints all play a crucial role in the distribution of forces in the joints and joint regions. These, in turn, are major determinants of the evolution and progression of osteoarthritis.

239

Ultimately it is the cumulation of the ongoing moment to moment movement and loading that the joints and periarticular structures are designed for that leads to the symptomatic primary generalized osteoarthritis predominantly involving the neck and back with associated degenerative disc disease and the variable combination of associated tendinitis, bursitis, and fasciitis of polypain. Therefore, adequate treatment of polypain requires a thorough understanding of how osteoarthritis, degenerative disc disease, tendinitis, bursitis, fasciitis, and associated pain are generated at all affected joint, spine, and periarticular sites at a functional level as related to the loading, structure, alignment, and biomechanics of these sites in a person's day to day activities.

The Ergonomic Interface Between Pain and Function

The knowledge of the interaction with the environment when sitting, lying, working, undertaking kitchen activities, doing household activities, working at the computer, performing desk work, holding, grasping squeezing, writing, talking on the telephone, and watching television provides the opportunity for joint and site specific treatment related to improving alignment, posture, biomechanics through ergonomic education, and appropriate accommodations and modifications of the environment or task performance. Such intervention also allows the opportunity to not only physically impact the immediate osteoarthritis process symptomatically but also to slow its progression especially in terms of potential joint damage and deformity. An appropriate ergonomics treatment program reduces pain intensity and severity and leads to improved pain processing by reducing peripheral and central sensitization which in turn leads to improved pain amplification, pain magnification, wind-up or temporal summation, and reduces referred pain through a process whereby less pain begets less pain and less pain begets reduced inflammation. By improving pain source intensity and severity, the pain gap narrows or the pain free reserve deepens and not only is there less pain for any increased demand on the joints, tendons, bursae, and fasciae but there is an increased ability to carry out activities without obvious or significant flare of symptoms and there is a more rapid and greater ability to recover from an exacerbation.

The fundamental ergonomic questions are: Are activities and lifestyle hurting the affected individual? If so, how can the impact be lessened? The answer to both these questions lies in the undertaking of a thorough, comprehensive medical assessment. Items to assess include: a thorough work history and work duties performed as well as work related disability; exercise and recreational sports activities; hand and upper extremity function; lower extremity function including walking ability; ability to get dressed; ability to bathe or shower; ability to drive; ability to participate and perform household duties and activities; hobbies; and recreational activities. The musculoskeletal examination must not only be thorough and comprehensive, but should provide a sense of dynamic musculoskeletal function in these settings specific to the patient. The ability to translate the results of the assessment into functional recommendations to reduce excess and/or abnormal joint and joint related structure loading and improve abnormal biomechanics and posture is another crucial component to successfully managing polypain.

The management of ergonomics in polypain centers around three concepts: 1) patient education; 2) improving the posture and biomechanics of joints and joint related structures in specific task oriented situations; 3) and physically altering the environment to allow improved posture and biomechanics. Patient education is central to the success of an ergonomic intervention program as ultimately it is the patient who must transfer the knowledge regarding ergonomic issues into the everyday environment. The power of such knowledge lies in its therapeutic benefit.

The process by which these interventions are accomplished are through: 1) accommodation, a process by which the interventions allows the task to be carried out to completion in the face of intervention; 2) or, modification, a process by which the elements of a task are reduced such that the task cannot be fully carried out despite ideal accommodation. Accommodations include changes in posture and/or biomechanics, changes in the environmental arrangement, use of orthotics, and changes in pattern or timing of activity. Modifications may include accommodations but also consist of a reduction in intensity, frequency, or duration of task related activity such that the activity cannot be completed despite accommodations or cannot be completed in timely way. As such, accommodations are preferable over modifications if functional activity is to be sustained. It is clearly desirable to reduce and eliminate, as possible, any existing modifications and to fully optimize any and all accommodations to preclude functional limitations in activities. Further, the degree of accommodation and/or modification is variable over time depending on symptoms and polypain activity. While each individual's environmental interactions are unique, there are some common areas shared by many patients with polypain.

Ergonomic Accommodations To Reduce Pain and Improve Function

The Sitting Environment

Despite spending good parts of our day in a seated position, it is astounding how few of us know how to sit in a biomechanically neutral position. Check it out, if you haven't already done this earlier when reading the section on orthotics for the neck. As you read this book, take a momentary break and consciously check out your body position and specifically your neck. The least likely position you are in at this moment is a neutral one whereby you are sitting upright with this book held at eye level

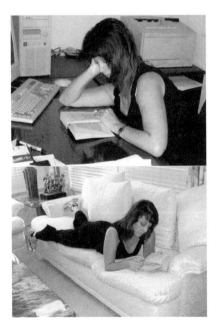

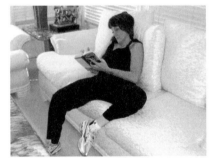

Figure 10.1:
Incorrect seating postures.

with virtually no neck flexion and absolutely no neck side tilt. Indeed, if you are sitting at a desk, you are likely bent forward with a significant neck flexion with your book on the desk and your head fairly closely buried into the book and likely leaning your head into one of your hands supporting your head by leaning on an elbow as depicted in Figure 10.1. If you are sitting on a couch or sofa, you are most likely sprawled out and leaning to one side with your neck bent forward and to the side. If you are lying and reading the book, you are most likely lying chest down and severely hyper-extending your neck. Unless you have been trained in ergonomics, biomechanics, and posture, it is natural to adopt these poor positions. While likely detrimental to all who sit in these positions, it unquestionably detrimental to those who have polypain.

General ergonomic recommendations for sitting for individuals with polypain include:

1) Sit in seats and chairs that are at a height to allow your feet to rest flat on the floor and your knees to be bent at about 90 degrees. If the seat is too high and your feet are off the floor, lower the chair seat, get another chair, or get a footstool. If the seat is too low, raise the seat or get a higher seat.

2) Be sure the seat pan is tilted downward from front to back about 5 degrees.

3) Be sure the seat pan is not too long or too short. It should allow your low back and upper buttock to comfortable reach the chair back and the front should end somewhere in the front third of the back of your thigh.

4) Make sure the chair back is supportive. It should be angled back at about 100 degrees from the seat pan. Sit back into the seat back as much as possible.

5) You should be able to do a pelvic tilt comfortably and appropriately against the seat back. Do pelvic tilts intermittently and any time if there are any new or increased symptoms such as fatigue or pain developing in the mid or low back area.

6) Wear your Smart Support Neck Collar with sitting activities as dis-

cussed in Chapter 8.

7) Sit vertically with your weight evenly distributed on your buttocks.

8) For prolonged sitting, use a footstool about several inches high. Elevating your legs on a footstool when seated appropriately adds pelvic tilt to reduce lumbar hyperextension and provide a more neutral posture for the low back.

8) Do not sit in chairs that are too tall or too short without accommodating the height.

9) Do not maintain a position that requires you to lean, twist, or bend causing your spine to go out of neutral alignment.

Appropriate seating postures on an office chair, dining chair and couch are depicted in Figure 10.2.

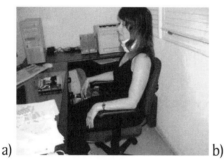
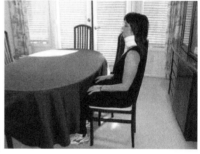

a)   b)

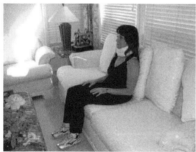

Figure 10.2: Appropriate seating postures: a) on an office chair; b) on a dining chair; c) on a couch.

c)

The Standing Environment

The upright standing position is another position in which appropriate ergonomics, biomechanics, and posture are critical in managing polypain. As discussed in Chapter 8, in regard to biomechanics and posture, findings and symptoms in individuals with polypain include: pain related to the lumbar spine due to osteoarthritis and degenerative disc disease noted in 97% of patients; hypermobility of the lumbar spine seen in 10%; thoracic rotoscoliosis with unbalanced alignment and loading of the lumbar seen in 96% of patients; leg length discrepancy with similar unbalanced alignment and loading seen in at least 48% of individuals; lumbosacral hyperextension seen in 88% of patients; iliotibial band tightness seen in 93% of patients; trochanteric bursitis seen in 39% of patients; angular deformities of the knees with valgus, knock-knee, type deformity observed in 93% of patients and varus, bowlegged, type deformity seen in 5% of patients; pes anserine bursitis seen in 19% of patients; subjective pain in the ball of the foot reported by 40% of patients with polypain; pain in the heel identified in 25%; pain in the sole identified in 20%; pain in the midfoot identified in 10%; pain in the toe proximal interphalangeal joints identified in 7%; osteoarthritic bony osteophytes of the first metatarsophalangeal joints noted in 58% of patients; loss of the metatarsal arch is noted in 95% of patients and loss of the longitudinal arch in 70% with total flat foot pes plano valgus in 33%; hallux valgus and cock-up toes present in 86% and 85% respectively; pain on examination of the metatarsophalangeal joint found in 51%; plantar fasciitis identified in 27% of patients; and deep Achilles bursitis found in 10%. All of these joints and joint related sites are impacted by standing and walking.

General ergonomic recommendations for standing for individuals with polypain include:

1) Wear your Smart Support Neck Collar.

2) Wear your sport shoes with an appropriately set up Universole or Winsole Arch Support System.

3) Stand vertical with body weight evenly distributed onto both feet.

4) Do pelvic tilts.

5) Do not lean, twist, or bend unnecessarily or for prolonged periods to

prevent the spine from shifting out of neutral alignment.

6) Minimize knee bending, kneeling, or squatting from a standing position.

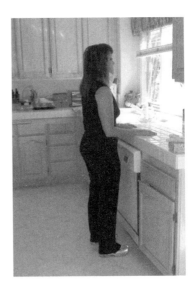

Figure 10.3: Neutral standing position.

The Walking Environment

The ergonomics, biomechanics, and posture related to walking is covered in the section describing the Integrated Daily Walking Program in Chapter 8. The elements of this program should be performed during any walking activity.

The Lying Environment

Approximately, one third of the 24 hour day is spent recumbent and sleeping. While not thought of typically as a time to be concerned about ergonomics, biomechanics, and posture, lying down is indeed another position in which abnormal loading and posturing of the spine readily develops. This is particularly important in individuals with polypain. The amount and type of support the spine requires greatly depends on the position of the head, neck, and body relative to the pillow and mattress.

General ergonomic recommendations for lying for individuals with polypain include:

1) Use your Smart Support Pillow as discussed in Chapter 8. Alternatively, if you are lying on the couch, you can lie on a supportive regular pillow while wearing the Smart Support Neck Collar to maintain your head and neck in a neutral, supported position.

2) Be sure you have an appropriate mattress in terms of cushioning and

support for sleeping. It is my experience that patients with polypain do best with a mattress that has a comfortable, cushioning pillow top of about 3-4 inches overlaying a firm, but not hard, supportive spring mattress. Mattresses comprised exclusively of foam, especially viscoelastic foam mattresses, offer insufficient support and my patients with polypain do poorly with these types of mattresses.

3) When lying on your back, if your low back remains hyperextended, place a small pillow under your knees to produce a mechanical pelvic tilt and reduce the lumbar hyperextension. This is shown in Figure 10.4a.

4) For all women and men with wide hips relative to their waist, when side lying, place a small pillow between your knees as shown in Figure 10.4b. This pillow will subconsciously be moved by you during sleep from between your knees to under your knees when you turn onto your back and back between your knees when you again turn onto your side.

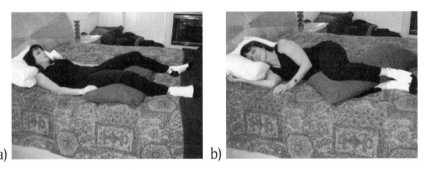

a)   b)

Figure 10.4: *Accommodations when: a) lying on the back; b) lying on the side.*

The Work Desk Environment

The major challenge of sitting at a desk is the desk itself. Virtually all desks have a fixed height with no ability to be adjusted. Thus, the ability to accommodate the chair and your body position in order to maintain neutral posture and biomechanics is critical, especially in regard to the neck, mid, and low back. Sometimes, however, even with the best of efforts at ergonomic accommodation, because of an individual's height, required posture, or biomechanics, it may be impossible to accommodate for the desk and the desk itself may need to be modified or replaced in order to prevent exacerbating polypain symptoms.

General ergonomic recommendations for working at a desk for individuals with polypain include:

1) Be sure to have a height adjustable office chair with an adjustable back for setting seat pan length and adjustable arm rest height.

2) Set up the chair ergonomics as above under accommodations for sitting and be attentive to the need for pelvic tilts.

3) Set the arm rests so your elbows rest directly on them without pushing your shoulders upward, causing your shoulders to sag, or making you lean forward to get your elbows to reach when you are seated in a neutral position. Hopefully, the arm rests are pretty close to the level of the desk top. This minimizes side leaning and uneven loading of the shoulder girdle and spine.

4) Wear your Smart Support Neck Collar.

The Computer Environment

One of the greater ergonomic challenges both in the home and work setting in our modern age of technology is working at a computer. In polypain, the joint regions most affected by computer work and keyboard use include the neck, mid and low back, as well as the hands and wrists. The prevalence of cervical and lumbar spine symptoms has been reviewed above. Polypain patients note subjective pain in the finger PIP joints in 36%, the wrists in 25%, the thumb base first carpometacarpal joints in 25%, the MCP joints in 22%, and the finger DIP joints in 12%. There are objective findings of osteophytes in the thumb base first carpometacarpal joints in 92% and DIP joints of the fingers in 74%. Alignment deformities due to osteoarthritis are seen in the DIP joints of the fingers in 95%, the thumb base first carpometacarpal joints in 92%, and the finger PIP joints in 88%. Objective joint pain is identified in the thumb base first carpometacarpal joints in 63%, PIP joints of the fingers in 25%, DIP joints of the fingers in 21%, and the thumb IP (thumb end knuckle) in 9%. Thus, in addition to improving the ergonomics, biomechanics, and posture of the spine during keyboard use, reducing the loading on the hands and wrists during keyboard use must be considered.

General ergonomic recommendations for working at a computer for individuals with polypain include:

1) Set up the ergonomics as above for working at a desk and be attentive to the need for pelvic tilts.

2) Let the Smart Support Neck Collar dictate your head and neck position, and arrange the keyboard, mouse, and video display monitor to accommodate the neutral position directed by your chair, desk set-up, and the Smart Support Neck Collar.

3) One of the great advantages of our computer era is that there are programs that make computer use less demanding. The most important computer program I can recommend to improve ergonomics while using a computer is voice recognition software. With a little training, you can use your voice to dictate notes and commands and greatly reduce keyboard and mouse use. Not only do you spare your hands and wrists, but you also maintain more neutral neck and low back posture not having to lean into the keyboard, mouse, and video display monitor.

4) Use a touchpad in place of a mouse to further reduce hand and wrist use.

The Telephone Environment

The next time you are holding a telephone handset, portable phone, or cell phone to your ear, take a moment and mentally observe your head and neck posture or, better yet, go look in a mirror. You will note your head and neck are actually side tilted in the direction of the telephone. Indeed, this adverse loading of the cervical spine is even more exaggerated when you use your shoulder to cradle the telephone. Given the universal involvement of osteoarthritis and degenerative disc disease in the cervical spine of individuals with polypain, clearly there is a need for optimizing the ergonomics of telephone use.

General ergonomic recommendations for using a telephone for individuals with polypain include:

1) Wear your Smart Support Neck Collar when talking on the telephone.

2) Use a telephone headset instead of holding a handset or use a speakerphone.

The Hand Use Environment

Individuals with polypain have significant subjective symptoms and objective findings of osteoarthritis involving the hands as detailed above in the section working with a computer. In addition to computer use, the hands are subjected to constant loading and use as we interact with the surrounding environment through fine motor manipulation, gripping, grasping, and holding. We use our hands to: manage self-care activities; manipulate buttons; pull zippers; push and pull clasps and snaps; open and close lids, bottles, and jar tops with pushing, pulling, turning, or twisting motions; turn faucets and knobs; flip light switches; hold and turn keys; hold pens and pencils for writing; tap computer keyboards; hold and tap computer mice; use remote controls; bathe and self-toilet; brush hair; grasp and turn a car steering wheel; hold and grasp clothing to dress; hold and pull or push shoes on and off; tie laces; hold and grasp cups; hold and manipulate food utensils; wash dishes; wash laundry; iron; grocery shop; vacuum; clean house; work in the yard or garden; and even hold this book. The presence of hypermobility of the hands and wrists in 72% of patients with polypain further adds to the increased risk of abnormal alignment, increased joint loading, or unexpected joint loading in the hands through use. The burden of this everyday hand use is compounded by work related activities that require additional hand use and loading. Clearly, there are many potential opportunities to improve hand use ergonomics, posture, and biomechanics.

General ergonomic recommendations for hand use for individuals with polypain include:

1) For handwriting, use a wide bodied or fat pen or pencil. This improves the load distribution especially with respect to the frequently involved thumb base first carpometacarpal joint. This is shown in Figure 10.5.

2) For items with a grip or handle, replace them with items with wider or fatter grips or handles, or pad the items with foam to increase the size of the grip or handle. The increased size produces a greater surface area to better distribute the forces on the hand joints.

3) Use a strap wrench device to open tight lids and jars to avoid loading the hand joints, especially the thumb base first carpometacarpal joint. This is demonstrated in Figure 10.6.

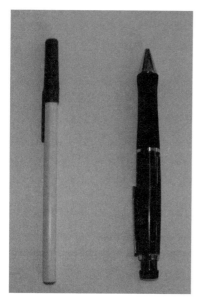

Figure 10.5: Wide bodied fat pen compared to regular pen.

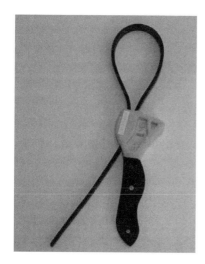

Figure 10.6: Strap wrench.

4) Avoid thumb based grip when possible to reduce loading the thumb base first carpometacarpal joint. If gripping, grasping, or holding is required for an activity, try gripping with your fingers keeping your thumb out of the way adjacent to your hand as shown in Figure 10.7.

5) Use voice recognition software for your computer as above.

6) Use a touchpad in place of a computer mouse.

7) Use a telephone headset in place of a handset.

The Driving Environment

Of all the activities we undertake throughout the day, perhaps none is more overlooked in terms of biomechanics and ergonomics than driving. Unlike regular chairs and working at a desk, a car seat offers significant limitations in adjustability to allow a neutral position. There is, other than a rare exception, no car seat that provides the ability to rest the driver's head and neck against the seat and headrest in a neutral position while maintaining the lumbar spine in a neutral position. The height of car seats cannot usually be optimally adjusted to provide appropriate elevation and tilt to allow the driver's low back to be in a neutral position. While driving, the driver's pelvic and

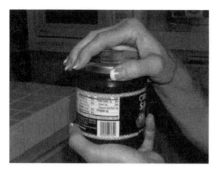 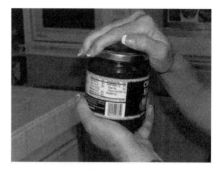

Figure 10.7: *Thumb based grip and same activity using non-thumb based grip*

spinal biomechanics are unbalanced given the right foot and leg controls the gas and brakes and the left foot and leg tries to find a comfortable spot or controls a clutch. The distance of the driver's arm to the steering wheel may not be commensurate with the distance of the seat needed for the driver's legs and feet to control the gas, brakes, and clutch, if present. This is further complicated by the seat height needed for the driver to see comfortably and safely out the front windshield. Then there is the issue of positioning the hands and arms to hold the steering wheel, which in turn loads the shoulder girdle, which in turn loads the cervical and upper thoracic spine as well as the hands, especially in the thumb base first carpometacarpal joints. Of course, driving induces neck motion in all directions with commensurate loading of the cervical spine. And naturally, we must not overlook the musculoskeletal demands of driving in reverse. Indeed, observe carefully, the next time you get in and out of the car, the degree of twisting your head, neck, mid, and low back undergo in addition to the uneven loading of the right compared to left side upper and lower extremities. Now, consider the excess abnormal loading brought on by driving the car for prolonged periods and/or repeatedly getting in and out of the car. Thus, there are many potential opportunities to improve car related ergonomics, posture, and biomechanics.

General ergonomic recommendations for driving in a car for individuals with polypain include:

1) Set up the car seat ergonomics as described under the accommodations for sitting above as close as possible to optimal given the limitations of your car seat and be attentive to the need for performing pelvic tilts.

2) Wear your Smart Support Neck Collar when driving only if you feel you can drive safely. As in other situations such as sitting or working at a desk, the Smart Support Collar, in my experience, helps improve cervical posture and biomechanics to reduce symptoms while driving as well. It facilitates neuromuscular re-education and the trained maintenance of improved posture and biomechanics even absent the collar in the long term. However, the issue of safe driving prevails when in the car. The collar does significantly restrict neck motion and should not be worn while driving unless you feel you can drive safely with it. You should never put yourself at increased risk of an automobile accident. As with all treatment, the decision to wear the Smart Support Neck Collar is based on a risk-benefit analysis. Reality dictates. Thus, if uncertain about using the Smart Support Neck Collar when driving, then do not use it when driving.

3) Set the arm rests, if present, so your elbows rest directly on them when you are seated in a neutral position. Hopefully, the arm rests are pretty close to a neutral position as reviewed regarding sitting at a desk. However, the car seat is limiting.

4) Avoid thumb based grip when possible to reduce loading the thumb base first carpometacarpal joint.

5) Minimize driving.

6) Minimize the frequency of getting in and out of the car.

The Purse Environment

Women's purses are amazing as to how much stuff they can hold. Unfortunately, all that stuff has weight. For shoulder slung purses this excess weight cause uneven loading of the shoulder girdle region. This in turn leads to uneven loading of the neck, mid, and low back. This is further exacerbated by the thoracic rotoscoliosis with unbalanced alignment and loading of the cervical, thoracic, and lumbar seen in 96% of patients with or without the accompanying leg length discrepancy seen in at least 48% of individuals with polypain.

General ergonomic recommendations for carrying a purse for individuals with polypain include:

1) Reduce the weight and size of the handbag.

2) Use a backpack type purse to center the load and more evenly distribute the weight.

Assesment of the Work Environment Is Vital

One of the major issues in the work setting is that standard ergonomic recommendations deal with work environment interaction with healthy, normal individuals. They do not factor in, nor account for, individuals with polypain or other musculoskeletal disease—despite the staggering statistic that over 43 million Americans have arthritis and rheumatic diseases; and, despite the fact that arthritis, back, and spine problems are the commonest cause of work disability. Clearly, all working individuals with fibromyalgia polypain should have a musculoskeletal assessment by a rheumatologist to determine the nature of the underlying osteoarthritis, degenerative disc disease, tendinitis, bursitis, fasciitis, pain, other musculoskeletal disease factors, and the biomechanical and postural risk factors contributing to symptoms and disease to provide for potential ergonomic accommodations and/or modifications to reduce symptoms and progression of disease. This type of evaluation also provides the opportunity to determine musculoskeletal appropriateness of a job with potential risk identification of ergonomic factors contributing to osteoarthritis, polypain, or other musculoskeletal factors for appropriate benefit-risk assessment by the employer and employee. This would help reduce progression of osteoarthritis and polypain. By anticipating and responding to ergonomic needs, such an evaluation would also help improve the liability of employers in identifying the evolution of natural disease which would have been mistaken for a work related event otherwise.

Chapter 11

Step 5: How Sleep Disturbances Adversely Affect Pain and Effectively Managing Them to Reduce the Hurt

"Weary with toil I haste me to my bed,
The dear repose for limbs with travel tired;
But then begins a journey in my head,
To work my mind when body's work expired..."
— William Shakespeare, Sonnet XXVII

Nearly one third of our lives is spent sleeping and this almost invariably is performed lying in a recumbent position. Yet, despite the obvious need to lie down and sleep, and despite the massive contribution of life time to undertake this requisite activity, there is no established consensus on the function or functions of sleep. Sleep is not a passive process. The brain and body are not at rest during sleep. It is a physiologically and behaviorally active, complex, and busy reversible behavioral state of perceptual disengagement from the environment with reduced and relative responsiveness to the environment. Many theories have been postulated as to why we sleep. These fall into one of three categories. Restorative theories hold that sleep restores tissue and biological processes in preparation for the next day, especially the brain, and particularly in the organization and consolidation of memory. Adaptive theories propose that sleep increases survival by causing us to cease physical activities at the most dangerous parts of the day and protect us from harm's way such as being attacked by predators looking to make a meal of us or injuring ourselves

255

in the dark of night. Energy conservation theories suggest that sleep induces low energy metabolism for the purpose of energy conservation.

The drive to sleep is a process of homeostasis, a process maintaining physiologic equilibrium, much like hunger, thirst, and the drive for sex. It is a need. To understand the effect of sleep disturbances on pain and how pain influences sleep, it is necessary to understand what sleep is all about.

Sleepiness and Fatigue Are Not The Same Things

It is critically important to recognize that sleepiness is not the same as fatigue. Sleepiness is the physiological state in which an individual would fall asleep if the circumstance allowed or despite the circumstances. Fatigue, on the other hand, is a symptom recognized as a sensation of exhaustion or lack of energy limiting the undertaking or performance of physical and/or mental activities. Fatigue is improved by rest. Sleepiness can only be relieved by sleeping, even if sleeping is delayed. Sleepiness however, can, but does not necessarily, lead to a sensation of fatigue. Fatigue does not lead to sleeping but the reduced activity levels of fatigued individuals may increase the likelihood of falling asleep.

SLEEPINESS ≠ FATIGUE

Figure II.I: Sleepiness is not the same thing as fatigue.

What Normal Sleep Is All About
Sleep Stages

Sleep is composed of two processes. The first process is that sleep occurs in various and sequential stages leading to two major states of sleep identified as Non-Rapid Eye Movement (NREM) sleep and Rapid Eye Movement (REM) sleep. NREM sleep is further subdivided into different stages. These states and stages are based upon a constellation of changes in brain electrical activity, muscle activity, and eye movement. The second process is that of sleep architecture. The stages of NREM sleep and REM sleep recur in a cyclical pattern lasting about 90-120 minutes each.

Stage W or Stage 0 sleep is the state of wakefulness. During the awake phase, eye movements can be rapid or slow and there is a high degree of voluntary muscle activity.

The onset of sleep can be determined by brain electrical activity as measured by electroencephalogram (EEG) within seconds of its occurrence. Despite the immediacy of its onset, individuals do not perceive the point at which they enter sleep. The latency to sleep onset, the time it takes to fall asleep after going to bed, is normally less than 15 minutes.

Stage 1 NREM sleep is the transition from wakefulness to sleep. It lasts only 1-7 minutes per sleep cycle and comprises 2-5% of total sleep time. During this stage the individuals are easily awakened and they do not perceive that they were asleep. A common finding of disrupted sleep is an increase in the amount of Stage 1, or light sleep.

Stage 2 NREM sleep is an intermediate level of sleep. Individuals are more difficult to arouse in this stage compared to Stage 1 NREM sleep. This stage lasts about 10-25 minutes per sleep cycle and comprises 45-55% of total sleep time.

Stage 3 NREM sleep lasts only a few minutes and is a transitional phase leading to stage 4 sleep. Stage 3 NREM sleep occupies 3-8% of total sleep.

Stage 4 NREM follows stage 3 NREM sleep. Stage 3 and 4 NREM sleep are collectively referred to as deep sleep or slow wave sleep (SWS). Stage 4 NREM sleep lasts about 20-40 minutes per cycle when present. It occupies 10-15% of total sleep time.

Subsequent to Stage 4 NREM sleep, there occurs a series of body movements followed by a sequential ascent through the lighter stages of sleep with a 1-2 minute phase of stage 3 sleep followed by a 5-10 minute period of stage 2 sleep accompanied by body movement followed by an ascent to the stage 1 NREM level. This is followed by REM sleep which is identified by the presence of eye movements and muscle paralysis during which there is an absence of voluntary muscle activity other than eye and ear muscles. The presence of a wakeful EEG in the face of sleep has caused this phase to be referred to as paradoxical sleep whereby the body appears externally paralyzed but is internally active. The three features of REM sleep: the wakeful EEG; the rapid eye movement; and absence of voluntary muscle movement do not necessarily occur at the same time. The ability to be aroused from REM sleep is variable. REM sleep lasts about 1-60 minutes, recurs through the night in 4-6 cyclic episodes, and constitutes 20-25% of total sleep. During REM sleep, the visual and auditory portions of the brain are activated. REM sleep is a time when vivid and rich dreaming occurs. Further, independent of the sexual content of dreams, REM sleep is a time of genital arousal with males developing erections and females developing increased vaginal lubrication and clitoral engorgement. Indeed, such erections in males may outlast the REM sleep phase. A younger male, in fact, may sustain an erection for nearly half the night and an older man in his sixties may also sustain an erection for nearly one quarter of the night. The issues surrounding male impotence and erectile dysfunction are indeed much more clearly defined by the observation of the presence of a morning erection or erections during REM sleep. The ability to develop and sustain an erection at these times clearly identifies the physical functioning of all the required parts and suggests psychosocial factors to be driving such erectile dysfunction.

REM sleep can be associated with elevated blood pressure, cardiac ischemia with impaired blood supply to the heart, cerebral ischemia with impaired blood supply to the brain, cardiac arrhythmias with changes in heart rhythm and other changes in heart rate, and breathing stoppages with short apneas or shallow breathing with hypopneas. The rapid eye movement phase of REM sleep predisposes to early morning heart attacks and stroke.

Sleep Architecture

Sleep architecture is the second process of sleep. It relates to the cycling of NREM sleep stages and REM sleep throughout the night. Normally, sleep is entered through NREM sleep. Subsequently, NREM and REM sleep alternate cyclically. Typically each cycle lasts 90-120 minutes with the first cycle being the shortest at 70-100 minutes. Typically, there are 4-6 REM episodes through the night with episodes increasing in duration as the night progresses with REM predominating sleep in the last third to half of the night. Stage 3 and 4 slow wave sleep predominate in the first third of the night and occupy less time in the second and third cycles and may not appear in subsequent cycles with stage 2 sleep taking up more time in later cycles. There may be brief episodes of wakefulness in later cycles usually developing near REM sleep transitions. These wakenings are brief enough as not to be remembered in general and comprise less than 5% of the sleep duration, thus yielding a 95% sleep efficiency. The emphasis toward slow wave sleep is related to the physiology of sleep initiation, how long the individual has been awake prior, and the sleep pattern. The prominence of REM sleep in the later cycles is felt to be a process driven by internal circadian rhythm (the body's internal clock). Figure II.2 displays a typical pattern of sleep architecture in a normal individual.

Length of Sleep

The length or duration of sleep is extremely variable between individuals as well as within any one individual. The factors impacting sleep duration include the obvious volitional component, internally driven and genetically determined components, and environmental components that may interfere with sleep. Further, the time when an individual goes to sleep in part determines the length of sleep due to circadian rhythms. The amount of sleep required by an individual is the amount of sleep needed

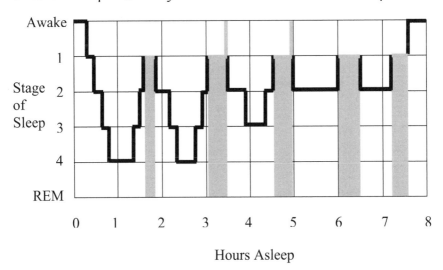

Figure II.2: Sleep stages and cycles for a typical night's sleep.

to prevent daytime sleepiness, ensure the ability to sleep through normal sleep cycles and architecture, and to prevent sleep related impairment in function when awake. This baseline amount of sleep need averages 7-8 hours. However, some individuals do well with less sleep and some need more. It is not the length of sleep that matters but rather that an individual sleep long enough to attain his or her basal sleep requirement. Failure to maintain the individual amount of requisite baseline sleep leads to sleep debt and the consequences of sleep deprivation.

Factors Affecting The Quality and Quantity Of Sleep
Age

Of all the factors affecting sleep stages and architecture, the most powerful is the contribution of age. The total duration of sleep declines with age. However, the character of sleep itself also changes relative to the total duration of sleep. The quantity of the slow wave sleep seen in stage 3 and 4 sleep, as a percentage of total sleep, diminishes as one gets older. By age 60, slow wave sleep may no longer be present. Sleep fragmentation with increased wakefulness intermixed with sleep is noted with aging, especially beyond the fifties. There may be extended periods of wakefulness that are actually recalled in addition to more frequent unrecalled wakenings. REM sleep remains relatively stable throughout adult life.

Another phenomenon noted with aging is the disruption of the normal sleep-wake cycle. Older adults do not exhibit the same responses to environmental cues or are exposed to fewer of them and display impaired circadian rhythms in regard to sleep-wake patterns. This causes the sleep-wake cycle in older individuals to advance with onset of the sleep cycle earlier in the day. This is known as advanced sleep phase syndrome. Thus, older individuals are sleepy earlier in the evening and waken too early. The earlier sleepiness, rather than motivating the individual to go to bed to sleep, causes the individual to doze or nap in the evening leading to difficulties falling asleep at the environmentally dictated bedtime and promoting early morning wakening.

Sleep Deprivation

An individual who tries to recover a prior sleep loss of one night or more demonstrates a sleep pattern with increased slow wave sleep during the recovery night. This is accompanied by an even deeper sleep than the baseline slow wave sleep would provide. On the other hand, REM sleep rebounds on later nights. Thus, total sleep deprivation preferentially induces recovery of slow wave sleep first, then REM sleep. When REM or SWS is specifically deprived, rebound is preferential to that specific stage of sleep on recovery.

Circadian Rhythms-The Body's Internal Clock

Another very significant factor impacting sleep stages and architecture is the issue of circadian rhythms. REM sleep is strongly influenced by circadian rhythms. Thus, if sleep is delayed until the early morning when REM sleep is at its peak, REM sleep will predominate and may even be noted at the onset of sleep. This type of sleep phase shift leads to a completely reversed sleep architecture. Sleepiness with impaired sleep stages and architecture are noted in shift workers, individuals with jet lag phenomenon, and individuals with delayed or advanced sleep phase shifts. Delayed sleep phase shifts occur when individuals go to sleep much later than normal or appropriate and waken in the late morning or early afternoon. Advanced sleep phase shifts occur when individuals go to bed too early in the evening and waken too early in the morning.

Drugs

Many drugs used to treat a large variety of diseases as well as recreational drugs have central nervous system effects that may adversely affect sleep and wakefulness and cause sleepiness and sedation. Sedating drug classes include benzodiazepines, alcohol, antiepileptic medications, antihistamines, antihypertensive medications especially beta blocker medications, many antidepressant drugs, antipsychotic medications, antiarrhythmic drugs, alcohol, nicotine, and opioids. Opioids produce sedation through their effects on mu and kappa receptors as reviewed in Chapter 7. NSAIDs may impair sleep efficiency with increased waking although sleepiness may also develop as a side effect. Both NSAIDs and opioids are reported subjectively to ultimately improve sleep quality in patients with pain through their benefits in controlling the pain. Other drugs may have stimulant effects interfering with normal sleep stages and architecture to reduce sleepiness and increase wakefulness and alertness. Such drugs include caffeine, amphetamines, modafinil, pseudoephedrine and phenylpropanolamine, cocaine, some antidepressants including the selective serotonin reuptake inhibitor (SSRI) group, Parkinson's disease medications, and corticosteroids.

Alcohol

In non-alcoholics, alcohol causes sedation, shortens sleep latency, and increases non-REM sleep with concomitant reduction in REM sleep in the early hours of sleep. Unfortunately, due to the rapid metabolism of alcohol, blood levels drop rapidly as sleep progresses. This leads to rebound sleep disruption with shallow light sleep and wakefulness accompanied by increased REM sleep and increased dream recall. The adverse alcohol related sleep effects may persist even after blood alcohol concentration falls and becomes undetectable.

Nicotine

The nicotine found in cigarettes and other tobacco products is sedating in low doses and stimulating in high doses. It increases sleep latency and nighttime wakenings and reduces total sleep time and REM sleep in particular in non-depressed individuals.

Primary Sleep Disorders

Primary sleep disorders such as narcolepsy and sleep apnea, by definition, affect the stages and architecture of sleep. Numerous medical disorders also impact sleep stages and are associated with sleep fragmentation and increased frequency of arousals.

The Consequences of Sleep Deprivation

From a clinical perspective, normal sleep is achieved when: 1) the quality of sleep as determined by the sleep stages and architecture; 2) the quantity or length of sleep; 3) and the timing of sleep within the 24 hour day are sufficiently appropriate to prevent daytime sleepiness, ensure the ability to sleep through subsequent normal sleep cycles and architecture, and preclude sleep related impairment in function when awake. Failure to attain the individually required quality, quantity, or timing of sleep through one night or cumulatively through multiple nights leads to sleep deprivation.

The significance of sleep deprivation is that it is associated with numerous adverse consequences. First and foremost amongst these complications is the development of excess daytime sleepiness with the propensity to fall asleep inappropriately during the day or requiring arousal stimulation to prevent falling asleep. This may be accompanied by a feeling of fatigue.

Impaired cognitive function is noted after acute and chronic sleep deprivation. Deficits include reduced ability to stay on task, impaired cognitive and motor processing speeds worsening with increasing complexity, impaired retention of newly learned skills, impaired short term memory, and impaired attention. It is not that the sleep deprived individual cannot perform cognitively or has a true loss of cognitive ability, but rather performance is slowed and there is increased difficulty with short term recall all of which is compensated for in the sleep deprived individual by accommodations to the pacing and cueing of the tasks. Similar cognitive impairment occurs from either cumulative partial sleep deprivation such as sleeping less than 6 hours nightly for 2 weeks or remaining awake for 24-48 hours straight.

Mood disturbances with negative mood and reduced motivation are noted in sleep deprived states. Individuals with sleep deprivation have an increased risk for depression, anxiety, panic, and substance abuse.

Sleep deprivation increases the risk of traffic accidents and work related accidents. Indeed, excessive sleepiness is reported to be the second leading cause of auto accidents and a major factor in truck accidents. Driving performance is impaired after as little as restricting one night's sleep to 5 hours.

Quality of life is impaired in sleep deprived individuals with impairment of family, social, and occupational functioning. These individuals reduce participation in pleasurable activities, take unplanned naps at home and work, and have impaired work productivity. These consequences lead to difficulty in maintaining a job, being promoted, as well as marital discord.

Neurological and behavioral changes noted in sleep deprived individuals include mild involuntary eye motions, tremor, slurring of speech, eyelid droop, and increased muscle reflexes. Sleep deprivation may adversely affect the respiratory system especially in those with pre-existing cardiopulmonary disease. Sleep deprivation alters immune regulation and impairs immune responses. Sleep deprivation leads to increased hunger and appetite with an increase in serum ghrelin, an appetite stimulating hormone, along with a reduction of leptin, an appetite reducing hormone. An increased risk of adverse cardiovascular events such as myocardial infarction is reported to develop with sleep limitation.

The proportion of individuals who sleep less than seven hours per day has increased from 16% to 37% in the past 40 years.

Insomnia:
The Inability To Sleep As Biologically Needed

Insomnia is a sleep disturbance characterized by an inadequate quality, quantity, or phase of sleep with difficulty initiating sleep, difficulty maintaining sleep, wakening too early, or sustaining poor quality or non-restorative sleep resulting in daytime related symptoms and impairment associated with sleep deprivation including sleepiness; fatigue; mood disturbances; cognitive impairment in the areas of short term memory, processing speed and retention of newly learned skills; physical motor impairment in the area of processing speed and reaction times; social impairment; occupational impairment; and/ or reduced pain thresholds. Insomnia is not the same as sleep deprivation. Insomnia leads to sleep deprivation. However, sleep deprived individuals become sleepy and are driven to sleep. Individuals with insomnia, are driven to stay awake and become sleep deprived without the normal drive to sleep as seen in sleep deprivation. In essence, insomnia is a state of hyperarousal making sleep more difficult.

Insomnia is a common experience with 95% of adults subjectively reporting having had it at some time in their lives. In most of these instances, the insomnia is transient or short term and is related to an identified cause such as: stress or other transient psychological disturbance; transient medical illness; transient stimulating medication effect; environmental changes such as change in sleeping environment, excessive ambient noise or unpleasant ambient temperature; change in schedule; or jet lag with a disruption of the synchronization of the body's internal clock relative to the new sleep schedule in the new location. Such insomnia resolves with resolution of the precipitating event and appropriate sleep management.

Chronic insomnia is variously defined as insomnia lasting greater than 3 weeks or one month or longer according to the diagnostic criteria of primary insomnia. Chronic insomnia can occur as a primary sleep disorder condition with no identified underlying medical or psychiatric cause. Within this category is primary or idiopathic insomnia which is characterized by a lifelong, childhood onset difficulty in achieving and maintaining sleep that may lead to sleep deprivation with reduced sleep efficiency. Other primary sleep disorders, sleep disorders with identified characteristic features, precipitating insomnia include: circadian rhythm disorders with altered sleep phases; restless legs syndrome; inadequate sleep hygiene; insufficient sleep syndrome secondary to excess environmental light and sound as well as what I refer to as "insomnia by proxy" which I characterize as insomnia caused by the insomnia or sleep disorder of your bed partner; altitude insomnia; central sleep apnea syndrome; and periodic limb movement disorder.

The remaining individuals with chronic insomnia have an underlying predisposing medical or psychiatric condition causing the insomnia. This group is classified as having secondary insomnia. The most common group of secondary causes of insomnia are psychiatric disorders. These include mood disorders such as depression, anxiety disorders, psychotic conditions such as schizophrenia, personality disorders, and other psychiatric conditions. In addition to psychiatric disorders causing chronic insomnia, chronic insomnia itself is a risk factor for the development of psychiatric disturbances that lead to depression and anxiety. Thus, insomnia begets depression and anxiety and depression and anxiety beget insomnia. Another major group contributing to chronic insomnia are general medical and neurological disorders and their treatments. Significant contributors to the insomnia in these conditions are pain such as seen in fibromyalgia polypain and psychological disturbances including depression, anxiety, and stress. Other factors may include medication related adverse effects, breathing difficulties including obstructive sleep apnea, bladder and bowel control difficulties, metabolic imbalances, and neurological conditions directly affecting sleep or indirectly through pain, cognitive impairment, organic brain syndromes, altered sensation, or movement disorders. Another large group contributing to insomnia comprises the effects of medications and other substances such as recreational drugs and alcohol. Sleep-wake schedule difficulties generally produce transient insomnia as noted above. When the schedule cannot be adjusted, however, chronic insomnia may result.

Understanding Non-restorative Sleep

Sleep deprivation and sleep disturbances in individuals with features of fibromyalgia polypain cause a poor quality or shallow sleep that is described as non-restorative. The sleep is unrefreshing and feels inadequate despite a reasonably normal duration. This non-restorative sleep also contributes to a distinctive fatigue independent from sleepiness. This fatigue is characterized by wakening in the morning feeling unrefreshed, followed by mid-day improvement in the fatigue, which is then followed by a worsening of the fatigue as the day progresses.

Chronic Daytime Napping Is Bad

Daytime napping is a process of undertaking sleep during the daytime, outside of the usual sleep time. Just like sleepiness is not the same as fatigue, napping is not the same as resting. Napping is a sleeping process, whereas resting is not. The drive for daytime napping is daytime sleepiness. Daytime sleepiness is due to sleep deprivation from insomnia as a general rule. However, there is a short term mid-afternoon normal circadian drive to sleep with associated declines in neurocognitive function and temperature. This is recognized as the mid-afternoon or post-lunch dip and drives the culturally driven mid-afternoon activities such as resting or taking a siesta. In Western cultures, it motivates the intake of stimulants such as tea or coffee. Absent sleep deprivation, generally, the mid-afternoon dip does not result in napping in younger or active individuals and the drive to sleep is self-limited. However, if given the opportunity to rest, especially to lie down, and especially as one gets older, this dip may result in a nap.

In the face of sleep deprivation, the drive to nap is to make up for lost quality and/or quantity of sleep. Thus, in the face of transient, short-term insomnia, daytime napping has no known negative consequences other than disrupting the daytime schedule. The goal in these cases is to consolidate sleeping back to the nighttime and eliminate the daytime napping once the trigger for the insomnia is eliminated. The consequences of daytime ongoing, chronic napping however are the development of altered sleep phases with shifting of the night-time sleep schedule and altered sleep quality and quantity during the nighttime sleep phase leading to insomnia and the attendant complications of sleep deprivation. In addition, daytime sleepiness and napping in older individuals has been associated with possible increased risk of depression, stroke, myocardial infarction, and possibly increased mortality.

The Interaction Between Poor Sleep And Chronic Musculoskeletal Pain

Individuals with chronic musculoskeletal pain report sleep disturbances or poor sleep in 50-90% of the group. Indeed, other non-musculoskeletal medical conditions manifesting with pain are also associated with impaired sleep. Of major significance to individuals with fibromyalgia polypain is the impact of sleep deprivation on pain thresholds. There is an abundance of supportive evidence in the medical literature correlating sleep disturbances with reduced pain thresholds and increased pain sensitivity. Indeed, introducing sleep disruption or deprivation in normal individuals leads to increased pain sensitivity. Disruption of slow wave stage 3 and stage 4 NREM sleep by wakeful EEG alpha wave sleep patterns has been strongly correlated with the symptoms of pain, cognitive impairment, fatigue, and negative mood seen in patients with symptoms and findings of polypain. In addition, patients with symptoms seen in polypain have protracted sleep latencies with increased time to sleep onset, reduced sleep efficiency with increased wakenings, decreased total sleep time, decreased slow wave sleep and decreased REM sleep, increased motor activity, and generalized restlessness during sleep. Thus, pain begets poor sleep and poor sleep begets pain through the reduction of pain thresholds. This leads to further reduction in the pain thresholds and propagation of the sleep disturbances.

This critically important relationship is depicted in Figure II.3.

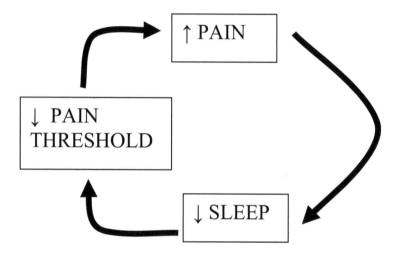

Figure II.3: *The relationship of pain and pain thresholds to sleep in polypain.*

The Interaction Between Sleep, Chronic Musculoskeletal Pain, and Psychological Issues

Of further significance to individuals with fibromyalgia polypain is the impact of sleep deprivation on the psychological health of the individual and the resulting effect on pain thresholds. There is a higher prevalence of psychological symptoms in those with symptoms and findings of fibromyalgia polypain compared to controls and these individuals have a greater number of lifetime psychiatric diagnoses compared to controls. The most frequent psychiatric disorders in these patients are anxiety, stress, and depression. Further, amongst patients with chronic musculoskeletal pain, there is an increased prevalence of depression and the psychiatric symptoms correlate with health-care seeking behavior and the perceived severity of the symptoms of pain. In chronic musculoskeletal disease, psychological status is a major determinant of health status along with physical functioning and the pain itself. There is clear evidence that anxiety, stress, and depression significantly affect the appreciation of pain and its presentation in polypain. Further, as discussed above, mood disturbances with negative mood and reduced motivation are noted in sleep deprived states and individuals with sleep deprivation have an increased risk for depression, anxiety, panic, and substance abuse. Thus, patients with polypain have mood disturbances characterized by stress, anxiety, and depression that are highlighted or exacerbated by sleep deprivation.

Individuals suffering from depressive disorders are inherently recognized as having sleep disturbances as part of their underlying condition. This is highlighted by the DSM-IV-TR criteria for major depressive disorder as noted in Chapter 12, Table 12.1 which identifies the associated sleep disturbances of insomnia or hypersomnia. Patients with major depression note difficulty falling asleep, frequent wakenings from sleep, early morning awakening, non-restorative sleep with a feeling of light or unrefreshed sleep, reduced total sleep time, unpleasant dreams, daytime fatigue, and daytime napping with or without excess daytime sleepiness. The abnormalities in sleep stages and architecture in major depression include prolonged sleep latency to fall asleep, increased frequency and duration of wakenings, and early morning wakening leading to sleep fragmentation and reduced sleep efficiency. Depressed patients have a reduced amount of stage 3 and 4 slow wave sleep and may demonstrate the same EEG wakening alpha wave intrusion into slow wave sleep as seen in chronic pain syndromes. Depressed patients also demonstrate REM sleep abnormalities with a reduced time to onset of REM sleep, longer duration of first REM period, and increased REM sleep contribution to total sleep.

Further, individuals suffering anxiety disorders and stress are also inherently recognized as having sleep disturbances as a part of their underlying condition. This is highlighted by the DSM-IV-TR criteria for the diagnosis of generalized anxiety disorder as noted in Chapter 12, Table 12.2 which identifies the associated sleep disturbances with features of difficulty falling or staying asleep or restless, unsatisfying sleep. These criteria also identify fatigue and irritability symptoms that may in part be due to the associated sleep disturbance. The abnormalities in sleep stages and architecture in patients with stress and anxiety include increased sleep latency with longer time to fall asleep, increased frequency and duration of wakenings after sleep onset, reduced total sleep time, and reduced sleep efficiency with increased wakening periods after sleep onset.

Thus, poor sleep begets depression, anxiety, stress, reduced pain thresholds, and pain; and depression, anxiety, and stress beget pain, reduced pain thresholds, and poor sleep. Ongoing poor sleep, depression, anxiety, and stress lead to additional further reductions in pain thresholds, increased pain, and further sleep impairment. In total, the poorer the sleep quality, architecture, and duration: the more the sleep disruption arising from pain and psychological disturbances such as depression,

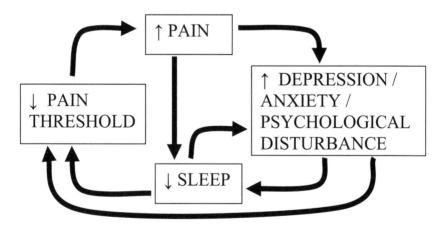

Figure 11.4: *The relationship of pain, pain thresholds, and psychological disturbances to sleep in polypain.*

anxiety, and stress; the lower the pain thresholds; and the greater the pain felt in polypain. This relationship is depicted in Figure II.4.

It appears the facilitation of pain through reduction of pain thresholds by sleep disturbances mediated by pain and psychological disturbances such as depression, anxiety, and, stress develops as a result of pain message processing in the brain where perception of pain occurs. Reduction of pain threshold develops through the affective, behavioral, and cognitive responses to the perceived pain and the impact of sleep disturbances on these areas. These responses cause various areas of the brain to generate a response to pain that is conducted through the descending modulation pathway back to the dorsal horn to reduce pain thresholds through central sensitization. Thus, reduced pain thresholds, pain amplification, and pain magnification driven by sleep disturbances in polypain arise in the higher levels of the central nervous system as a response which heightens pain sensitivity and reduces pain thresholds by sending signals through spinal cord pain pathways to the spinal pain message areas to reduce pain thresholds.

The Evaluation of Sleep And Fatigue In Fibromyalgia Polypain

A complete and detailed sleep history and evaluation is a necessary component of the comprehensive and thorough evaluation undertaken in patients with poylpain. The sleep history must include: the time the patient goes to bed; how long it takes to fall asleep; the frequency, duration, and reason or reasons for recalled wakenings and ability to return back to sleep from these wakenings; the time the patient awakens; the time the patient gets out of bed to start the day; the presence of morning and/or daytime fatigue; the presence of morning and/or daytime sleepiness; whether napping takes place, and if so, when, for how long, and what is the outcome; medication, food, and fluid intake in the evening and night and especially closer to bedtime; activities undertaken at bedtime, sleeping rituals including watching television, working on the laptop, reading, or doing paperwork in bed; sleeping conditions including noises, lights, temperature, bed partner, mattress, pillows under the neck, and other body supports. It is important to determine the accuracy of the subjective reporting given that individuals with insomnia may have distorted or incorrect perceptions of their sleep. Formal sleep studies such as polysomnography (study of electrical brain wave activity and eye movements during sleep and possibly other physiologic variables), tests for sleepiness such as the multiple sleep latency test, and actigraphy tests for recording movement are generally not needed in assessing the sleep disturbance of polypain unless a sleep-related breathing disorder is suspected, the insomnia or sleep disturbance remains unexplained, or the sleep issues are unresponsive to appropriate and thorough treatment.

Based on self-reporting, the study data from Chapter 4 reveals the presence of sleep disturbance in 90% of patients with polypain. The data identifies

Clinical Sleep Feature	Clinical Concerns in Fibromyalgia Polypain	Possible Sleep Factors Affected
Increased Sleep Latency to Fall Asleep	Pain / Psychological disturbances / Poor sleep hygiene / Insufficient sleep / Other insomnia conditions	Impaired quality Reduced quantity Sleep phase shift
Increased Number of Wakenings	Nocturia / Pain / Psychological disturbances / Insufficient sleep / Age / Other insomnia conditions	Impaired quality with fragmentation Reduced quantity with reduced sleep efficiency
Early Wakening	Depression / Age / Insufficient sleep / Other insomnia conditions	Impaired quality with reduced NREM and/or REM sleep Reduced quantity
Morning Sleepiness	Frequent wakenings	Impaired quality with fragmentation Reduced quantity with reduced sleep efficiency
Morning Fatigue Wakening Unrefreshed	Pain Psychological disturbance	Impaired quality with reduced or interrupted deep, slow wave sleep
Daytime Sleepiness	Pain / Psychological disturbances / Insufficient sleep / Age / Other insomnia conditions	Impaired quality Reduced quantity
Daytime Napping	Daytime sleepiness	Impaired quality Reduced quantity Sleep phase shift

Table II.I: Sleep difficulties in polypain and their clinical correlations.

significant abnormalities of sleep quality and quantity in polypain including prolonged sleep latency, fragmented sleep, reduced sleep efficiency, less than 8 hours total sleep nightly in half the group, and an unrefreshed and non-restorative sleep with morning fatigue in almost half the group. The most common reason individuals with polypain waken from sleep is nocturia (getting up at night to urinate). The next commonest reason is pain followed by, in descending order of frequency: reasons unknown; noise or light; flushing or sweats; nightmares or dreams; psychological stress; intruding thoughts; and cough. Table II.I outlines clinical sleep difficulties in polypain and their clinical correlations.

The pain of polypain begets poor sleep which in turn begets reduced pain thresholds with concomitant increased appreciation of pain. Thus, poor sleep begets pain and pain begets poor sleep. However, in addition to the identified sources of pain in polypain of primary generalized osteoarthritis predominantly involving the neck and back with associated degenerative disc disease and the variable combination of associated tendinitis, bursitis, and fasciitis as well as the psychological disturbances that may impact sleep, any additional sleep disturbance not specifically caused by polypain may also adversely affect sleep independently. Such unrelated insomnia further contributes to reduced pain thresholds in polypain and increases the appreciation of the active pain sources in polypain. This is depicted in Figure II.5.

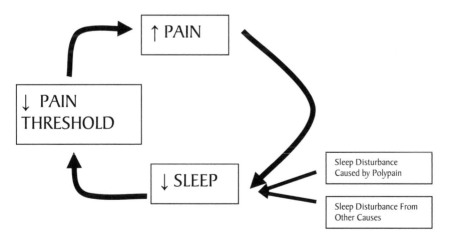

Figure II.5: *The relationship of pain and pain thresholds to any sleep disturbance in polypain.*

The Fibromyalgia Polypain Wellness Core Sleep Management Program:
Getting A Good Night's Sleep

The approach to sleep management in polypain re-emphasizes the need for proper, thorough, and comprehensive assessment to determine the characteristics of any related sleep disturbance, to assess for contributing factors and other disorders not specifically related to polypain that contribute to the sleep disturbance, and to develop an appropriate understanding upon which to base treatment decisions. Only through such evaluation can the rheumatologist be sufficiently informed and knowledgeable to be able to provide needed patient education in order that patients be able to fully participate in their own care and make truly informed decisions regarding treatment. As with managing any and all components of polypain, intensive follow-up regarding sleep related issues with appropriate evaluation of progress to provide optimal benefit from a properly designed treatment program is of crucial importance.

The Polypain Wellness Core Sleep Management Program forms part of the more comprehensive Polypain Wellness Core Program. In addition to their contributions to the symptoms and findings in polypain: the polypain sources of pain consisting of primary generalized osteoarthritis predominantly involving the neck and back with associated degenerative disc disease and the variable combination of associated tendinitis, bursitis, and fasciitis; the reduced pain thresholds from adverse pain processing generated by increased nociception; and the psychological disturbances related to stress, anxiety, and depression contribute specifically to the sleep disturbances identified in polypain. Thus, the fundamental and basic treatment for the disrupted sleep stages and architecture in polypain requires treatment with all the elements of the Polypain Wellness Core Program. Therefore, the Polypain Wellness Core Sleep Management Program incorporates: the pharmacologic intervention to control site specific pain symptoms, pain processing abnormalities, and psychological disturbances; biomechanical and postural intervention through exercises including the Integrated Daily Walking Program, orthotics, neuromuscular re-education, and weight control including the Rule of Thirds Polypain Weight Loss Program; ergonomic intervention through appropriate accommodation and modification; and psychological support and counseling.

The specific sleep related interventions comprising the Polypain Wellness Core Sleep Management Program component of the Polypain Wellness Core Program begins with the implementation of appropriate sleep ergonomics and sleep hygiene. This is the foundation upon which the Polypain Wellness Core Sleep Management Program is built. The successful management of the sleep disturbances and disruptions of polypain can only occur in the presence of appropriate sleep ergonomics. Equally important is the need to incorporate appropriate joint and joint related alignment, posture, and biomechanics as detailed in the Polypain Wellness Core Program and specifically the components that relate to sleep biomechanics and posture in regard to the Polypain Wellness Core Sleep Management Program. Finally, these treatment elements must be appropriately incorporated before the consideration of adding or modifying sleep medications. In the management of the sleep disturbances of polypain, medications are never enough. However, in some instances, the sleep disturbances of polypain may be adequately treated through the Polypain Wellness Core Program and all its components along with the sleep ergonomics, biomechanics, and posture components of the Polypain Wellness Core Sleep Management Program such that sleep specific medications may not be required at all points of treatment.

Sleep And The World Around You

1) A bed has only two purposes: sleeping and having sex (absent a medical recommendation otherwise).

2) If you are in bed, you should be falling asleep, sleeping, or having sex. Otherwise get out of bed. If you wish to remain in bed, plan on doing one of these three activities (absent a medical recommendation otherwise).

3) A bedroom is not an office, library, TV room, kitchen, mail sorting zone, debating site, or argument zone. Therefore, a bed is not an office chair, reading carousel, office desk, television lounger, kitchen table, or debating podium. Do not watch television, read, drink, eat, argue, or ruminate in bed when lying down to sleep.

4) TV is not a sleeping aid. It does not cause or induce sleepiness. Indeed, late night programming is adult-oriented and is stimulating, not sedating.

5) Maintain a relatively consistent sleep schedule regarding bedtime and waking time.

6) Avoid eating and drinking before bedtime and at least 4 hours before bedtime, especially if you waken at night to urinate.

7) Avoid stimulants known to cause insomnia at least 4 hours before bedtime. Such stimulants include caffeine such as found in coffee, tea, and cola; chocolate; over-the-counter stimulant drugs such as the decongestants pseudoephedrine and phenylpropanolamine; as well prescribed or recreational medications that act as stimulants.

8) Avoid alcohol. If you do drink alcohol, avoid drinking at least 4 hours before bedtime.

9) Avoid smoking. If you do smoke, avoid smoking at least 4 hours before bedtime.

10) Avoid exercising before bedtime unless it is related to sexual activity.

11) Do not struggle to fall asleep. If you cannot fall asleep within 15 minutes of going to bed, get out of bed. After getting out of bed, do something active. Go watch television sitting on the couch or lounger (not in bed), read on the couch (not in bed), work on the computer, do desk work, or do housework until you are sleepy - not tired - but sleepy. Once you are sleepy enough to fall asleep within 15 minutes, go back to bed to sleep. Do not fall asleep while doing these activities.

12) Do not nap during the daytime.

13) For purposes of sleeping, the bedroom should be fairly dark such that light does not disturb you, fairly quiet such that sound does not disturb you, and should be cool enough requiring that you cover up with at least a sheet or light comforter.

14) If you suffer from "insomnia by proxy", the above measures are vital for your bed partner. If not sufficient, be sure your bed partner gets appropriate medical intervention. Reconsideration of the sleeping arrangements may be necessary if "insomnia by proxy" is not managed sufficiently.

15) During the daytime, spend time outdoors or in natural light, especially later in the afternoon and early evening.

Sleep Biomechanics and Posture

These strategies have been discussed in Chapter 8 as part of the Polypain Wellness Core Biomechanics and Posture Program. General ergonomic recommendations for sleeping for individuals with polypain have been reviewed in Chapter 10 and include:

1) Use your Smart Support Pillow. Alternatively, you can lie on a supportive regular pillow while wearing the Smart Support Neck Collar to maintain your head and neck in a neutral, supported position.

2) Be sure you have an appropriate mattress in terms of cushioning and support for sleeping. It is my experience that patients with polypain do best with a mattress that has a comfortable, cushioning pillow top of about 3-4 inches overlaying a firm, but not hard, supportive spring mattress. Mattresses comprised exclusively of foam, especially viscoelastic foam mattresses, offer insufficient support and my patients with polypain do poorly with these types of mattresses.

3) When lying on your back, if your low back remains hyperextended, place a small pillow under your knees to produce a mechanical pelvic tilt and reduce the lumbar hyperextension. This is shown in Chapter 10, Figure 10.4a.

4) For all women and men with wide hips relative to their waist, when side lying, place a small pillow between your knees as shown in Chapter 10, Figure 10.4b. This pillow will subconsciously be moved by you during sleep from between your knees to under your knees when you turn onto your back and back between your knees when you again turn onto your side.

Medication to Manage Sleep

The sleep disturbances found in polypain clinically fall into one of two major categories for purposes of sleep medication intervention. The first category relates to sleep disturbances associated with impaired sleep stages and architecture. The sleep disturbances in this category reveal reduced sleep efficiency with increased wakenings, decreased total sleep time, disruption of stage 3 and 4 slow wave sleep with wakening alpha wave intrusion, decreased stage 3 and 4 slow wave sleep, decreased REM sleep, increased motor activity, and generalized restlessness during sleep. These features lead to increased frequency of wakenings, morning fatigue with feeling unrefreshed or unrested, morning sleepiness, daytime sleepiness, daytime napping, and symptoms of sleep deprivation. The sleep medications impacting this category of sleep disturbance are known as sleep modifiers. These medications predominantly impact the quality and quantity of sleep without causing significant sleepiness at bedtime.

The second category of sleep disturbances relates to increased sleep latency with taking greater than 15 minutes to fall asleep. This leads to decreased total sleep time, decreased sleep efficiency, decreased stage 3 and 4 slow wave sleep, and decreased REM sleep. This also causes morning fatigue with feeling unrefreshed or unrested, morning sleepiness, daytime sleepiness, daytime napping, and symptoms of sleep deprivation. The sleep medications that predominantly impact increased sleep latency are known as sleep inducers and they directly affect sleepiness at bedtime.

Sleep Modifiers

The medications comprising the sleep modifier group are the antidepressant medications consisting predominantly of the sedating tricyclic antidepressant (TCA) medications and the muscle relaxant cyclobenzaprine (Flexeril) which has a chemical structure similar to the tricyclic antidepressants. See Chapter 7 for a thorough review on the antidepressant medications in managing polypain. The TCAs and cyclobenzaprine provide analgesic benefit through improved pain message processing directly and primarily, independent of psychological effect, as well as secondarily through their benefit in treating psychological disturbances and sleep disruption. Just as the analgesic benefit is noted to occur at doses lower than full antidepressant doses, similarly, the benefit to the sleep disturbance is also noted at less than antidepressant doses. The ability to use less than full antidepressant doses to manage the pain and sleep disturbances in polypain allows for a reduced risk of side effects or adverse reactions, especially medication related residual morning sedation or cognitive impairment. Indeed, it is my experience that patients with polypain are uniquely sensitive to the sleep modifying benefits of the sedating TCA medications and cyclobenzaprine as well as the potential risk of morning sedation or cognitive impairment. These physiological circumstances provide the opportunity for successful management of the sleep disturbances of polypain with much lower than typical TCA antidepressant doses.

Further, unlike sleep inducers, sleep modifiers should be taken well before bedtime to ensure adequate drug levels to impact the sleep process itself. In patients with polypain, my experience suggests taking sleep modifiers about 2 hours before bedtime to optimize benefit. Table II.2 displays the sleep modifier and sleep inducer medications, their properties, and usual dosing at night for sleep management in polypain.

The sedating TCAs are considered hypnotic sedatives. They have been reported to improve sleep quality with decreased sleep latency, decreased wakenings, and improved sleep efficiency. Reduction in REM sleep has been noted with most sedating TCAs. With regard to slow wave stage 3 and 4 sleep, some studies have shown benefit with increased slow wave sleep and reduced wakening alpha wave intrusion into stage 3 and stage 4 NREM sleep, but other studies have not confirmed these changes. More consistent is the finding that TCAs increase the slow wave activity during the early phases of sleep as seen in stage 2, 3, and 4 sleep. Thus, the sedating TCAs have been shown to directly improve most of the abnormalities of sleep stages and architecture identified in patients with symptoms and findings of polypain.

This improvement in sleep stages and architecture correlates with improvement in pain, pain thresholds, and well-being. Amitriptyline (Elavil), in low doses ranging from 10-50 mg daily, has been shown to improve: pain, sleep, and global well-being; improve pain thresholds; and reduce tender point counts. Cyclobenzaprine, in doses ranging from 10-40 mg daily, shows improvement in pain, sleep, global well-being, and fatigue.

Sleep Inducers

The medications comprising the sleep inducer group are also categorized pharmacologically as hypnotic or sedative drugs. These sleep inducing hypnotic drugs exhibit similar neurotransmitter effects and act on the gamma-aminobutyric acid$_A$ (GABA$_A$)-benzodiazepine receptor complex. Gamma-aminobutyric acid (GABA) is an important sleep inducing neurotransmitter in the brain. Based on their pharmacologic properties, the sleep inducer medications can be further categorized into a benzodiazepine, Valium-like, group and a non-benzodiazepine, non-Valium-like, group. The benzodiazepine hypnotics include flurazepam (Dalmane), triazolam (Halcion), temazepam (Restoril), quazepam (Doral), clonazepam (Klonopin), diazepam (Valium) and chlordiazepoxide (Librium). The non-benzodiazepine hypnotics include zolpidem (Ambien), zaleplon (Sonata), and eszopiclone (Lunesta). As these medications are used to induce sedation and sleep, they should be taken at bedtime.

Sleep inducer, benzodiazepine class medications improve sleep quality not only by reducing sleep latency but they also decrease the frequency of wakenings with less sleep fragmentation and improved sleep efficiency resulting in improved total sleep time. REM sleep may be reduced. Unlike the sleep modifiers, benzodiazepines suppress slow wave sleep. This is of

Sleep Group	Medication	Onset of Action	Duration of Action	Typical Dose
Sleep Modifier				
	Amitriptyline (Elavil)	Rapid-Intermediate	Short-Long	10-100 mg.
	Cyclobenzaprine (Flexeril)	Rapid-Intermediate	Short-Long	5-20 mg.
Sleep Inducer				
Benzodiazepine	Flurazepam (Dalmane)	Rapid	Intermediate-Long	15-30 mg.
	Triazolam (Halcion)	Rapid	Intermediate	0.125-0.25 mg.
	Temazepam (Restoril)	Intermediate	Intermediate-Long	15-30 mg.
	Quazepam (Doral)	Rapid-Intermediate	Long	7.5-15 mg.
	Clonazepam (Klonopin)	Rapid	Long	0.5-3 mg.
	Diazepam (Valium)	Rapid	Long	2-10 mg.
	Chlordiazepoxide (Librium)	Rapid	Long	10-25 mg.
Non-Benzodiazepine	Zolpidem (Ambien)	Rapid	Short	5-20 mg.
	Zaleplon (Sonata)	Rapid	Short	5-10 mg.
	Eszopiclone (Lunesta)	Intermediate	Intermediate	1-3 mg.

Table II.2: Sleep modifier and sleep inducer medications, their properties, and usual dosing at night for sleep management.

concern in polypain in view of the impairment of slow wave sleep due to the polypain itself. In this regard, it is notable that zolpidem does not adversely affect slow wave sleep and should be considered as a first choice sleep inducer in polypain because of this property.

It should be anticipated that sleep inducers that inherently have lesser effects on sleep modification should have no significant impact on pain thresholds when used exclusively and absent a sleep modifier in patients with polypain. Indeed, zolpidem has been shown to improve sleep and possibly fatigue but had no effect on pain.

Management of Sleep Medication in Polypain

In view of the sleep disturbances identified in patients with polypain, the reduced pain thresholds with increased nociception, and the psychological disturbances identified in polypain, the sleep modifier medications in low doses are initial drugs of choice in managing the disordered sleep of polypain. As noted, the sleep modifiers also demonstrate benefit to the prolonged sleep latency, and as such may be the only medication needed to manage the constellation of sleep abnormalities of polypain. However, if prolonged sleep latency remains despite all appropriate interventions with sleep ergonomics, biomechanics, posture, and optimal dosing of an effective sleep modifier, then consideration to adding a sleep inducer to the sleep modifier should be given. In view of the lack of adverse impact on slow wave sleep, zolpidem should be the initial sleep inducer drug of choice absent a contraindication to its use.

In the presence of symptoms of pain and psychoaffective disturbances with ongoing sleep disruption not improved by the Polypain Wellness Core Program, sleep modifying and sleep inducing medications should be introduced as early as possible as appropriately indicated in a parallel treatment track in concert with: optimal biomechanical and postural intervention through exercises, orthotics, neuromuscular re-education, and weight control; the Polypain Wellness Core Sleep Management Program ergonomics, biomechanics, and posture components; ergonomic intervention through appropriate accommodation and modification; and psychological support including medication and counseling. The sleep modifying and sleep inducing medications are introduced either as an adjunct to specifically and directly treat issues related to sleep and pain processing independent of their effects on psychological issues or TCAs may primarily treat the associated psychological disturbances with concomitant benefits in managing sleep disturbances and pain processing.

Absent a contraindication to using sleep modifying and sleep inducing medications, the selection of sleep modifying and sleep inducing medication is based upon a benefit-risk analysis looking at such factors as severity and extent of sleep disturbances, pain severity and extent relative to pain thresholds, disease severity and extent including severity and extent of psychological disturbances, functional impairment, the outcome of prior treatments, co-morbid medical conditions, concomitant medications, complication risk, compliance, convenience, and cost. As always, reality dictates.

When choosing a sleep modifier or sleep inducer based on the above criteria, the lowest dose, fastest acting, shortest lasting, and least potent should be selected that is anticipated to meet the needs of treatment. In the management of polypain, sleep modifiers and sleep inducers are introduced for one or more of three components of polypain. They are used to directly treat sleep disturbances, and sleep modifiers are used to improve nociception and pain processing and may also be used to treat depression. Thus, dosing of sleep modifying and sleep inducing medications is highly dependent on the purpose for which the sleep modifying and sleep inducing medications are being used. However, under-treating the patient to reduce risk carries no benefit but only risk of complications from treatment as well as allowing progression of symptoms given that: poor sleep begets pain; pain begets poor sleep; pain begets pain; poor sleep begets depression, anxiety, and stress; depression, anxiety, and stress beget reduced pain thresholds and poor sleep; all of which lead to additional further reductions in pain thresholds, further sleep impairment, and psychological disturbance.

Furthermore, patience is required as it takes time to build up a consistent sleep medication response and, once achieved, for the sleep modifying and sleep inducing medications to optimally interact with the underlying sleep impairment, aberrant pain processing, and psychological disturbances. Absent an adverse reaction or contraindication otherwise, a sleep modifying or sleep inducing medication should be slowly titrated to the highest dose needed up to an appropriate maximal dose for the purpose it was introduced to obtain a maximal response or to absolutely rule out lack of efficacy if a lower dose does not produce a maximal response.

In the face of an adverse reaction, lack of efficacy, or inadequate response at the safest maximal dose, the sleep modifying or sleep inducing medication under consideration should be discontinued and replaced with one of another of the sleep modifying or sleep inducing medication group, absent any contraindication, and the same process should be undertaken with the new sleep modifying or sleep inducing medication. In the face of medication induced morning sedation or cognitive impairment and in the face of a positive response otherwise, the sleeping medication should be taken even earlier before bedtime absent a contraindication or adverse effect or should be replaced by a drug from the same group with a shorter duration of action. In the face of a dose escalation adverse reaction and in the face of a positive but inadequate response, the dose should be reduced to the safest tolerated level at which a positive response is noted and absent any contraindication a second medication of the same group may be cautiously added and the same process should be undertaken to introduce and dose adjust the new sleep medication. Similarly, in the face of a positive but inadequate response at a maximal dose of a sleeping medication, absent any contraindication, a second medication of the same group may be cautiously added and the same process should be undertaken to introduce and dose adjust the new sleep medication. However, in my experience this is rarely indicated in polypain and usually suggests that other elements of the Polypain Core Sleep Management Program are not in place, not being complied with as prescribed, an unidentified factor contributing to polypain has not been identified, or a new component contributing to polypain has developed.

Treatment with sleep modifying and sleep inducing medications is further complicated by the fact that they are used in parallel with other treatment modalities that are being adjusted at the same time and treatment benefit, as well as complications, need to be assessed against the background of the treatment effects and complications of these other medications and any potential interactions between them. Further, in view of the selective benefit of TCA type medications in treating sleep disruption and pain processing independent of depression and at lower doses than needed to treat depression, side effects seen at higher doses as needed to treat depression with tricyclic type medications are avoided or minimized.

The benefits of sleep modifying and sleep inducing medications in managing the components of polypain must be balanced by their potential adverse effects. See Chapter 7 for a complete discussion of adverse effects associated with the sleep modifier TCA medications. Many, but not all, of the adverse effects of the sleep inducing medications are mediated by their hypnotic and sedative actions. Generally, adverse reactions to hypnotic medications are rare ranging from 1-5 per 10,000 doses taken. All sleep inducers cause central nervous system depression as the mechanism by which they cause sedation and sleepiness. While this effect is desired therapeutically to improve sleep, the presence or persistence of the central nervous system depression outside of sleep leads to dose related adverse effects including sedation, dizziness, cognitive impairment, impaired alertness, memory impairment, ataxia with motor function impairment especially with unsteadiness with walking, and falls. These adverse reactions are compounded by other sedating medications.

Benzodiazepines may also induce agitation, anxiety, emotional lability, depression, seizure, slurred speech, and fatigue. Benzodiazepines have muscle relaxing and anti-anxiety effects which can be used to therapeutic benefit. Benzodiazepines may worsen narrow angle glaucoma. In depressed suicidal patients, benzodiazepines may possibly increase the risk of suicide. Dependency may occur necessitating gradual tapering upon discontinuation. Benzodiazepines may be addictive in individuals with known substance abuse.

Zolpidem has similar central nervous adverse effects as the benzodiazepines and in addition carries an increased risk of somnambulism – sleep walking, that in fact may not be recalled by patients but is recognized by activities they did while sleep walking resulting in otherwise unexplained changes to the surroundings on wakening. Zaleplon has similar central nervous system adverse effects as the benzodiazepines. Eszopiclone has similar central nervous side effects as the benzodiazepines as well a similar risk of addiction in substance abusers and suicide in suicidal depressed individuals.

Ramelteon (Rozerem) is a more recently available sleep inducing medication. It is characterized as a melatonin receptor agonist stimulating melatonin receptors in the brain. It is reported to reduce sleep latency without significant other effects on sleep quality and architecture. In addition to the side effect concerns of sleep inducer medications as a group, ramelteon may raise prolactin levels and lower testosterone levels. It is also contraindicated in patients taking the antidepressant fluvoxamine. Further investigation is needed to determine the role of ramelteon in the management of the sleep disturbances of polypain.

The addition of sleep modifying and sleep inducing medications in the management of the disturbances of sleep stages, architecture, and quantity in polypain should be considered: 1) only in the presence of a comprehensive polypain management program with implementation of at least the Polypain Wellness Core Program; 2) only in the presence of the sleep ergonomics, sleep hygiene, sleep biomechanics, and posture elements of the Polypain Wellness Core Sleep Management Program; 3) and absent a contraindication to using sleep modifying and sleep inducing medications based upon a thorough benefit-risk analysis that includes consideration of the nature and severity of the sleep disturbances and their contribution to reduced pain thresholds, psychological disturbances, fatigue, cognitive impairment, functional impairment, and other sleep disturbance related symptoms as well as the outcome of prior treatments. Awareness and vigilance are critical in monitoring patients for potential adverse effects of treatment and this is accomplished through intensive follow-up with appropriate and comprehensive evaluation of progress and monitoring of treatment risk in terms of co-morbid medical conditions, concomitant medications, complications, compliance, convenience, and cost relative to treatment benefit. Reality dictates. Be aware of the Law of Unintended/Unrecognized Consequences.

Thus, the Polypain Wellness Core Sleep Management Program is a comprehensive subset of the Polpain Wellness Core Program that treats the sleep disturbances of polypain. These sleep disturbances have adverse effects on the pain of polypain and pain message processing. They also adversely affect the psychological disturbances of polypain including depression, stress, and anxiety. Furthermore: poor sleep begets pain, depression, anxiety, and stress; and pain, depression, anxiety, and stress beget poor sleep. This leads to further reductions in pain thresholds and poorer sleep, both of which lead to additional further reductions in pain thresholds and further sleep impairment. The Polypain Wellness Core Sleep

Management Program incorporates sleep ergonomics, hygiene, biomechanics, posture, and, as appropriately indicated, sleep modifier and sleep inducer medication to improve these sleep disturbances and consequently improve pain thresholds with concomitant reduction in pain symptoms and improvement in psychological well-being.

Chapter 12

Step 6: Psychological Problems Create More Pain: How To Recognize Them and Life Skill Strategies to Alleviate Them

"For everything there is season, a time for everything under the sun.
A time to be born and a time to die; a time to plant and a time to reap.
A time to kill and a time to heal; a time to break and a time to build.
A time to weep and a time to laugh; a time to mourn and a time for dance.
A time to cast stones and a time to gather stones; a time to embrace and a
time to refrain.
A time to seek and a time to lose; a time to be silent and a time to speak.
A time to love and a time to hate; a time for war and a time for peace.
[…] And I saw that there is nothing better than that man rejoice in his
deeds, for that is his portion…"
                    —Ecclesiastes 3:1-22, Book of Ecclesiastes

The relationship of psychiatric, psychological, and psychosocial disturbances to pain, especially chronic pain, and more specifically chronic musculoskeletal pain such as occurs in polypain, is significant. Chronic musculoskeletal pain is not a simple one dimensional process whereby something that causes pain is perceived as the same pain by all who experience it. Rather, chronic pain is a complex, highly nuanced, multidimensional, and highly individualized experience driven and controlled by the mechanisms that generate pain from the source of pain and process pain messaging to set pain thresholds.

Psychological and Psychosocial Problems Are A Two-Way Street

The current paradigm of healthcare focuses attention on the biomedical model. In this traditional model, pain develops and evolves from something that can be seen, touched, or physically identified. Psychiatric, psychological, or psychosocial factors are considered secondary outcomes of a primary physical illness causing pain. In other words, all identified psychological problems and psychosocial disturbances are felt to arise from the pain of the underlying physical illness. As the psychological and psychosocial issues are considered to be dependent on the physical condition affecting the individual, all attention is, therefore, directed to the physical issues. This healthcare model fails to consider the concept that psychological and psychosocial disturbances may exist as distinct and separate conditions from the physical condition of the individual and independently contribute to and alter the symptoms and outcome of the pain process. While there is a strong expectation bias of healthcare professionals to recognize that chronic pain is associated with psychological and psychosocial problems such as depression and anxiety, the understanding is unidirectional with pain identified as the cause of the psychological issues.

There is virtually no recognition that psychological disturbances driven by pain independently contribute to and alter the presentation and outcome of that pain. There is also no recognition that psychological processes present independent of the condition producing pain contribute to and alter the presentation and outcome of that pain. Thus, the bias of the current traditional approach leads to significant limitations in the understanding of the relationship of chronic pain to symptoms, treatment, and outcome. Most importantly, psychological and psychosocial disturbances that are either unrecognized/undiagnosed or under-recognized/under-diagnosed in the setting of chronic pain lead to the attribution of symptoms and behavioral responses to incorrect causes. This ultimately leads to treatment failure, worsening symptoms, functional limitations, and disability.

Psychological and Psychosocial Disturbances in Fibromyalgia Are Common

Psychological distress is a common and significant feature of fibromyalgia. Psychological disturbances occur in a significantly higher prevalence in those with fibromyalgia compared to controls. Increased scores are noted on the Minnesota Multiphasic Personality Inventory (MMPI), a psychological health status instrument. However, these results may be partly biased on the depression, hypochondriasis, and hysteria scales as the chronic pain of fibromyalgia itself yields positive responses to pain and somatic symptoms and does not necessarily differentiate between physical and psychological symptoms. Patients with fibromyalgia have a greater number of lifetime psychiatric diagnoses compared to controls, especially mood disorders such as depression and anxiety disorders, with a threefold increase over control patients. Fibromyalgia patients are reported to have major depression in 20-30% and anxiety disorder in 10-20% at the time of assessment. The clinical features of sleep disruption, fatigue, and psychomotor changes commonly identified in patients diagnosed with fibromyalgia are also present in individuals with diagnostic criteria for major depressive episode as well as generalized anxiety disorder as seen in Tables 12.1 and 12.2.

Thus, there is significant overlap in the clinical features of depression, anxiety, and fibromyalgia. This most likely results in a severe underestimation of the true prevalence of psychological disturbances in patients with fibromyalgia at the time of assessment as the symptoms of depression, stress, anxiety, somatization, and other psychological processes are wrongly attributed to the diagnosis of fibromyalgia rather than correctly attributed to the psychological diagnosis that more correctly accounts for the symptoms. When this attribution bias is partly eliminated by looking at lifetime diagnoses of psychological disorders, including when fibromyalgia was not present as a diagnosis, the prevalence rate of psychological conditions rises dramatically. A prior diagnosis of psychiatric disorder is identified in 90% of patients eventually diagnosed with fibromyalgia. A lifetime diagnosis of major depression is noted in 68% - 86% of fibromyalgia patients. A lifetime diagnosis of anxiety disorder is identified in 60% of individuals with fibromyalgia. Furthermore, psychiat-

A. Five (or more) of the following symptoms have been present during the same 2-week period and represent a change from previous functioning; at least one of the symptoms is either (1) depressed mood or (2) loss of interest or pleasure.

   (1) Depressed mood most of the day, nearly every day, as indicated by either subjective report (e.g., feels sad or empty) or observation made by others (e.g., appears tearful)

   (2) Markedly diminished interest or pleasure in all, or almost all, activities most of the day, nearly every day (as indicated by either subjective account or observation made by others)

   (3) Significant weight loss when not dieting or weight gain (e.g., a change of more than 5% of body weight in a month), or decrease or increase in appetite nearly every day

   (4) Insomnia or hypersomnia nearly every day

   (5) Psychomotor agitation or retardation nearly every day (observable by others, not merely subjective feelings of restlessness or being slowed down)

   (6) Fatigue or loss of energy nearly every day

   (7) Feelings of worthlessness or excessive inappropriate guilt (which may be delusional) nearly every day (not merely self-reproach or guilt about being sick)

   (8) Diminished ability to think or concentrate, or indecisiveness, nearly every day (either by subjective account or as observed by others)

   (9) Recurrent thoughts of death (not just fear of dying), recurrent suicidal ideation without a specific plan, or a suicide attempt or a specific plan for committing suicide

B. The symptoms do not meet criteria that includes a manic component.

C. The symptoms cause clinically significant distress or impairment in social, occupational, or other important areas of functioning.

D. The symptoms are not due to the direct effects of a substance (e.g., a drug of abuse, a medication) or a general medical condition (e.g., hypothyroidism).

E. The symptoms are not accounted for by Bereavement.

Table 12.1: DSM-IV-TR diagnostic criteria for major depressive episode. (Adapted from American Psychiatric Association. Diagnostic and Statistical Manual of Mental Disorders, Fourth Edition, Text Revision. Washington, DC: American Psychiatric Association; 2000. Reprinted with permission.)

A. Excessive anxiety or worry (apprehensive expectation), occurring more days than not for at least 6 months, about a number of events or activities (such as work or school performance).

B. The person finds it difficult to control the worry.

C. The anxiety or worry are associated with three (or more) of the following six symptoms (with at least some symptoms present for more days than not for the past six months).

    (1) restlessness or feeling keyed up or on edge
    (2) being easily fatigued
    (3) difficulty concentrating or mind going blank
    (4) irritability
    (5) muscle tension
    (6) sleep disturbance (difficulty falling or staying asleep, or restless, unsatisfying sleep)

D. The anxiety and worry are not about another psychological disturbance or its features.

E. The anxiety, worry or physical symptoms cause clinically significant distress or impairment in social, occupational, or other important areas of functioning.

F. The anxiety is not due to the direct effects of a substance or medication, a general medical condition with anxiety-like symptoms or exclusively related to another psychiatric condition.

Table 12.2: DSM-IV-TR diagnostic criteria for generalized anxiety disorder. (Adapted from American Psychiatric Association. Diagnostic and Statistical Manual of Mental Disorders, Fourth Edition, Text Revision. Washington, DC: American Psychiatric Association; 2000. Reprinted with permission.)

ric disorders including depression, anxiety, stress disorders like posttraumatic stress disorder, and sexual and physical abuse are identified in 75% of dysfunctional fibromyalgia patients. A past history of increased abusive physical and emotional trauma and childhood sexual abuse has been reported in patients with fibromyalgia and has been reported to adversely affect coping mechanisms. Sexual and physical abuse in women with fibromyalgia, while not appearing to occur more frequently than in control groups, correlates with increased severity of fibromyalgia symptoms. Somatization, the expression of physical complaints not fully explained by a medical or psychiatric disorder or the direct effects of a substance is noted in 14% of patients with fibromyalgia at the time of assessment and a lifetime diagnosis of somatization is noted in 23%. Posttraumatic stress disorder is an anxiety disorder characterized by exposure to a traumatic event that is re-experienced in thoughts, dreams, or emotions with avoidance of experiences triggering these thoughts, dreams, or emotions through social withdrawal and estrangement accompanied by anxiety symptoms or hypervigilence. Symptoms of posttraumatic stress disorder have been identified in 57% of fibromyalgia patients. Cognitive coping mechanisms in

Psychiatric/Psychosocial Disturbance	Prevalence
Pre-existing diagnosis of psychiatric disorder	90%
Lifetime psychiatric diagnoses	3 times higher than controls
Depression	
At the time of assessment	20-30% (Likely Underestimated)
Lifetime diagnosis major depression	68%-86%
Anxiety/Stress	
At the time of assessment	10-20% (Likely Underestimated)
Lifetime diagnosis anxiety/stress	60%
Post-traumatic stress disorder	57%
Somatization	
At the time of assessment	14%
Lifetime diagnosis somatization	23%
Sexual abuse	Not increased, but worse symptoms
Physical/Emotional Abuse	Not increased, but worse symptoms
Coping Mechanism/Personality/Behavior	
Catastrophizing	
Pessimism	
Learned helplessness	
Dependence and passivity	
Denial of life problems and attributing psychosocial problems solely to physical illness	

Table 12.3: *Psychiatric, psychological, and psychosocial disturbances in fibromyalgia.*

fibromyalgia patients identify catastrophizing which correlates with poorer pain control, pessimism, learned helplessness, dependence and passivity, and denial of life problems attributing psychosocial issues solely to fibromyalgia. The psychiatric and psychosocial disturbances identified in fibromyalgia are shown in Table 12.3.

Individuals With Fibromyalgia Polypain Are Frequently Aware of Their Psychological Turmoil

Based on self-reporting, the study data from Chapter 4 reveals the presence of self-reported stress and anxiety in 91% of patients with polypain and depression in 89%. My own experience with polypain patients clearly shows a relationship between pain and symptom quality and quantity that correlates with the presence and severity of the psychological disturbance.

The Interaction Between Psychiatric, Psychological, And Psychosocial Trouble and Chronic Musculoskeletal Pain

In chronic musculoskeletal pain disorders, psychological status is a major determinant of health status along with physical functioning and the pain itself. The psychiatric and psychosocial disorders identified in fibromyalgia correlate with healthcare seeking behavior, the perceived severity of the symptoms of pain and fatigue, and perceptions of environmental stress. Clearly, anxiety, stress, depression, and other psychological disturbances and conditions are significant components of fibromyalgia. These psychological states, in turn, significantly affect the appreciation of pain and its presentation in fibromyalgia. Of major significance to individuals with polypain, which includes all individuals diagnosed with fibromyalgia, is the adverse impact of psychological and psychosocial disturbances on pain thresholds. Most importantly, this unfavorable impact on pain results directly from the presence of psychological and psychosocial disturbances independent of whether these disturbances are induced by pain itself or other non-pain related factors that affect the psychological and psychosocial balance of the individual. Furthermore, the perceived severity of pain negatively impacts the psychological and psychosocial state of the individual.

Thus, psychological and psychosocial disturbances beget pain and pain begets psychological and psychosocial disturbances. Ultimately, psychological and psychosocial disturbances beget further psychological and psychosocial disturbances through their effect on pain. While the details of the mechanism of how stress, anxiety, depression, and other psychological disturbances and psychosocial disruption modulate pain are not precisely known, it is known that cognitive modulation of pain by distraction or attention stimulates several brain areas and brain related pain activity is stimulated by hypnotic suggestions directed at intensifying the perception of a painful stimulus. It is also clear that patients with chronic widespread musculoskeletal pain, as seen in polypain, display impairment in the descending modulation pathway, a central nervous system mechanism that modulates the severity of a painful stimulus as reviewed in Chapter 6. Thus, it appears the facilitation of pain by psychological disturbances such as anxiety, stress, and depression arises somewhere in the higher levels of the central nervous system as a cognitive behavioral response which heightens pain sensitivity and reduces pain thresholds by sending signals through spinal cord pain pathways to the spinal pain message areas to reduce pain thresholds. The understanding that psychiatric, psy-

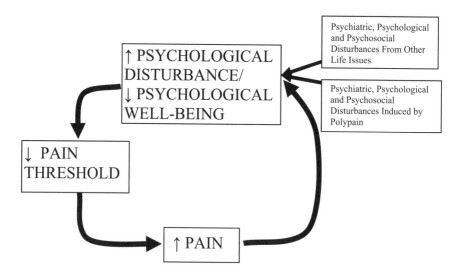

Figure 12.1: *The fundamental relationship of psychiatric, psychological, and psychosocial disturbances to pain and pain thresholds in polypain.*

chological, and psychosocial disturbances contribute independently to chronic musculoskeletal pain symptoms and behavioral responses and that chronic musculoskeletal pain impacts pain behavioral responses leads to the recognition that the traditional biomedical model is inadequate to address these interrelationships and that a more encompassing biopsychosocial model better explains and accounts for these processes. The fundamental relationship between psychiatric disorders, psychological, and psychosocial disturbances and polypain is depicted in Figure 12.1.

In addition, psychological disruption may have other effects that impact pain processing such as disrupting sleep as reviewed in Chapter 11 and affecting physical functioning such as producing muscle tension or inappropriate physical posturing that may directly impact the pain arising from the musculoskeletal symptoms.

Behavioral Coping Factors: Reacting To Pain
Pain Suffering and Pain Behavior

Chronic musculoskeletal pain as seen in fibromyalgia polypain does not develop in a vacuum. It evolves and presents symptoms in individuals with a pre-existing identity and an established psychiatric, psychological, and social construct. The diagnosis of fibromyalgia conjures up many superimposed emotions and fears simply by virtue of the stigma of the label alone. These are based on the many uncertainties and unknowns of having a chronic, lifelong, painful musculoskeletal disease with no known cause, no specific treatment, a poor prognosis, and the potential to impact functional activities and well-being. The diagnostic label of fibromyalgia and chronic musculoskeletal pain itself significantly impacts this underlying self-image and, conversely, this self-image impacts the physical, psychological, and social responses to the diagnoses of fibromyalgia and chronic musculoskeletal pain.

While the sensation of pain in polypain is driven and controlled by the mechanisms that generate pain from the primary generalized osteoarthritis predominantly involving the neck and back with associated degenerative disc disease and the variable combination of associated tendinitis, bursitis, and fasciitis and modulated by the pain itself, sleep disturbances, and psychological disturbances in setting pain thresholds, the experience of pain extends well beyond the perception of the pain to the highly complex and individualized responses to the sensed pain. These responses affect the emotional, social, familial, occupational, recreational, spiritual, psychological, and physical aspects of the individual's well-being. These responses are commonly recognized as pain distress or suffering, and pain behavior. Pain suffering incorporates the negative emotional and physical responses to the perceived pain and pain behavior identifies the actions taken in response to the perceived pain. Pain suffering and pain behavior result in ongoing psychological and psychosocial disruption, and in the face of maladaptive coping responses as seen in fibromyalgia, lead to increasing psychological and psychosocial distress which ultimately lower pain thresholds and worsen the perception of pain. How individuals with chronic pain cope with their symptoms correlates with the perception of pain severity, physical functioning, level of functional disability, and psychological adaptation. These associations of pain suffering and pain behavior to pain perception are depicted in Figure 12.2.

Pain behavior encompasses a large variety of actions taken by the individual in response to perceived pain. These include physical responses to the pain itself, taking medications, seeking health care, altering daily activities, avoiding physical activities, and claiming disability. The physical responses to pain are the most obvious to another observer. These include verbalization of the presence of pain with descriptors that include the sensory quality, the affective impact, subjective severity qualifiers, and pattern identifiers. Other verbal responses include altered tone, altered volume, moaning, grunting, or sighing. There may be changes in respiration with breath holding, rapid breathing, panting, or irregular breathing. Various facial expressions may be seen including the frequently observed grimacing. Typical non-verbal physical responses to pain include: withdrawal; guarding with slow, stiff, interrupted movements; rubbing an area perceived as painful or a different area; grasping an area perceived as painful or a different area; sucking; licking; pinching; digging or biting around the perceived area of pain or another area; avoidance of use; holding an area stiff; repeated bending in an area perceived as painful; and limping in the case of pain in the low back and lower body. The potentially beneficial results of rubbing, grasping, sucking, licking, pinching, digging, biting, or repeatedly moving an area perceived as painful or an area remote to that site are found in the pain modulation that occurs through the elevation of pain thresholds induced by such activity as reviewed in Chapters 2 and 6.

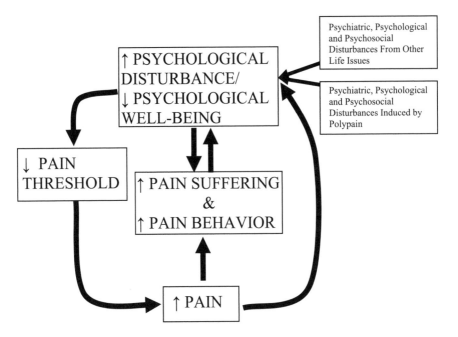

Figure 12.2: *The relationship of pain suffering and pain behavior to psychiatric, psychological, and psychosocial disturbances in polypain.*

Pain Coping Factors

Pain coping factors are critical components to setting the psychological balance that determines pain thresholds as well as pain behavior and pain suffering. Just as chronic pain is a complex, highly nuanced, multidimensional, and highly individualized experience driven and controlled by the mechanisms that generate pain from the source of pain and that process pain messaging and set pain thresholds, pain coping mechanisms are also complex, highly nuanced, multidimensional, and highly individualized responses to perceived pain that lead to adaptive or maladaptive behavior identified through pain suffering and pain behavior.

Pain coping is determined by cognitive-emotional strategies based on cognitive problem and conflict solving skills and abilities, the physical abilities of the individual to carry out these cognitive-emotional responses, and the social setting of the individual to allow expression of the cognitive-emotional strategies. Thus, a strategy to deal with perceived pain may be considered highly adaptive for one individual and maladaptive for another. In fact, in any one individual, an adaptive behavior in one domain may be maladaptive in another leading to value based trade-offs. For instance, if bed rest is needed to recover an exacerbation of low back related symptoms, but the patient cannot afford the lost wages of time off and does not undertake the bed rest because of this, then the behavior is maladaptive to the treatment of the low back issue and is positively adaptive to the social issues. Thus, pain behavior and pain suffering are highly contextual and not only vary from individual to individual but vary as any one individual's circumstances changes.

Cognitive-emotional strategies commonly used in dealing with chronic pain include confrontive coping, distancing, self-control, seeking social support, accepting responsibility, escape avoidance, problem-solving, and positive reappraisal. In patients with chronic musculoskeletal pain, coping strategies that include higher levels of dependency and anger correlate with higher levels of pain and depression and lower functional activity. The physical and social expressions of cognitive-emotional coping strategies include distracting attention, reinterpreting pain sensation, the use of coping self-statements, ignoring pain sensations, catastrophizing, praying or hoping, and increasing activity level.

Distraction is a strategy that involves thinking about more pleasant things than pain while ignoring pain involves not paying attention to the pain. Reinterpreting pain leads to a distancing of the recognition of pain. Use of positive self-statements relies on the use of statements that anticipate a better outcome. There is no clear evidence that distraction, ignoring pain, reinterpreting pain, or positive self-statements are useful strategies in positively coping with pain or pain related function.

Passive prayer involving asking for deliverance from pain correlates with increased pain severity and disability. It is not clear if this effect is due to prayer being invoked by individuals with more pain and disability or if in fact passive prayer has a maladaptive coping component in chronic pain. On the other hand, positive, guiding prayer leads to acceptance of chronic pain.

The lack of pain specific coping mechanisms to produce positive adaptive responses that actually improve pain or function in chronic musculoskeletal pain is likely related to the fact that much of the psychological disturbance and disruption seen in patients with chronic musculoskeletal pain is primarily due to psychiatric, psychological, and psychosocial disturbances from other life issues and not predominantly caused by the pain itself. However, these psychological and psychosocial disturbances from other life issues have significant impact on pain thresholds and increase the perception of pain leading to maladaptive coping behaviors that incorrectly assume the pain is the major driving force behind the psychological and psychosocial disturbances. Thus, coping efforts are wrongly directed to dealing with pain as a cause of psychological problems rather than as a result of independent psychological problems. This is another example of where correlation is not causation.

Catastrophizing is a negative cognitive-emotional response leading to faulty correlations and misinterpretations. It is characterized by pessimism and assumes the worst possible outcomes. Catastrophizing patients tend to: 1) over-generalize and assume that a process or outcome of one event may apply to other unrelated events; 2) personalize causes and outcomes rather than relating them to the processes by which they occur; 3) and selectively abstract by focusing on the negative components of things. They exhibit negative thoughts related to pain including negative self-statements, negative social acceptance, and impose self-blame. These cognitive distortions lead to maladaptive behaviors such as inappropriate activity levels, dependency, and non-compliance to treatment. Catastrophizing strongly correlates with pain, function, disability, and depression in chronic pain including fibromyalgia. It also predicts long-term depression in chronic musculoskeletal pain.

Self-efficacy is a measure of the confidence of an individual to achieve a certain outcome or activity. The greater the self-efficacy, the harder the individual will work, the more likely the individual will persevere, and less anxiety will be present in the efforts expended to achieve set goals. Greater self-efficacy is associated with less pain behavior, a lesser adverse impact on functional activities, lower pain levels, and less depression. A more generalized belief in the ability to affect personal outcomes evolves from learned behavior that correlates personal effort to its effect on outcomes. A strong belief that that personal efforts to change things will be successful is identified as an internal locus of control. When outcomes are perceived as outside a personal sphere of influence, this is identified as an external locus of control. In chronic musculoskeletal pain, a stronger internal locus of control is associated with lower levels of pain, lesser psychological disturbance, and better response to treatment. More specifically, in patients with fibromyalgia, an internal locus of control correlates with less pain, less psychological disruption, and improved functional ability. However, there is an increased prevalence of an external locus of control in patients with fibromyalgia compared to other chronic pain conditions including musculoskeletal pain. This is associated with increased pain severity, increased disability, and increased psychological disturbance.

Helplessness develops in circumstances in which individuals do not believe their efforts will affect an outcome. They perceive an external locus of control. While chronic musculoskeletal pain may cause physiological functional impairment, patients who feel helpless and hopeless develop functional impairment in excess of that impairment and enter into a progressive spiral of learned helplessness whereby the increased perception of impairment leads to further helplessness, hopelessness, and resignation leading to a worsening perception of functional ability in a progressive downward spiral. Learned helplessness correlates with more severe pain, higher levels of functional impairment, and greater depression in chronic musculoskeletal pain.

A lack of self-efficacy, an external locus of control, and helplessness lead to the emotional responses of sadness, shame, and guilt. In the face of chronic pain, they also lead to the maladaptive cognitive distortions of self-victimization, self-blame, reduced self-esteem, and negative self-identity. There is a natural tendency for us to view ourselves in a favorable, self-enhancing manner which is identified as a self-serving bias. This self-serving bias is significantly negatively impacted in patients with chronic musculoskeletal disease as their lives are increasingly occupied by the physical symptoms and the consequences of these symptoms on their psychological, emotional, social, familial, occupational, recreational, and spiritual well-being. This is especially magnified in fibromyalgia in which unknown elements regarding cause, treatment, and prognosis offer no rationale to reconcile the symptoms. Thus, a patient's pre-existing self-identity increasingly becomes intertwined with the chronic pain and its manifestations in a process in which the underlying self-identity is progressively subjugated and patients identify themselves in the context of the pain and its effects.

Emotions, Fear, and Pain

Emotions represent another element of expressive behavior. Emotion requires: an emotion inducing stimulus accompanied by physiological responses in various body systems such as sweating and increased heart rate; and a cognitive label based on perceptions and learned experience attached to the emotional response identifying the emotion leading to the behavioral expression of that emotion physically, both non-verbally and verbally. The basic emotions have been identified as happiness-joy, interest-excitement, surprise, sadness, anger, disgust, contempt, fear, shame, guilt, and love. Furthermore, emotions can be categorized as positive, such as happiness-joy, interest-excitement, surprise, and love or negative such as sadness, anger, disgust, contempt, fear, shame, and guilt. In patients with chronic pain, the negative emotions comprised of sadness, shame, disgust and guilt are accounted for by co-existing depression. Anger and contempt are accounted for by the associated anxiety.

The negative emotional experience of fear, while associated with depression and anxiety, appears to arise separately. The chronic musculoskeletal pain of fibromyalgia polypain is associated with fear based on the fundamental experience of pain, modified by learned experience incorporating life experiences, beliefs, and perceptions. Such fear includes the fear of the pain itself, the physical threat of pain to well-being, the psychological disruption, the impact of pain of functional ability, and the potential and real social losses. In a disorder with unknown cause, unknown treatment, and poor prognosis, such as fibromyalgia, there is also the fear of the unknown. Fear, anger, and sadness are emotions that correlate with the affective components of chronic pain. In chronic pain, the

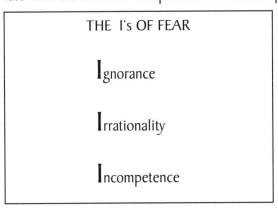

THE I's OF FEAR

Ignorance

Irrationality

Incompetence

Table 12.4:
The basis of fear.

presence of fear is a theme that unites pain from the anticipation of the experience, through the pain experience itself, and the psychosocial response to the pain.

Evolution, genetics, psychology, and life experience all play a role in determining what we fear and our threshold for that fear. Fundamentally, however, fear develops because there is a lack of knowledge or understanding of the circumstance or its outcome. In essence, fear is driven by three I's – ignorance, irrationality, and incompetence as seen in Table 12.4. Ignorance refers to not knowing all there is to know about an issue because such information or evidence does not exist, is not available, or is not sought. Irrationality is a process whereby available information or evidence is not analyzed rationally or logically leading to unfounded assumptions, inappropriate bias, distortions of known facts, faulty correlations, and incorrect conclusions. Incompetence refers to a lack of ability to obtain otherwise available information or a cognitive inability to process such information correctly. In fibromyalgia, ignorance and irrationality play a significant role in generating fear because it is a disorder with unknown cause, unknown treatment, and unknown but poor prognosis.

Social Cognitive Coping Factors: Relationships, Society, And Pain
Pain-Behavior-Related Social Adaptation

Pain behavior identifies the actions taken in response to perceived pain which includes the physical responses that identify elements of pain suffering as well as the behavioral responses to perceived pain in the social, familial, occupational, recreational, and spiritual realms of the individual's well-being. These responses, in turn, significantly affect the emotional, social, familial, occupational, recreational, spiritual, psychological, and physical aspects of the individual's well-being. Pain behavior reflects the end result of the pain coping factors that set the psychological balance that determines pain thresholds. Furthermore, depending on how adaptive or maladaptive the pain behavior is, the behavior itself determines future pain behavior and pain suffering through its effect on psychological and psychosocial factors directly, as well as through its subsequent influence of the psychological and psychosocial factors on pain thresholds and ultimately pain perception.

Pain-behavior-related social adaptation to chronic musculoskeletal pain is dependent upon: 1) the perception of the pain severity; 2) the physiological impact of the pain process upon function; 3) the psychological state independent of pain and as affected by pain; 4) the behavioral and coping mechanisms available; 5) the social circumstances of the individual; 6) and the industrial-legal context of the pain such as whether it is in some way related to work or an accident. Pain behavior and the attendant social responses can range any where from complete avoidance/withdrawal to thoroughly solicitous/activity-seeking. How adaptive or maladaptive the pain-behavior-related social response is, is specific to not only the overall physical and psychological state of the individual at a given point in time but also to the pain behavior being assessed. As in the example earlier, if bed rest is needed to recover an exacerbation of low back related symptoms, but the patient cannot afford the lost wages of time off and does not undertake the bed rest because of this, then the solicitous/activity seeking behavior of working is maladaptive to the treatment of the low back issue and is positively adaptive to the social issues. Similarly, if time off from a weight-bearing job is needed to recover an exacerbation of knee related symptoms and the individual is subsequently able to return to work but refuses because of inadequate coping mechanisms or fear, then the avoidance/withdrawal behavior is adaptive to the knee symptoms initially but later maladaptive to the social work issue. Clearly, cognitive factors in pain behavior social adaptation to chronic musculoskeletal pain are highly fluid in terms of time and context and the ideal balance between avoidance/withdrawal behavior and solicitous/activity-seeking behavior must constantly be re-evaluated and adjusted. This balance is shown in Figure 12.3. Failure to adapt uniformly leads to maladaptive social behavior which in turn negatively impacts the psychological state and behavioral coping mechanisms of the individual. This ultimately leads to a reduction in pain thresholds with increased perception of pain which, in a vicious cycle, leads to further maladaptive pain behavior.

The outcome of pain behavior significantly affects the emotional, social, familial, occupational, recreational, spiritual, psychological, and physical aspects of an individual's well-being. Conversely, the emotional, social, familial, occupational, recreational, spiritual, psychological, and physical aspects of the individual's well-being significantly impact pain suffering and behavior. Thus, for any particular level of perceived pain, individuals with chronic musculoskeletal pain exhibit a large range of individualized and situation specific responses identified as pain suffering and pain behavior. The influence of these external factors in modulating pain suffering and pain evolves through a process of operant conditioning. Through operant conditioning, pain suffering and pain behavior are conditioned by either positive or negative reinforcement. Positive reinforcement occurs when there is a desired, pleasing secondary gain from the pain behavior. Negative reinforcement occurs when there is a desired reduction or limitation of an unpleasant state through the pain behavior.

In the social context, attention-getting from friends and family, or economic gain from receiving disability or other compensation payments positively reinforces the value of the chronic pain and directly motivates this type of pain-behavior-related social adaptation. Similarly, avoiding undesirable but expected or socially appropriate work, household responsibilities, or legal obligations which an individual is capable of undertaking in the face of chronic pain serves as negative reinforcement of pain behavior social adaptation by enhancing the value of the chronic pain. Indeed, these behaviors may directly conflict with the biopsychosocially appropriate pain behavior of undertaking activities to reduce pain and improve well-being. The rewards gained by pain behavior lead to further reinforcement of the behavior which in turn drives the emotional, social, familial, occupational, recreational, spiritual, psychological, and physical aspects of the individual's well-being in a self-perpetuating cycle. The adverse pain behaviors lead to perpetuation of the sick role and distancing of social relationships, and fail to reinforce the appropriate and ex-

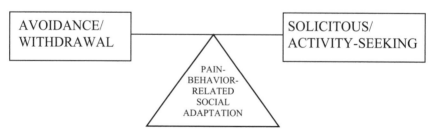

Figure 12.3: *The balance between avoidance/withdrawal and solicitous/activity-seeking pain behavior related to social adaptation.*

pected pain-behavior-related social adaptation.

Furthermore, the pain behavior may become detached and indepen-dent of the actual pain present as determined by the pain generators and pain thresholds. There is little relationship between the perceived pain level and pain behavior identifying functional impairment, but there is a strong association of pain behavior to psychosocial factors. Indeed, pain behavior may persist long after the pain itself is controlled. This is the basis of malingering, a condition in which external incentives cause a patient to produce symptoms that are not fully attributable to a general medical condition.

Social Relationships and Pain Behavior

In the setting of marital and spousal relationships, the presence of an anxious and concerned spouse, in and of itself, causes pain patients to report higher levels of pain. The concern and anxiety displayed by the supportive spouse develops in direct response to pain behavior displayed by the patient. Pain patients are less likely to persist in painful physical effort and report more pain in the presence of a sympathetic, anxious spouse. Chronic pain patients report increased sensitivity to a painful stimulus when sympathetic anxious spouses are present at the time of testing. In essence, a solicitous spouse who responds with anxiety and concern to the underlying pain behavior becomes an enabler of adverse pain behavior. By modifying the social situation in an attempt to be sympathetic, the enabling spouse in fact undertakes behavior that both positively reinforces adverse pain behavior and negatively reinforces the avoidance of healthy pain behavior. Spousal criticism also leads to psycho-logical distress and poorer coping responses in the setting of chronic pain. On the other hand, chronic pain patients who report high levels of satisfaction with their marriages have less depression.

In a similar manner, sympathetic healthcare providers may also become enablers of adverse pain responses and behaviors. The provision of pas-sive treatment by healthcare providers in which the patient is not actively involved in the treatment process or participating in self-management pro-motes avoidance/withdrawal behavior to limit functional activities to avoid pain and encourages the appearance of impairment. Such treatment also promotes solicitous/activity seeking behavior to obtain increasing amounts of healthcare support through excessive dependence on healthcare providers.

Social support in the form of a network of social relationships in chronic musculoskeletal pain is associated with lesser physical disability and reduced levels of depression. However, the character of the perceived support plays a significant role in the benefit of that support. If the support is perceived as helpful, there is lesser depression and if the support is considered problematic, there is increased depression.

The Influence of Social Support

The influence of external social factors such as spousal support, social network supporters, or healthcare providers upon pain suffering, pain behavior and pain-behavior-related social adaptation is highly dependent upon the recognition of the highly individual and situation specific factors described above that influence pain behavior. The provision of supportive sympathy may provide positive benefits in terms of the acceptance of avoidance/withdrawal behavior that in fact may ultimately benefit musculoskeletal pain because of diminished activity and use. However, such behavior may permit patients to be viewed and accepted as more impaired than they physiologically are. The benefits of sympathetic support are significantly diminished by the consequences of enabling: 1) the source of pain to be inadequately treated; 2) worsening pain thresholds; 3) the progression of the underlying cause of pain; 4) impaired coping mechanisms; 5) and inappropriately excessive social, familial, occupational, and recreational limitation. Ultimately, the enabling of maladaptive pain behavior leads to increased psychological and psychosocial disturbance that leads to reduced pain thresholds and increased pain perception as well as further maladaptive pain behavior in response, all of which leads to further enabling of the negative behavior in a reinforcing, self-perpetuating cycle. Patients with fibromyalgia underestimate their physical abilities and are at particular risk for this course.

The character and quality of external social support received from sources such as spousal support, social network supporters, or healthcare providers is highly predictive of pain, pain behaviors, and outcomes. In the management of fibromyalgia, cognitive behavioral therapy programs include education, coping skills training, cognitive and behavioral retraining, relapse prevention, education, pacing activities in terms of time and intensity, incorporation of scheduled activities that are pleasurable, developing problem solving skills, improving communication skills, and improving sleep hygiene and sleep related behavior. Additional components may include relaxation training, stress management, biofeedback, meditation, exercise, physical therapy, or occupational therapy. Healthcare support that includes these elements of cognitive behavioral therapy in patients with fibromyalgia leads to improvement in pain, tender point counts, stiffness, stress, distress, functional ability, sleep, mood including depression and anxiety, and general health assessment. In contrast, healthcare support consisting of providing attention only but without specific behavioral interventions shows no improvement in pain and other fibromyalgia symptoms. Thus, sympathetic, concerned support is enabling to pain and adverse pain behavior whereas support consisting of graded physical, psychological, and psychosocial goals leads to a reduction of adverse pain behavior which in turn leads to improved psychological well-being which then leads to improved pain thresholds and ultimately to a reduction in perceived pain which leads to further negative reinforcement of the maladaptive pain behavior.

Sex and Pain Behavior

Sexual desire and sexual activity are often impaired in the setting of chronic musculoskeletal pain. Fatigue and pain are identified as the major reasons for limiting sexual intercourse from a mechanical standpoint. Impaired sexuality correlates not only with pain and levels of physical disability, but psychological factors such as depression. Thus, sexual activity in sexual relationships my be limited or curtailed for both physical and psychological reasons. Psychological and social factors independent of the actual pain itself may also reduce the desire for sexual interaction in relationships. In this social conditioning context, the avoidance of unwanted sexual activity creates an avoidance/withdrawal pain behavior that negatively reinforces and enhances the value of the pain itself.

Functional Impairment, Activity Limitation, and Disability Are Not the Same Things

The relationship between a source of pain, the perception of that pain, and the pain-behavior-related social adaptation referred to as disability is complex and poorly correlated. Pain is a symptom that arises from a disease process that induces physical and/or physiological changes that are identified by the body as pain. Impairment identifies the physical loss or abnormality of a body part or body function physically, physiologically, or psychologically. Musculoskeletal pain related impairment is a pain behavior that refers to a physical, physiological, or psychological limitation or loss of musculoskeletal function such as altered range of motion, reduced strength, or pain limited function. Physical, functional, or activity limitation relates to a restricted ability to perform activities of daily living such as sitting, standing, walking, lying, dressing, bathing, and so forth and when related to pain is another pain behavior. Disability is a social construct identifying a compromised ability to participate in expected societal roles and, in the context of pain, is a pain-behavior-related social adaptation. Pain and the attendant pain behaviors of impairment, activity limitation, and disability are linked, complementary, and interdependent insofar as in the presence of a valid, quantified source of pain and pain threshold in a given psychological state and psychosocial circumstance there is an expected and limited range of normal behavioral response to that pain in terms of impairment, activity limitation, and disability.

However, psychological state and coping factors alter pain perception and pain behaviors and the effect may be discordant by selectively reinforcing certain responses over others. Thus, the impact of the psychological state and coping factors may disproportionately add bias in favor of any one or more of the components of pain, impairment, activity limitation, and disability. This leads to the situation whereby impairment, and/or activity limitation, and/or disability are discordant to and inconsistent with the perceived pain and expected responses to the pain, and psychological and coping factors independently contribute to the observed responses. In other words, the presence of pain and symptoms alone do not automatically account for impairment; the presence of impairment does not automatically account for activity limitation; and the presence of activity limitation does not automatically account for disability as shown in Figure 12.4. This leads to the situation whereby inconsistencies in the physical and physiological issues of pain and pain perception relative to patient identified physical impairments, functional activity limitation, and disability can only be reconciled by identifying and addressing the psychological state and psychosocial coping factors adversely impacting these components.

Individuals with chronic musculoskeletal pain exhibit a large range of individualized and situation specific responses identified as pain suffering and pain behavior for any particular level of perceived pain. Social cognitive factors related to economic gain from receiving disability payments, other entitlement compensation rewards, reduction in industrial or work related participation, and litigation with potential financial gain such as might be related to work or an accident act to reinforce the social value of the chronic pain and directly promote pain-behavior-related so-

SYMPTOMS ≠ IMPAIRMENT

IMPAIRMENT ≠ ACTIVITY LIMITATION

ACTIVITY LIMITATION ≠ DISABILITY

Figure 12.4: *Lack of direct association between pain, impairment, activity limitation and disability.*

cial adaptation in the form of disability. In patients diagnosed with fibromyalgia, most report that the chronic pain and fatigue adversely impacts their quality of life and impairs their ability to work. Disability is reported to occur in 9-44% of patients with fibromyalgia. Factors predicting the development of disability includes the patient's perception of disability and function, perception of pain, psychological disruption with mood disturbances, coping skills, associated litigation, and educational achievement.

Perceptual Cognitive Coping Factors: Perception And Pain
The Role of Bias

Perceptions and beliefs are the substrate that provide the context against which thinking, emotion, and behavior evolve. Perceptions and beliefs develop from the thinking or cognitive processes that control how we acquire information, how we process that information, how we understand that information, how we retain that information, and how we express that processed information. These processes are under the influence of genetic, physical, physiological, psychological, and psychosocial factors that introduce bias. Bias is the tendency to interpret or analyze information beyond what the facts or logic would support. Bias is the measure of how much and by what mechanisms subjectivity deviates from objectivity or relativity from truth. It is a construct used to support the bridge between what we do not know or understand to the knowledge and understanding we actually have. As such, our perceptions and beliefs are controlled and influenced by the biases we learn and hold.

While many different biases account for specific perceptions and beliefs, these biases usually arise from a consistent set of processes that can be identified by the acronym BIAS, as shown in Figure 12.5. Bad reasoning describes the analysis of information using faulty logic to create unfounded or false correlations and conclusions. Ignorance refers to not knowing all there is to know about an issue because such information does not exist, is not available, or is not sought. Assumptions are the use of non-existent facts, distortion of known facts, or the irrational alteration of the significance or order of known facts. Selectivity identifies the selection of limited data, arguments or correlations to fit a predetermined conclusion or understanding despite the sum of such data, arguments, and correlations weakening or negating that conclusion or understanding. Simply put, bias allows us to believe things that are not actually true or factual simply because we cling to the credibility or believability of information that fits our personal needs and understandings.

Not only does bias influence the development of perceptions and beliefs, but it also acts to reinforce them. Our perceptions and beliefs are held very tightly and through the process of belief bias we are willing to distort and alter our logical thought processes to support our belief systems. Through the process of belief perseverance, we bias our thinking processes to the point that we are unwilling to give up our beliefs despite obvious evidence to the contrary. Furthermore, the presence of bias influences the behaviors and actions taken in response to established perceptions and beliefs in order to support these beliefs. For instance, confirmation bias identifies the process by which we actively and selectively seek information that supports our beliefs and avoid seeking information that discounts or disproves our beliefs. Bias plays a significant role in the expression of pain suffering and pain behavior, especially in pain-behavior-related social adaptation such as when there are inconsistencies in the physical and physiological issues of pain and pain perception relative to patient identified physical impairments, functional activity limitation, and disability.

Processes Leading To BIAS

Bad Reasoning

Ignorance

Assumptions

Selectivity

Figure 12.5:
The elements of bias.

Social Learning

Social learning plays an important role in the development of cultural beliefs and perceptions that lead to the expression of pain suffering and pain behavior. Individuals learn about attitudes, beliefs, perceptions, and responses to pain from family and the social environment to which they are exposed. Such learning starts in childhood and evolves as a life-long experience subject to reinforcement or modification. While such learning can be adaptive and serve a protective function such as learning to avoid painful experiences and learning how to treat pain when it arises, it can similarly lead to maladaptive pain suffering and pain behavior. The process by which learning occurs by the observation of the experience of others is called modeling. Modeling significantly influences the description of pain, its impact on the individual, and the coping responses. Such modeling can be conditioned by the experience of watching others in pain. Children of chronic pain patients emphasize pain associated responses and display more health complaints and health seeking behavior compared to other children. Maternal behavior impacts the pain perceptions of their children. Modeling also explains the cultural variations noted in pain suffering and pain behavior.

Spirituality and Religion

Spirituality, religion, and practices of faith such as prayer are perceptual cognitive areas that significantly impact pain suffering and pain behavior including pain-behavior-related social adaptation. Spirituality involves the process of transcendence beyond the existential self to connect with other people, places, and powers to find faith, meaning, and purpose in life to give life itself context. Religion is a means by which an individual relates to an external higher power, such as G-d, by framing beliefs, values, and answers and providing practices for how to establish such a relationship. A survey of religious influence in the United States shows that 94% believe in G-d or a higher power and, for 60%, prayer is a significant part of daily life. Furthermore, 60% report that faith is their most important influence. In terms of individuals who are sick, 30-35% report praying for their own healing in addition to seeking standard medical care. In a survey of hospitalized patients, 94% ranked spiritual health as important as physical health, 73% indicated that they prayed daily, and

42% stated they participated in faith-healing practices.

Religious commitment is associated with significant health benefits. The perception of spirituality and belief in religion in individuals with pain correlates with lesser pain. On the other hand, passive prayer involving asking for deliverance from pain correlates with increased pain severity and disability. This correlation occurs either because individuals with more pain and disability are more likely to invoke prayer or passive prayer may induce a maladaptive coping component in chronic pain leading to increased symptoms and disability. Positive, guiding prayer leads to acceptance of chronic pain. Prayer, combined with group support, education, and counseling is associated with reduction in pain, fatigue, and functional impairment in moderately severe rheumatoid arthritis.

The beneficial effects of transcending spirituality and guiding prayer are found in the provision of hope, reduction of anxiety and depression, improved coping mechanisms including use of denial and projection, finding meaning and purpose, and enhanced social networking. The evidence suggests that religious practices such as passive prayer without accompanying spirituality and belief do not improve pain or associated impairments and disability and may lead to worsening of symptoms. On the other hand, gaining knowledge and power from spiritual transcendence and religious self-empowerment leads to reduction in pain and disability. The enabling of such adaptive pain behavior leads to decreased psychological and psychosocial disturbance that leads to increased pain thresholds and decreased pain perception which results in further adaptive pain behavior in response with further reinforcement of the beneficial aspects of spiritual transcendence, all of which leads to further enabling of the positive behavior in a reinforcing, self-perpetuating cycle.

The Interaction Between Coping Factors, Psychosocial Problems, And Chronic Musculoskeletal Pain

Behavioral coping factors, social cognitive coping factors, and perceptual cognitive coping factors significantly influence pain suffering and pain behavior in chronic musculoskeletal pain. These coping factors directly affect the psychological and psychosocial condition of the individual. Their influence on pain suffering and pain behavior leads to alterations in the psychological and psychosocial state of the individual. Conversely, pain suffering and behavior influence the behavioral, social, and perceptual cognitive coping factors through conditioning and learning mechanisms. Thus, underlying psychological and psychosocial disturbances such as depression, anxiety, and stress in polypain are exacerbated and promoted by maladaptive coping responses leading to maladaptive pain suffering and pain behaviors which lead to increasing psychological and psychosocial distress and poorer coping. The worsening psychological and psychosocial state ultimately lowers pain thresholds and worsens the perception of pain. This leads to a progressive worsening spiral of increasing psychological and psychosocial disruption, poorer coping strategies, descending pain thresholds, and increasing perception of pain. In essence, maladaptive cognitive coping begets psychological and psychosocial disturbances, maladaptive pain suffering and pain behavior, further maladaptive coping, and ultimately increased pain. Adaptive coping strategies and improved psychological well-being reverse this spiral to ultimately improve pain thresholds and reduce pain. These biopsychosocial relationships are depicted in Figures 12.6a and 12.6b.

The Fibromyalgia Polypain Wellness Core Psychological Management Program: Pain Relief From Inner Peace

The approach to the management of the psychiatric, psychological, and psychosocial disturbances in polypain re-emphasizes the need for proper, thorough, and comprehensive assessment to determine the presence and nature of psychiatric conditions and psychological and psychosocial impairments whether or not specifically related to polypain and to develop an appropriate understanding upon which to base treatment decisions. Only through such evaluation can the rheumatologist be sufficiently informed and knowledgeable as to be able to provide needed patient education in order that patients be able to fully participate in their own care and make truly informed decisions regarding treatment. As with managing any and all components of polypain, intensive follow-up regarding psychiatric, psychological, and psychosocial disturbances with appropriate evaluation of progress to provide optimal benefit from a properly designed treatment program is of crucial importance.

The Polypain Wellness Core Psychological Management Program forms part of the more comprehensive Polypain Wellness Core Program. In addition to their contributions to the symptoms and findings in polypain, the polypain sources of pain, the reduced pain thresholds from adverse pain processing generated by increased nociception, and the sleep abnormalities contribute to the psychiatric, psychological, and psychosocial disturbances identified in polypain. Thus, the fundamental and basic treatment for the psychiatric, psychological, and psychosocial disturbances in polypain requires treatment with all the elements of the Polypain Wellness Core Program. Therefore, the Polypain Wellness Core Psychological Management Program incorporates the pharmacologic intervention to control site specific pain symptoms and pain processing abnormalities; biomechanical and postural intervention through exercises including the Integrated Daily Walking Program, orthotics, neuromuscular re-education, and weight control including the Rule of Thirds Polypain Weight Loss Program; ergonomic intervention through appropriate accommodation and modification; and the Polypain Wellness Core Sleep Management Program.

The specific psychological related interventions comprising the Polypain Wellness Core Psychological Management Program component of the Polypain Wellness Core Program begins with the implementation of adaptive cognitive coping and pain behavior. This is the foundation upon which the Polypain Wellness Core Psychological Management Program is built. The successful management of the psychiatric, psychological, and psychosocial disturbances of polypain can only occur in the presence of appropriately adaptive cognitive coping and pain behavior. The treatment elements needed to accomplish correct adaptive cognitive coping and pain behavior must be appropriately considered and optimized before the

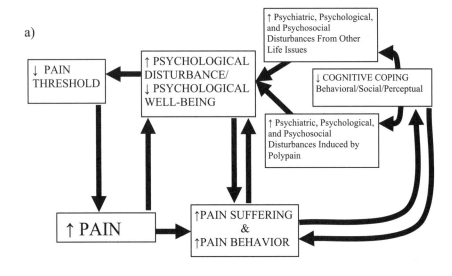

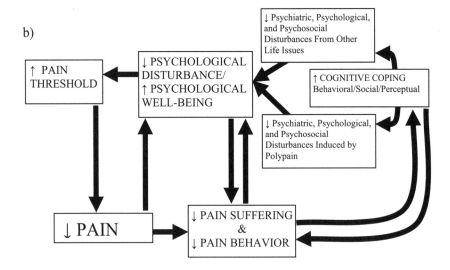

Figure 12.6: *The biopsychosocial relationship of pain suffering and pain behavior to psychiatric, psychological, and psychosocial disturbances in polypain: a) Poor coping with increased pain suffering and pain behavior; b) Good coping with reduced pain suffering and pain behavior.*

consideration of adding or changing psychiatric medications. The psychiatric, psychological, and psychosocial disturbances of polypain may be adequately treated through the Polypain Wellness Core Program and all its components along with the adaptive coping and pain behavior components of the Polypain Wellness Core Psychological Management Program. In the management of the psychiatric, psychological, and psychosocial disturbances of polypain, medications are never enough and also may never be needed.

Optimum Behavioral Coping Strategies to Relieve Pain
The Oxygen Mask in the Airplane Philosophy

Whenever we go on an airplane, the routine before take-off is fairly standard. The flight attendant reviews how to use the seat belt and tells us what to do in case the oxygen mask deploys. Usually, we hear the words, but don't give them much thought as the process is fairly routine. Yet, the part about the oxygen mask is very telling. Aside from being told how to put on the mask, we are instructed as to when to put it on. In particular, we are told that if we are traveling with children or others who need assistance, we must first put the oxygen mask on ourselves before we help others who depend on us. Of course, this is at first discordant with our intrinsic desire to help our children and other needy loved ones above our own safety and well-being. Yet, on closer analysis, the logic of the recommendation becomes obvious. A lack of oxygen will quickly cause us to lose consciousness and eliminate the ability to help any one else. Our efforts at being selfless and self-sacrificial become not only counterproductive, but dangerous, and potentially fatal to those that need us.

The message is very clear. In order to help others, you must help yourself first. This is neither selfish nor exclusively self-serving. To the contrary, by looking after yourself and your well-being you improve the well-being of those around you. This Oxygen Mask in the Airplane Philosophy of looking out for your well-being to benefit yourself, and by extension, those around you is crucial in the management of polypain as well.

1) FORGIVE YOURSELF.

It is not your fault you have polypain. You did not choose to be in pain. Do not blame yourself for your symptoms unless you knowingly make maladaptive choices. Forgiveness is a transforming process that allows you to take the necessary steps to place your pain into a context that recognizes the reality that not everything is under your control. It allows you to accept that not everything goes the way you plan or anticipate. It allows room for learning what you don't know. It allows you to reject things that won't or don't work. It allows you to make realistic appraisals of your symptoms in terms of diagnosis and treatment. It permits your pain suffering and pain behavior to be consistent with the physiological processes and psychosocial circumstances. Most importantly, it allows you to make rational benefit-cost/risk decisions in which potential negative outcomes are considered and readily accepted, if they occur, leading to the ability to make appropriate changes to move forward. Forgiving yourself also allows you to accept the negative emotions associated with chronic pain such as sadness, anger, disgust, contempt, fear, shame, and guilt in order to understand them and develop adaptive coping strategies to lessen and eliminate their impact. The act of forgiveness is one of the most truly liberating human experiences and is a fundamental and foundational component in the process of psychological healing.

2) YOU ARE NOT A VICTIM – DO NOT TREAT YOURSELF AS ONE.

The symptoms of polypain arise from: 1) primary generalized osteoarthritis predominantly involving the neck and back with associated degenerative disc disease and the variable combination of associated tendinitis, bursitis, and fasciitis; 2) the reduced pain thresholds from adverse pain processing generated by increased nociception, the associated sleep abnormalities and the psychiatric, psychological, and psychosocial disturbances identified in polypain. They arise from a combination of genetic predisposition acted upon by a conducive environmental setting. The genetic component is not under your control. The environmental component cannot be under your control until you are sufficiently educated in the understanding of the relationship of the environmental factors to the pain and your responses to it. Even subsequently, there may arise obstacles and limits to managing the environmental components that are not under your control. Thus, none of the predisposing factors are your fault or arise out of anything you knowingly did. Self-victimization can only develop in the setting of making knowingly negative choices that lead to worsening of symptoms or maladaptive pain suffering or pain behavior. Thus, it is crucial that that the diagnosis or symptoms of polypain not be used as an excuse to avoid coping with or to negatively cope with life conflicts. Do not allow pain to become a focus of escape from psychosocial conflicts, from avoiding function, or from attaining the things you desire.

3) THE REALITY PRINCIPLE ENDOWS THE NEED FOR TRANSFORMATIONAL ACCEPTANCE.
Polypain occurs in the context of the individual and the life of the individual. Treatment of polypain is ultimately dictated by the discrete and highly individualized, unique factors impacting the presence of joint and joint related disease that are related to: genetic predisposition; and the individual's unique pattern of usage, adverse biomechanics, and adverse ergonomics and posture from moment to moment coupled with the individual's highly situation specific factors that affect psychological well-being and sleep. These are constantly subject to trade-offs and patients are faced with moment to moment, day to day, and long term decisions as to what the ideal balance is for their highly individual and specific circumstances. The basic requirement to undertake such rational and informed decision making is the development of acceptance of the diagnosis of a chronic disease process and all that it encompasses. That does not mean accepting just to learn to live with it, to validate maladaptive pain suffering and behavior, or to withdraw from worldly affairs such as seen in a terminal illness. Instead, acceptance should be a transformative and transcendental process whereby you develop a new definition and a new self-construct of yourself in the context of you and polypain. Do not be defined by your disease.

By accepting the new paradigm, you can acknowledge your value in that setting and engage the world accordingly. Without acceptance, such engagement is flawed and leads to maladaptive coping and disproportionate dependency. The process of developing acceptance is not a devaluation of yourself, but rather a revaluation of you and your worthiness. Acceptance leads to the ability to make reasoned and rational healthcare choices rooted in the reality of the current time and circumstance and allows for more valid appraisals of benefits and costs/risks of treatments in the larger context of you as a whole person. It facilitates the ability to find needed accommodations that permit life's activities to continue and avoid modifications that require changes or restrictions in those activities as much as possible. It helps avoid settling for short-term relief of pain at the expense of long-term disease progression and functional limitation. Fundamentally, acceptance allows you to get on with your whole life sooner rather than later with less impairment, less activity limitation, and less disability.

4) DEVELOP AND DEFINE YOUR CONCEPT OF SELF WITH VALUE AND MEANING BEYOND POLYPAIN AND ITS PROCESSES.

There is a natural self-serving bias that drives us to see ourselves in a positive and favorable light. The benefits of maintaining high self-esteem and self-worth include better sleep, more independence, more persistence with challenging tasks, less loneliness, and greater happiness. On the other hand, low self-esteem correlates with unhappiness, despair, and frustration. By establishing and maintaining appropriate self-esteem, we provide the substrate by which we self-actualize and achieve what we potentially could. This only develops, however, once our more fundamental needs are met including physical and psychological well-being.

The presence of a chronic disease process may feel extremely consuming. This is particularly true of a chronic disease process that is associated with: symptoms of pain due to primary generalized osteoarthritis predominantly involving the neck and back with associated degenerative disc disease and the variable combination of associated tendinitis, bursitis, and fasciitis; reduced pain thresholds from adverse pain processing generated by increased nociception, associated sleep abnormalities, and the psychiatric, psychological, and psychosocial disturbances; as well as possible related functional impairments such as occurs in polypain. In addition to the impact of the symptoms, the individualized, integrated treatment elements of polypain add to the overwhelming nature of polypain. The entire process may stretch and divert your coping mechanisms to the point where all your physical and psychological efforts are invested into the disease and you lose your existing sense of self-identity and become defined by the polypain itself. Consequently, the pursuit of things beneficial to self-development are increasingly ignored and replaced by the pursuit of things related to polypain exclusively. This inevitably leads to adverse pain suffering and pain behavior as well as psychological and psychosocial disturbances.

Thus, it is vital to develop a realistic cognitive appraisal of how polypain affects your sense of self and to develop understanding and cognitive coping skills to define your self-concept in the face of polypain rather than allowing polypain to define your self-identity. This not only prevents the potential reduction of self-worth and self-meaning that polypain may engender but also provides for enhancement of your self-concept in redefining your self-identity by positively incorporating the issues related to polypain.

Furthermore, it is crucial to continue defining and refining your self-concept inclusive of polypain as you would pursue this absent the presence of polypain. Pursue your new self. Make time for your self-pursuits. In this regard, it is important to distinguish self-development and self-pursuit activities from selfish behavior to which such conduct may be erroneously ascribed. Selfish behavior occurs at the expense of others to benefit oneself. Self-development and self-actualization, to the contrary, are undertaken to benefit the individual and those supporting that person. Remember, "me first" is not the same as "me only". As taught by the Oxygen Mask in the Airplane Philosophy, it is not selfish or narcissistic to pursue your own well-being as the benefits extend well beyond you. The accomplishment of this healthy integration of your whole person requires that you self-actualize as optimally as you can. This requires self-efficacy as discussed earlier, self-esteem, self-love, self-respect, self-validation recognizing your own merits, self-identity, self-empowerment, and self-acceptance. By ensuring the integrity of these elements, the psychological and psychosocial impact of polypain is minimized and favorable pain suffering and pain behavior follows and you and those around are benefited by that work.

5) Do not be a slave to polypain and do not be imprisoned by it.
This naturally follows by avoiding victimization and pursuing the concept of self. However, it only occurs if you actually make time for yourself. In other words, you must have "me" time to pursue your self.

6) Pursue happiness, surprise, and things of interest.

Positive emotions such as happiness, interest, surprise, and love are not simply the absence of negative emotions such as sadness, anger, disgust, contempt, fear, shame, and guilt. While positive and negative emotions interact with each other to form an emotional balance, emotions are acted on selectively and independently by specific psychological and psychosocial circumstances at a particular point in time upon an individual's inherited genetic predisposition to those emotions. Thus, happiness is not the same as not being sad, but rather a higher state of positive emotional fulfillment.

The heritable, genetic component of happiness appears to contribute about 50% of the total measure of an individual's happiness level. In other words, we are born with a certain predisposition to happiness which is up or down adjusted based on psychological and psychosocial circumstances. Furthermore, there is a superimposed natural drive to achieve a positive emotional state through the day in normal individuals with positive mood levels increasing after awakening, peaking at mid-day and falling off in the later evening whereas negative emotions remain fairly flat with a rise in the late evening. Ultimately, however, happiness is relative. We set cognitive threshold levels for determining the point we become happy. Falling below that threshold leaves us unhappy. Rising above that threshold makes us happy; however, the happiness is short lived as the new level of happiness sets the new threshold to maintain that happiness and sets the new level by which we subsequently define happiness. Similarly, events that are unhappy reduce happiness threshold levels and it is from this lower level that we have to rise above in order to feel happy. These thresholds change throughout the day, change in response to varying psychological and psychosocial circumstances, and change by the cognitive strategies we use to compare happiness relative to others. In essence, we adapt to our current level of happiness which then becomes the new baseline from which we have to then rise higher to consider ourselves happy again. Thus, happiness is a perpetual pursuit and should be sought for the emotional, social, psychological, and physical benefits it brings.

When the emotional balance shifts in favor of happiness, people see the world as a safer place and are more decisive and more accommodating. Happiness correlates with healthier adaptation, coping, and cognitive benefit. Happiness also correlates with high self-esteem, optimism, close relationships, good sleep, pursuit of engaging work, leisure activities, and exercise. Happiness in the form of job satisfaction, financial security, and using one's skills to self-advantage correlate with reduced psychological distress and pain in individuals with chronic pain. Through the cognitive restructuring of pursuing and achieving increased levels of happiness, the significant psychological disturbances of polypain such as depression, anxiety, and stress are mitigated and favorably adaptive pain suffering and pain behavior evolve. Ultimately, happiness, surprise, and interest lead to improved pain thresholds and lesser pain perception.

7) DISCARD NEGATIVE EMOTIONS.

In addition to pursuing the positive emotions of happiness, surprise, and interest, there is great benefit in discarding the negative emotions that correlate with depression, anxiety, and stress by further shifting the emotional balance in favor of the positive emotions.

8) EMBRACE KNOWLEDGE, UNDERSTANDING, AND ENLIGHTENMENT FOR TRULY INFORMED, FREE WILL DECISION MAKING.

It is vital for you to have as complete an understanding as possible of how your symptoms develop and the factors that modulate them. Learn everything you can. However, this is not enough by itself. It is also crucial that you learn what it is that you don't know and what is not known. This level of understanding leads to enlightenment. The more thorough your understanding and enlightenment, the more useful is the information available regarding the issues impacting the course of disease and symptoms. The effectiveness of any treatment program not only depends on its appropriateness and anticipated effectiveness but also significantly on the patient's ability and willingness to fully comply with the recommendations. This is especially true in patients with chronic musculoskeletal diseases including those diagnosed with fibromyalgia. The ability and willingness to comply with treatment recommendations correlates with the knowledge and understanding of how symptoms and disease develop and what factors modulate them, how treatment is anticipated to interact with and provide benefit to these processes, and at what cost or risk. Further, with knowledge, understanding, and enlightenment you are more able to modulate the environmental interactions and coping factors related to pain suffering and pain behavior seen in polypain.

With respect to treatment, nothing is without risk. In order to undertake truly informed, free will decision making, it is necessary for you to be as knowledgeable, rational, capable, and enlightened as possible. Armed with these tools of understanding, treatment decisions can be made to optimize the benefit versus cost-risk ratio. Furthermore, by embracing these tools, you foster critical coping strategies including forgiveness, acceptance, self-concept, happiness, and suppress victimization and negative emotions, especially fear.

This ability to directly, effectively and freely participate in your own care is in and of itself is therapeutic. However, there is a further benefit from such knowledge, understanding, and free will decision making that relates to the presence of these elements unto themselves. The cognitive processing of these elements has a direct effect on the processing of the pain information itself by providing input into the descending modulation pathway from the brain to the dorsal horn causing elevation of pain thresholds with a reduction in the intensity of pain appreciated. Thus, knowledge, understanding, and enlightenment are empowering in allowing you to comprehend the polypain process: to make free will, truly informed decisions regarding treatment; to develop adaptive pain suffering and pain behavior strategies; and to directly mitigate pain severity. Such is the immense power of knowledge, understanding, and enlightenment.

9) Do not let fear control you.

Fear is negative emotion driven by ignorance, irrationality, and incompetence. To discard this negative emotion and relinquish its hold, the most powerful strategies are to embrace knowledge, rational understanding, and enlightenment and exercise truly informed, free will decision making.

10) You are not helpless.

You do need to learn what to do, how to do it, and why. To this end, it is notable that passivity fails. You cannot rely upon passive interventions exclusively such as using medications only without biomechanical or ergonomic interventions or count on passive psychological support such as sympathy or encouragement without actually changing your coping skills or behavioral responses. Nor can you count on prayer to help you unless the results of that prayer lead you to participate actively in the treatment program. Passive participation in the assessment and treatment phase of polypain dooms treatment to failure.

As noted, the Polypain Wellness Core Psychological Management Program incorporates pharmacologic intervention, biomechanical and postural intervention, orthotics, neuromuscular re-education, weight control, ergonomic intervention through appropriate accommodation and modification, and sleep management. The treatment program is highly individualized and comprehensive, and requires active participation by you to be successful. You must actively participate in the implementation of all components of the program and be knowledgeable in the circumstances and situations in which various elements need to be applied. Furthermore, adaptive coping and pain behavior strategies can only be implemented by you. Thus, you must be an active participant in the entire process.

To avoid passivity, a significantly effective cognitive strategy is to set time and place based goals with measurable objectives to achieve those goals and strategies for goal revision depending on the response. The development of such goals and objectives requires realistic appraisals based on knowledge, understanding, and enlightenment coupled with positively adaptive coping strategies to effectively implement these goals and objectives.

Social Coping Adaptation Skills to Maximize Healthy Relationships and Minimize Pain
The Three Fundamental Principles Of Healthy Relationships

The need for interdependent relationships and attachments is another fundamental human need. Indeed, close, satisfying relationships are rated as a necessary component for happiness and to give meaningful context to life. Our need for relationships influences our self-esteem and as such influences the quality and quantity of our social behavior to increase our acceptance into relationships and establish deep attachments. Close relationships correlate with physical health and happiness. Increased survival and reduced occurrence of premature deaths have been noted in individuals with marital, close family, or close friend relationships. Positive, supportive marriages promote health whereas marital strife does not.

Just the ability to share painful feelings correlates with better health.

The Fundamental Principles of Healthy Relationships requires the recognition and understanding of three basic principles:

Principle 1: The units of any interdependent relationship consist of you as yourself, the other party as a distinct entity and the interaction between the two of you as a unique and distinct bonded entity that has an independent and fused component contributed by both of the partners. This first principle recognizes the uniqueness of each member of the relationship and the need to maintain and promote each individual self. It also identifies a distinct, unified, bonded component that brings together certain elements of each of the individuals to create new elements through the combination of what each member offers the other as well as providing a synergy by which one member strengthens the other's weaknesses and enhances the other's strengths.

Principle 2: If you chose to live in your own world, be prepared to live alone; if you choose to live in the world with others, be prepared. Relationships are obligations that you undertake not only to better yourself, but also to better your partner and to ensure the bond of the relationship provides value, meaning, and strength beyond yourself.

Principle 3: To change others, you must change yourself. You cannot control others directly. However, you can control others indirectly through your actions within a relationship, for better or for worse. The goal is to better your partner and the relationship through self-improvement. This leads to a ripple effect whereby a positive impact on your partner and the relationship leads to further benefit to you and enhances the value, meaning, and strength of the relationship further.

I) Assess your relationships with a Relationship CAT Scan.

The core of any positive relationship requires the development and maintenance of the strategies that allow the partners the ability to interact effectively and with benefit. To achieve such beneficial and effective inter-action, a productive and mutually rewarding close relationship must es-tablish and maintain clear, unambiguous, knowledgeable, rational, and non-rhetorical communication. You must eliminate as much as possible the components of BIAS described earlier. This entails competently ex-pressing yourself in consideration of your partner's receptive ability to comprehend accurately what it is you are trying to convey. Whether by verbal or nonverbal means, you have to say what you mean, mean what you say, and say it to be understood. Your partner has an identical obligation. This is particularly true for expressions of pain. Your experience of pain, pain suffering, and pain behavior is unique and specific to your physical make-up, innate physiology, and your unique psychiatric, psychological, and psychosocial circumstances. Your ability to com-municate the character of your symptoms and the impact of your symptoms upon your physical and psychological function not only requires knowledge, understanding, and enlightenment in the con-text of yourself but also in the context of how your partner will process that information based on your partner's circumstances, knowledge, understanding, and enlightenment.

A mutually rewarding, close relationship also requires accountability to ensure each partner is responsible to the other. The establishment of the unified, bonded component that defines the uniqueness of the rela-tionship obliges the need for such accountability. It is through such ac-countability that the interdependence of the individuals to form a unique relationship can develop.

A worthy and mutually beneficial relationship also requires trust that each partner is predictably and reliably committed to the relationship and to the other partner.

These three elements: communication, accountability, and trust, form the basis of the Relationship CAT Scan and its acronym as displayed in Figure 12.7. As no relationship can be successful without a full commitment to these fundamental components, it is crucial that all relationships be assessed to determine the presence and quality of these elements.

Components of the Relationship CAT Scan

Communication

Accountability

Trust

Figure 12.7:
The relationship CAT Scan.

Successful communication, accountability, and trust are key fundamental tools of relationships that, when employed correctly, benefits the partners in helping fulfill one another's needs and wants while at the same time enhancing the bonded component of the relationship providing increased psychological benefit. The support garnered from such communication, accountability, and trust enables beneficially adaptive pain suffering and pain behavior. In polypain, that translates into improved pain thresholds, lesser perceived pain, better participation and compliance to treatment, and improved function.

2) Ensure your relationships contain the basic FACTS.

The symptoms and challenges of polypain should not inure you to the plight of those around you, but rather make you more aware, sensitive, and understanding that nobody and no situation is perfect and that humans and their relationships always need tending and mending. While communication, accountability, and trust are foundational to healthy, supportive relationships, they are subject to the fallibility of human cognitive ability. In other words, despite their best intentions, people make mistakes. To deal with such mistakes, it is crucial to add two more elements to make relationships run smoothly. These are the need to forgive others and the need for development of self-concept in the face of relationships.

a) Forgive others.

It is not anyone else's fault you have polypain. Nobody who cares about you wishes you to be in pain. Do not blame others for your symptoms unless you are knowingly forced to make maladaptive choices. As discussed, forgiveness is a transforming process that allows you to take the necessary steps to place your pain into a context that recognizes the reality that not everything is under your, or anyone else's control. Like forgiving yourself, forgiving others allows you to make realistic appraisals of your symptoms related to diagnosis and treatment, to establish context appropriate pain suffering and pain behavior, and to experience the power of psychological healing. It also allows you to place into context the support offered by your social relationships. In a relationship endowed with appropriate communication, accountability, and trust, it is a given that your partner's support is intended to be beneficial to you and vice versa. Yet, even the best of intentions may suffer a lack of knowledge, understanding, enlightenment, or ability to appropriately implement the support needed. The consequence may be a less than adequate outcome or even an adverse outcome. Forgiving others allows you to accept these outcomes when they occur, to make rational decisions regarding such potential negative outcomes, and allows you the ability to make appropriate changes to move forward. Forgiving others also allows you to accept the negative emotions associated with adverse relationship issues such as sadness, anger, disgust, contempt, fear, shame, and guilt in order to understand them and develop adaptive coping strategies to lessen and eliminate their impact upon the relationship. The ability to forgive implicitly identifies your recognition and acceptance that no one and no situation is perfect. This recognition leads to humility and the ability to express gratitude and appreciation of the value of your partner's contribution to the relationship. The act of forgiving another person is another one of the most truly liberating human experiences and is a fundamental and foundational component not only in the process of psychological healing but also in the development and maintenance of healthy, supportive, mutually rewarding relationships.

B) Self-concept must include the recognition of relationships.

Ultimately, as noted in the Three Fundamental Principles of Relationships, what you put into a relationship not only helps define the relationship, but also influences your partner and your partner's contribution to the relationship. In the face of polypain, it is crucial to continue defining and refining your self-concept inclusive of polypain as well as your established relationships. Pursue your relationships by pursuing your self-concept. To this end, you must recognize how you can improve yourself and your contribution to the relationship as well as how you can improve your partner and your partner's contribution to the relationship through your self-improvement.

Thus, the basic components of a functional relationship consist of forgiveness, accountability, communication, trust and self-concept. As shown in Figure 12.8, these components form an acronym that identify the FACTS of a relationship.

Figure 12.8:
The FACTS of a relationship.

> ## FACTS of a Relationship
>
> **F**orgiveness
>
> **A**ccountability
>
> **C**ommunication
>
> **T**rust
>
> **S**elf-concept

3) Promote happiness, surprise, and interest.

Happiness depends in part on the presence of close, satisfying relationships. Furthermore, positive, satisfying relationships are an important source of happiness. Thus, the pursuit of happiness, surprise, and things of interest in the context of relationships is important to the establishment and maintenance of these relationships; and they, in turn, provide increasing positive emotional returns of happiness, surprise, and interest. Satisfying relationships provide the opportunity to further enhance the benefits to behavior, pain, and pain thresholds bestowed by the successful pursuit of happiness.

4) Love and allow yourself to be loved.

In relationships where love is shared, recognize the need to give it as well as to receive it. To love and to be loved is a transcendental experience that provides purpose in our being and gives meaning and context to our existence. Love is a powerfully positive emotion that is even more resilient and enduring than happiness. It is an inherent substrate for deep, affectionate commitment and attachment as well as intimacy. While relationships can exist on many planes, love in a relationship is a catalyst to elevate relationships to a transcendent plane. Such relationships promote improved health and survival. Like happiness and other positive emotions, the love from a healthy, rewarding relationship provides cognitive restructuring and mitigates the significant psychological disturbances of polypain such as depression, anxiety, and stress and favors adaptive pain suffering and pain behavior. Ultimately, love leads to improved pain thresholds and lesser pain perception.

5) INSPIRE YOUR PARTNER AND BE INSPIRED BY YOUR PARTNER.

Inspiration is a positive driving force that leads to: adaptive coping; reduction in fear; improved pursuit of self; enhanced positive emotions including happiness, surprise and interest; and the pursuit of knowledge, understanding, and enlightenment. In the context of relationships, inspiring your partner benefits the relationship through Principle 3 of the Fundamental Principles of Healthy Relationships whereby an inspired partner is better prepared and more able to contribute beneficially to the relationship.

6) IN SEXUAL RELATIONSHIPS, HAVE SEX.

Sexual relationships require sexual contact to maintain not only that component of the relationship, but to maintain the relationship as a whole, as sexual activity is a part of that relationship. Therefore, have sex as often as the relationship requires and ensure that it is as pleasant and satisfying as needed to satisfy the partners of the relationship. In the context of polypain, accommodations may be required to physically accomplish some sexual activity, but such accommodations should not preclude mutually satisfying sexual involvement. This will be explored further in Chapter 13.

7) RECOGNIZE AND ELIMINATE THE ENABLING OF ADVERSE PAIN SUFFERING AND PAIN BEHAVIOR.

Perceptual Cognitive Coping Skills to Alleviate Pain

I) UNDERSTAND THE IMPACT OF BIAS.

The cognitive processes and appraisals involved in the development of perceptions, beliefs, and expectations are subjectively influenced and weighted by bias. Bias leads us to interpret or analyze information beyond what the facts or logic would support. In the setting of chronic pain, adverse bias leads to pain suffering and pain behavior beyond that expected for the known physiological, psychiatric, psychological, and social circumstances for an individual at any one particular time. It is important to recognize the influence of such bias. For instance, bias towards reducing symptoms through excess avoidance leads to maladaptive psychological and social behavior favoring impairment, limitation, and disability. Conversely, bias towards excessively maintaining activity at the expense of symptoms leads to maladaptive psychological and social behavior favoring pain and disease progression. Worse, bias is self-serving in that biased beliefs beget biased behavior reinforcing maladaptive pain suffering and pain behavior. Bias is enslaving and constrains free will decision making.

Thus, it is critical to recognize the elements that contribute to bias as identified by the acronym BIAS as described earlier and apply them to enhance the significance of your knowledge and understanding objectively, to highlight your enlightenment by allowing you to learn what you don't know, and to learn to accept the limits of your knowledge and rationale. By understanding bias and its impact, you are able to make more realistic, context sensitive, situation specific appraisals of pain behavior to determine its adequacy and appropriateness and to incorporate evidence-based changes.

2) EMBRACE SPIRITUALITY.

Spirituality involves the process of transcendence beyond the existential self to connect with other people, places, and powers to find faith, meaning, and purpose in life to give life itself context. Seek it. Embrace it. Find a means of relating to an external higher power, such as G-d. In this world, find meaning and purpose in life through faith, love, and forgiveness. These transcendent activities lead to hope. Through hope, the process of healing and recovery can be maximized.

3) DO NOT SIMPLY LEARN TO LIVE WITH IT.
Learn, challenge, accommodate, and overcome. Embrace all available strategies to reduce the impact of chronic pain.

4) *MINIMIZE THE ADVERSE IMPACT OF INDUSTRIAL/FINANCIAL/LEGAL ISSUES.*

5) *CARPE DIEM. (SEIZE THE DAY.)*

Psychological Therapy

Psychological therapy, known as psychotherapy, is a cognitive, psychological, and emotional interaction between a trained, socially sanctioned psychological healer and a psychologically distressed sufferer. The introduction of psychotherapy in the management of the psychiatric, psychological, and psychosocial disturbances associated with polypain should be considered: 1) only in the presence of a comprehensive polypain management program with implementation of the Polypain Wellness Core Program; 2) only in the presence of the best possible implementation of the behavioral, social, and perceptual cognitive self-management strategies of the Polypain Wellness Core Psychological Management Program; 3) and in the presence of ongoing psychiatric, psychological, and/or psychosocial disturbances with associated maladaptive coping leading to ongoing adversely affected pain thresholds, pain suffering, and pain behavior. In undertaking psychotherapy, it is critical for the psychotherapist to acknowledge and understand the influence on pain of psychiatric, psychological, and psychosocial factors associated with life issues independent and not specifically related to polypain as well as the factors contributed to and driven by the polypain process itself.

In general, there are multiple psychotherapeutic approaches to managing psychiatric illnesses, psychological disturbances, and psychosocial disruption that occur across life's spectrum. They are selected based upon thorough medical and psychological assessment providing a benefit-cost/risk analysis appropriate for the condition under consideration and the psychological and social circumstances of the individual. In the management of psychiatric, psychological, and psychosocial disturbances specific to chronic musculoskeletal pain as seen in fibromyalgia polypain, the best studied and most promising psychotherapeutic treatment is cognitive behavioral training. Cognitive behavioral therapy is based on the premise that pain suffering and pain behavior are affected by an individual's cognitive coping and perceptual interpretation of symptoms as reinforced by environmental and societal influences. Its use originates from traditional psychotherapy in the management of psychiatric conditions such as anxiety and depression.

Cognitive behavioral therapy programs are generally multidisciplinary involving integration of mind and body to restructure maladaptive and counterproductive coping strategies. The fundamental components of cognitive behavioral therapy programs include education, coping skills training, cognitive and behavioral retraining, and relapse prevention. Skills addressed in fibromyalgia cognitive behavioral therapy programs include education in what is known regarding symptoms of fibromyalgia, pacing activities in terms of time and intensity, incorporation of scheduled activities that are pleasurable, developing problem solving skills specific to fibromyalgia issues, improving communication skills regarding fibromyalgia issues, and improving sleep hygiene and sleep related behavior. Additional components may include relaxation training, stress management, biofeedback, meditation, exercise, physical therapy, or occupational therapy. Many of these features have been incorporated into the behavioral, social, and perceptual cognitive self-management strategies of the Polypain Wellness Core Psychological Management Program.

Studies of cognitive behavioral therapy in fibromyalgia have identified improvement in pain, tender point counts, stiffness, stress when stress management is incorporated, distress, functional ability, sleep, mood including depression and anxiety, and general health assessment. Improvements in pain or function have been reported to be sustained up to 30 months following completion of a program. In two studies reporting benefit of cognitive behavioral therapy, outcomes that were both statistically and most importantly, clinically meaningful, were noted in 25% and 42%. However, other studies in which cognitive behavioral therapy was compared to a group receiving the same amount of attention consisting primarily of education but no specific behavioral interventions showed no improvements in pain and other fibromyalgia symptoms compared to the attention-only group.

The therapeutic value of cognitive behavioral therapy in managing fibromyalgia is significantly enhanced by the knowledge and understanding of the mechanism of chronic musculoskeletal pain imparted by the Polypain Model. The understanding of the source of pain and how pain thresholds are modulated through pain processing leads to highly specific and targeted areas on which to focus cognitive behavioral interventions. Furthermore, in order to provide benefit, cognitive behavioral therapy must involve interventions that are not passive and require active involvement of the individuals to achieve objectives and goals through their active participation and work. The behavioral, social, and perceptual cognitive self-management strategies of the Polypain Wellness Core Psychological Management Program provide the foundation for effective cognitive behavioral treatment in the management of fibromyalgia and chronic musculoskeletal pain.

Medication to Manage Psychiatric, Psychological, and Psychosocial Disturbances

The introduction of psycho-active medications in the management of the psychiatric, psychological and psychosocial disturbances associated with polypain should be considered: 1) only in the presence of a comprehensive polypain management program with implementation of at least the Polypain Wellness Core Program; 2) only in the presence of the best possible implementation of the behavioral, social, and perceptual cognitive self-management strategies of the Polypain Wellness Core Psychological Management Program; 3) and in the presence of ongoing psychiatric, psychological, and/or psychosocial disturbances with associated maladaptive coping leading to ongoing adversely affected pain thresholds, pain suffering, and pain behavior despite actively being managed by appropriate psychotherapeutic intervention. While the discussion of psycho-active medications for specific psychiatric, psychological, and psychosocial disturbances is beyond the scope of this chapter, several crucial points about the use of such medications for these circumstances are notable.

As reviewed in Chapter 7, antidepressant medications may reduce pain and raise pain thresholds by improving pain processing in the dorsal horn of the spinal cord leading to reduced central sensitization, by altering neurotransmission in other parts of the brain as part of their antidepressant effect with stimulation of these areas leading to the stimulation of brain areas involved in pain processing causing further reduction in pain through descending pain modulation, and may have beneficial effects not only on mood but also on the cognitive-behavioral aspects and disrupted sleep patterns related to pain. In addition to the tiered or serial addition approach to the use of NSAIDs, acetaminophen, and opioids, in the management of pain and pain processing, antidepressant medications should be introduced as early as possible as appropriately indicated in a parallel treatment track in concert with the Polypain Wellness Core Program including the behavioral, social, and perceptual cognitive self-management strategies of the Polypain Wellness Core Psychological Management Program to specifically and directly treat issues related to pain processing independent of their effects on psychological issues and sleep. When antidepressant medications are also considered appropriate to treat psychiatric and psychological issues in polypain, the selection of medication must consider not only the psychiatric and psychological issues, but also the pain modulating benefits of the medication as well as the effect of the medication on sleep. Absent a contraindication to using an antidepressant, the selection of antidepressant is based upon a benefit-risk analysis looking at such factors as pain severity and extent relative to pain thresholds, disease severity and extent including severity and extent of psychological disturbances, severity and extent of sleep disturbances, functional impairment, the outcome of prior treatments, co-morbid medical conditions, concomitant medications, complication risk, compliance, convenience, and cost. As always, reality dictates.

When choosing an antidepressant or other psycho-active medication based on the above criteria, the lowest dose, fastest acting, shortest lasting, and least potent should be selected that is anticipated to meet the needs of treatment. In the management of polypain, antidepressant or other psycho-active medications are introduced for one or more of three components of polypain. They are used to directly treat to improve nociception and pain processing, to manage sleep disturbances, and to treat psychiatric, psychological, and psychosocial disturbances. Thus, dosing of antidepressant or other psycho-active medications is highly dependent on the purpose for which the antidepressant or other psycho-active medications are being used. However, under-treating the patient to reduce risk carries no benefit but only risk of complications from treatment as well as allowing progression of symptoms given that psychiatric, psychological, and psychosocial disturbances beget pain and pain begets psychiatric, psychological, and psychosocial disturbances with further reductions in pain thresholds.

Patience is required as it takes time to build up a consistent antidepressant or other psycho-active medication response and once achieved for the antidepressant or other psycho-active medication to optimally interact with the underlying psychiatric, psychological, and psychosocial disturbances and aberrant pain processing. Absent an adverse reaction or contraindication otherwise, antidepressant or other psycho-active medications should be slowly titrated to the highest dose needed up to an appropriate maximal dose for the purpose it was introduced to obtain a maximal response or to absolutely rule out lack of efficacy if a lower dose does not produce a maximal response. In the face of an adverse reaction, lack of efficacy, or lack of response at the safest maximal dose, the antidepressant or other psycho-active medication under consideration should be discontinued and replaced as appropriate with one of another of the antidepressant or other psycho-active medication group absent any contraindication and the same process should be undertaken with the new antidepressant or other psycho-active medication.

Treatment with antidepressant or other psycho-active medications is further complicated by the fact that they are used in parallel with other treatment modalities that are being adjusted at the same time and treatment benefit as well as complications need to be assessed against the background of the treatment effects and complications of these other medications and any potential interactions between them.

The addition of antidepressant or other psycho-active medications in the management of the psychiatric, psychological, and psychosocial disturbances associated with polypain should be considered by the criteria noted above as well as absent a contraindication to using antidepressant or other psycho-active medications based upon a thorough benefit-risk analysis that includes consideration of the nature and severity of the psychiatric, psychological, and psychosocial disturbances as well as their contribution to reduced pain thresholds, sleep disturbances, fatigue, cognitive impairment, functional impairment, pain suffering, and pain behavior as well as the outcome of prior treatments. Awareness and vigilance are critical in monitoring patients for potential adverse effects of treatment and this is accomplished through intensive follow-up with appropriate and comprehensive evaluation of progress and monitoring of treatment risk in terms of co-morbid medical conditions, concomitant medications, complications, compliance, convenience, and cost relative to treatment benefit. Reality dictates. Be aware of the Law of Unintended/Unrecognized Consequences.

Thus, the Polypain Wellness Core Psychological Management Program is a comprehensive subset of the Polpain Wellness Core Program that treats the psychiatric, psychological, and psychosocial disturbances impacting the symptoms of polypain. These psychiatric, psychological, and psychosocial disturbances have adverse effects on the pain of polypain and pain message processing. They also adversely affect the sleep disturbances of polypain. They result in maladaptive coping and adverse pain suffering and pain behavior. Furthermore, psychiatric, psychological, and psychosocial disturbances beget pain; pain begets psychiatric, psychological and psychosocial disturbances; pain begets pain; pain begets adverse cognitive coping; adverse cognitive coping begets psychiatric, psychological and psychosocial disturbances which in turn beget pain with further reductions in pain thresholds. The Polypain Wellness Core Psychological Management Program incorporates behavioral, social, and perceptual coping self-managed cognitive behavioral training and, as appropriately indicated, psychotherapy, antidepressant, and other psycho-active medication to improve these psychiatric, psychological, and psychosocial disturbances. This leads to improved pain thresholds with concomitant reduction in pain symptoms and improvement in psychological well-being, pain suffering, and pain behavior.

Chapter 13

Step 7: Sex Reduces Pain: Approaches to Bring Pleasure Back Into Your Life

"The natural man has only two primal passions, to get and beget."
—William Osler

Sex is a fundamental aspect of life. Sexual behavior comprises the integration and unification of biological, physical, psychological, social, and perceptual-spiritual components of our self-concept and our relationships that motivates pleasurable and rewarding sexual activity. It is a fundamental physiological drive like hunger, thirst, and sleep but significantly more nuanced by psychological and social factors. Despite the near universal participation by adults in sexual activity and the recognition by patients that issues relating to sex and sexual function are important, the topic is mostly ignored by healthcare providers. Polypain is a complex, highly nuanced, multidimensional, and highly individualized experience. It is driven and controlled by the mechanisms that: 1) generate pain from the source of pain; 2) process pain messaging to set pain thresholds; 3) result in sleep disturbances with their related complications; 4) and are associated with psychiatric, psychological, and psychosocial disturbances, that affect behavioral, social, and perceptual coping which ultimately impacts behavior. In view of the near-ubiquitous nature of sexual activity in adults, it should be expected that sexual function could be adversely affected by these components as well as medications used to treat polypain that may have sexual side effects. Conversely, sexual difficulties may adversely impact the pain and other elements of polypain. Thus, the evaluation of sexual function is another critical component in the assessment of patients with polypain.

Normal Sexual Response:
What You Need To Know
The Biology of Sex Is Consistently the Same

The sexual response cycle has been identified to consist of four stages. These stages comprise excitement, plateau, orgasm, and resolution. The excitement phase is further subcategorized into desire and arousal phases.

In both men and women, sex starts in the brain. In response to sensory inputs based on touch, smell, taste, sound, sight, thoughts, fantasy, or hormonally driven drivers, sexual excitement through the stimulation of desire is initiated. The threshold for desire and subsequent arousal is highly individual and situation specific related to: 1) physical, psychological, and psychosocial health; 2) prior learning, perceptions, and beliefs; 3) social factors such as social setting and relationship factors; 4) and the conduciveness of the environment. The sexual desire leads to neurologic activation in the brain which in turn leads to sexual arousal with increased blood flow to the genital areas. In men, the increased blood flow leads to penile erection along with increase in the size of the testes and thickening and tightening of the scrotum. The testes are pulled by muscles closer into the body. In women, the increased blood flow leads to vaginal transudation of slippery, clear fluid that lubricates the vagina for penile motion, neutralizes the otherwise normally acid conditions within the vagina, and facilitates survival of sperm. The labia swell and the clitoris enlarges and develops increased sensitivity to touch and pressure. The inner two-thirds of the vagina expands. A woman's nipples often become erect and the breasts may enlarge due to increased blood flow. Sexual flushing involving the chest, back, neck, and breasts are noted in about 25% of men and 50-75% of women.

The plateau phase consists of ongoing sexual arousal. The duration of this phase is highly variable depending on orgasmic control; and physical, psychological, and social factors conducive to sexual activity. In men, the head of the penis swells further in size with deeper flushing coloration. In women, the outer third of the vagina swells, narrowing the opening by at least 30%. The labia continue to swell and become a deeper red or purple color. The clitoris retracts toward the pubic bone, disappears under the clitoral hood, and is not visible but remains sensitive to stimulation of the tissue overlying it. Breast swelling continues with further breast enlargement that obscures the earlier nipple erection and the areola enlarges. In both men and women, muscle tension increases along with heart rate, breathing, and blood pressure.

Orgasm is a total body response consisting of the release of accumulated sexual tension and represents the shortest phase of the sexual response cycle. In men, orgasm begins with contractions that push semen into the urethra at which point ejaculation is inevitable. This is followed by contractions of the urethra, penis, and muscles at the base of the penis and pelvic floor leading to ejaculation with of spurts of semen. Orgasm starts with a sensation of warmth, pressure, or throbbing associated with ejaculatory inevitability followed by sharp, intensely pleasurable contractions of the muscles of the genitals and pelvic floor with a fluid rush or shooting sensation with ejaculation. In women, orgasm begins as an intensely pleasurable sensation starting in the clitoris, spreading to the pelvic floor, and from there to the entire body. It is accompanied by muscular contractions of the uterus, vagina, and pelvic floor muscles. In both men and women, the sexual flush peaks with orgasm. In both men and women the genital and pelvic floor muscles contract intensely at 0.8 second intervals for the first 3 to 5 contractions and in men this leads to the spurting of semen. As orgasm continues in both men and women, the intensity and frequency of contractions diminish and taper off. Women may experience 3 to 15 contractions and men may experience the same or less. In both men and women, the total body response comprising orgasm includes high levels of muscle tension in the entire body including the face leading to various uncontrollable facial expressions, contortions, moaning, or other vocalizations of intense of sexual arousal. Body rigidity and muscle spasms or cramps in the hands and feet may accompany late plateau and orgasm.

The final phase of sexual response is resolution. During this time, the post-orgasm sexual tension gradually diminishes and the physical and physiologic changes that developed during the earlier phases return to their prior baseline for both men and women. It is a period of physical and mental well-being and relaxation. The duration of this phase is highly variable depending on physical, psychological, and social factors. During the resolution phase, men enter a refractory phase during which another orgasm and ejaculation is not physiologically possible. The duration of this refractory phase may last minutes to hours during which time men must return to the excitement and arousal phases before achieving a new plateau phase in order to have a new orgasm. Women, on the other hand, have no refractory phase and are capable of multiple orgasms in a conducive setting within very short intervals as they can sustain the plateau level sexual phase between orgasms. Women will ideally achieve an orgasm 50 to 70% of the time with sexual intercourse, if that is their goal, and absent an orgasm will frequently experience physical and psychological satisfaction from a prolonged plateau phase.

The Psychological and Social Aspects of Sex Make the Experience Different

Normal sexual response requires the complex and coordinated integration of environmental, psychological, neurological, vascular, and hormonal events. As such, sex and sexual function should be viewed from the biopsychosocial perspective. While biologically, the events occurring during sexual activity are the same, there is a great deal of variation in the overall experience of any one personal sexual act compared to another. Desires, needs, circumstances, physical health, psychological well-being, and relationship issues all factor into the experience of sex. In a partnered, intimate relationship, the experience of sex is further complicated by the desires, needs, circumstances, physical health, psychological well-being, and relationship issues of the partner.

Sexual Responses Even Occur During Sleep

Independent of the sexual content of dreams, rapid eye movement (REM) sleep is a time of genital arousal with males developing erections and females developing increased vaginal lubrication and clitoral engorgement. Concerns regarding male impotence and erectile dysfunction are indeed much more clearly defined by the observation of the presence of a morning erection or erections during REM sleep. The ability to develop and sustain an erection at these times clearly identifies normal physical and physiologic sexual function and narrows the issues of such erectile dysfunction to sex environment, psychiatric, psychological, and psychosocial factors.

How Sex Varies With Age

The experience of sex changes with age. This is particularly notable during the middle adulthood transition years starting in the forties and referred to as midlife. Midlife in women develops in two phases. The first corresponds to the transition to menopause accompanied by fluctuating hormone levels; declining ovarian function; altered menses; age and hormone related changes in the anatomy and biology of sexual response; evolving sexual beliefs, perceptions, and expectations; and evolving social dynamics regarding relationships. The second midlife phase is a chronological, age related transition developing in the fifties with menopausal changes more completed or fully completed and the evolution of more specific age related changes related to anatomical, physiological, and psychological aging processes.

In a survey of women aged 45 to 55 years, 62% noted no change in sexual interest, 31% reported a decline, and 7% reported an increase in sexual interest with most of the latter group having new partners. In a survey of sexual satisfaction in women aged 45 and older comparing current sexual satisfaction to past levels, 49% were less satisfied.

The hormonal changes of menopause include reductions in the levels of estrogen and androgens such as testosterone. Estrogen deficiency leads to vaginal, clitoral, and genital atrophy, with thinning of tissues, reduced elasticity, reduced genital blood flow, and vaginal dryness with many women reporting impaired vaginal lubrication with sexual excitement and arousal. This leads to delayed or blunted sexual arousal responses with more time and stimulation needed for adequate lubrication for penile entry and thrusting. There is reduction or loss of the sex flush, reduction or loss of the increase in breast and nipple size, decreased pleasurable genital sensitivity, and increased genital and nipple pain sensitivity to touch. While normal testosterone levels in women facilitate sexual desire and arousal, and subsequent orgasm, low levels of androgens do not correlate specifically with sexual dysfunction. Reduced sexual desire or libido, however, is a common sexual dysfunction complaint in midlife.

In men, midlife changes are more subtle and gradual. These changes have been attributed to reduced testosterone production which begins in the mid-fifties. However, no acute drops in sex hormone production occur similar to a woman's menopause. In men, testosterone is critical for sexual function by driving libido and in the ability to develop and maintain a firm erection. A below normal deficiency of testosterone in men leads to loss of libido and impotence with inability to develop an firm erection sufficient for vaginal penetration. About 5% of men greater than sixty years of age note changes of a male menopause with symptoms of weakness, fatigue, reduced appetite, reduced libido, reduced sexual function, irritability, and cognitive difficulty due to below normal levels of testosterone. Yet, most midlife and older men do not have below normal levels of testosterone despite lower levels than earlier years and do not gain benefit from additional testosterone intake. They may, however, have reduced sensitivity to the effects of testosterone.

At age forty, 40 percent of men report impairment in sexual function and an additional 10% note sexual difficulties for each additional decade that follows. Changes noted include reduced libido, erectile dysfunction, impaired ejaculation, difficulties with orgasm, and reduced sexual satisfaction. After the age of fifty-five, erections take longer to develop and require more intense stimulation, are less firm, easier to lose, and are more difficult to regain. There is less elevation of the testes and this testicle retraction develops slower during the arousal and plateau phases. The volume of semen ejaculated is diminished along with the intensity of ejaculation. The refractory period lengthens. As with women in midlife, the sex flush diminishes as does muscle tension with arousal.

With regard to age, sexual activity appears to remain relatively stable during midlife but declines in frequency are noted after age sixty-five with 18% of men and 33% of women stopping sexual activity with their partners. The duration of marriage also correlates with declines in sexual frequency. Amongst couples married two years or less, having sex three times weekly or more occurs in 45%, sex between one to three times weekly in 38%, and between once a week to once a month in 11%. When married between two to ten years, only 27% are having sex three times weekly or more, 46% are having sex one to three times weekly, and 21% are having sex between once weekly and once monthly. Amongst couples married ten years or more, having sex three times weekly or more occurs in 18%, between one to three times weekly in 45%, between once weekly and once monthly in 22%, and less than once monthly in the rest. Importantly, amongst married couples, both men and women reported that satisfaction with the quality of their sex lives correlated with the frequency of sexual activity with 89% satisfaction rates in both men and women undertaking sex three times a week or more and only 32% of men and women were satisfied with their sex lives if having sex once monthly or less. Of course, this data does not say whether frequent sex is the source of satisfaction or if satisfied, nurturing, supportive, healthy couples are more likely to have sex. However, frequent sex and sexual satisfaction go together.

Why We Need Sex

The obvious short answer is because we are biologically driven to it because of the release and pleasure we derive. Yet, the psychological and social overlay upon sexual activity leaves sexual behavior to be defined in contexts that are relevant in explaining why we wish to experience sex. Thus, while normal, healthy sex is a basic biological drive, the need for sexual activity is rooted in the purpose for which one undertakes the sexual activity. Ultimately, normal, healthy sexual activity is undertaken for the pleasure it brings, however, the biopsychosocial context in which people undertake sexual activity falls into one of three categories.

As shown in Table 13.1, the most common type of sexual activity is the need for biological release of accumulated sexual tension. It stimulates desire and arousal by various psychological, biological, hormonal, and genital mechanisms. This type of sexual drive is experienced more often by men than women and accounts for the most frequent source of sexual activity drive. This drive leads to self or partnered sexual activity. However, when partnered, this type of sexual activity is not partner specific.

In the context of satisfying, healthy, nurturing partnered relationships which are not solely for casual sex encounters but in which sex is part of the broader relationship, an important element is intimacy. This involves the presence of a healthy and nurturing relationship, as described in Chapter 12, in which self-disclosure and the sharing of intimate and private details about ourselves to our partner enhances and strengthens the relationship and allows the partner to reciprocate. Thereby, intimacy strengthens the bond, permits deeper intimacy, and enhances passion. This drive for intimacy leads to a type of sexual experience in which sexual excitement and arousal is specifically induced by the desired partner of the relationship. Women seem to experience this stimulus for sexual activity more often than men.

Finally, sex is a biological tool for purposes of reproduction. The motivation for this sexual activity is social, cultural, spiritual, and survival based. Sex is periodically undertaken solely for this purpose.

Sexual Desire and Sexual Arousal Are Two Different Things

Sexual desire is a brain mediated process whereas the development of sexual arousal responses are not dependent on the brain and can occur by direct genital stimulation through nerve reflexes in the spinal cord. Thus, while sexual desire always leads to some degree of sexual arousal, non-desire stimulated sexual arousal may or may not lead to sexual desire.

Furthermore, all sexual encounters do not necessarily lead to or require an orgasm for sexual activity to be acceptable and the acceptability of this varies with the type of sex undertaken. For biological release sexual

Type of Sex	Purpose	Stimulus	Frequency of Experience in Males (M) and Females (F)	Participants	Relative Frequency of All Sex Encounters
Biological Release	Biological Release of Accumulated Sexual Tension	• Psychological • Biological • Hormonal • Genital	M>>F	Self or Partnered but Not Partner Specific	Frequent
Relationship Intimacy	Partner Based Intimacy	• Psychological • Relationship Affirmation, Bonding, and Enhancement	F>M	Partnered and Partner Specific	Often
Procreation	Social Duty	• Social • Cultural • Spiritual • Survival	F=M	Partnered and Partner Specific	Periodic

Table 13.1: The biopsychosocial contexts of sexual activity.

activity in both men and women, the drive and goal is ultimately to achieve an orgasm. In sex for procreation, orgasm for both partners is preferable but the minimum goal is male orgasm as female orgasm, while helpful, is not necessary. In relationship intimacy based sexual activity, a satisfying sexual experience is the goal and this may or may not include achieving an orgasm, particularly by the female partner.

Problems With Sex Are Common
Sexual Dysfunction Is Prevalent In General

When surveyed in general, sexual dysfunction is reported frequently by men and women. Sexual difficulties are reported by approximately 50% of patients seen in primary care. Amongst healthy, married couples 40% of men and 63% of women note sexual problems according to one survey and another survey of adult sexual behavior identified sexual dysfunction in 43% of women and 31% of men. Sexual difficulties progress in frequency with age. Sexual dysfunction is also correlated with a large spectrum of medical illnesses including diabetes mellitus, atherosclerosis, pituitary gland tumors, chronic renal disease, and chronic cardiac disease. It is associated with psychological and psychosocial disturbances including depression and marital difficulties. In the rheumatic diseases, a loss of sexual interest is noted in up to half the patients.

Sexual Dysfunction Is Associated With Pain

Pain and fatigue are reported as the major reasons for reduced sexual satisfaction and physical limitation of sexual activity in patients with chronic musculoskeletal pain related to arthritis. The impaired sexual function correlates with greater physical disability, depression, anxiety, adverse coping mechanisms, and pain. In patients identified as having chronic pain, sexual dissatisfaction is noted by 50-67% with a 77-78% reduction in the frequency of sexual activity reported. In the chronic pain setting, 28% of men are noted to have erectile dysfunction. In women, low sexual desire is noted in 36% with orgasmic difficulty in 40%. In a survey of premenopausal women diagnosed with fibromyalgia, it was noted that the physiological aspects of excitement and orgasm were similar to healthy women but the fibromyalgia group had reduced sexual desire and satisfaction, more body pain, and reduced genital sensitivity. Psychological distress, but not pain, correlated with sexual dysfunction. Other studies have reported pain, anxiety, and depression to correlate with sexual dysfunction in patients. In women with fibromyalgia, relationship satisfaction is a strong predictor of satisfactory sexual function. Based on self-reporting, the study data from Chapter 4, identify the presence of reduced libido with reduced sexual interest or desire in 66% of responding patients with polypain.

Why Sex Becomes Unsatisfactory Or Difficult
The Causes of Sexual Dysfunction in General

In a study of the normal, general population, women with identified sexual dysfunction noted the problems to include a lack of interest in sexual activity in 33.4%, inability to achieve orgasm in 24.1%, lack of pleasure from sex in 21.2% , painful intercourse in 14.4%, performance anxiety in 11.5%, and problems with lubrication in 10.4%. In the men with sexual dysfunction, the problems included premature ejaculation in 28.5%, performance anxiety in 17%, lack of interest in 15.8%, erectile dysfunction in 10.4%, inability to achieve orgasm in 8.3%, lack of pleasure from sex in 8.1%, and painful intercourse in 3%.

In women, it appears that psychiatric, psychological, and psychosocial factors are the predominant issues impacting sexual function. This, of course, follows from the understanding that sexual desire is a brain mediated event whereas sexual arousal is a physiological process. In women, sexual desire and satisfaction correlate with past and current psychological health status, emotional well-being, physical well-being, self-image, positively rewarding past sexual experiences, and positive relationship expectations. The effect of midlife and associated hormonal changes on sexual function has been discussed earlier.

Sexual dysfunction in women also correlates with overall health. Chronic diseases that are associated with impaired sexual function include chronic musculoskeletal pain, arthritis, rheumatologic diseases, multiple sclerosis, chronic renal failure, cancer including breast cancer and chemotherapy for breast cancer, and diabetes. Both prescription and over-the-counter medications can affect the components of the sexual response. These include medications that may affect brain neurotransmitters involved in the sexual response such as antidepressant medications and other psychoactive medications, medications that affect blood flow

Category	Causes	Specific Issues
Psychiatric Psychological Psychosocial	• Psychiatric	• Depression • Anxiety • Other Psychiatric Conditions
	• Psychological	• Behavioral Coping Factors • Social/Relationship Coping Factors
	• Social Behavioral	• Perceptions • Beliefs • Expectations
	• Performance Anxiety	• Men and Women
	• Loss of Sensate Focus	• Men
Environmental	• Environment/Circumstance Not Conducive for Sex	
Hormonal Midlife	• Loss of Estrogen in Women • Reduced testosterone effect in men	
Health Issues	• Disease	• Arthritis Conditions • Diabetes Mellitus • Neurological Conditions • Chronic Renal Failure • Diabetes • Cancer • Cardiovascular Disease • Hypertension • Obesity • Hyperlipidemia
	• Medications	• Antidepressants • Opioids • Antihypertensives • Cardiovascular Medications • Alcohol • Recreational Drug Use • Oral Contraceptives (Women)
	• Sleep disorders	• Availability for sex
	• Smoking	
Age	• Age related declines in function and frequency	
Reduced Genital Sexual Sensitivity	• Age • Opioid Medication	
Sexual Dysfunction by Proxy	• Lack of Available Partner • Partner with Sexual Dysfunction • Sexual Relationship Psychological/Social Behavioral Issues	
Bicycle Seat	• Men	

Table 13.2: Mechanisms of sexual dysfunction in men and women.

such as cardiovascular and blood pressure medications, medications that cause vaginal dryness or impede vaginal lubrication in response to sexual arousal, analgesic medications such as opioids that may reduce genital sexual sensitivity, alcohol, and other recreational drugs.

In men, as in women, it appears that psychiatric, psychological, and psychosocial factors are the predominant issues impacting sexual function. Psychological status such as the presence of depression correlates with sexual dysfunction as do levels of emotional satisfaction, levels of general happiness, and the presence of emotional problems or stress. Erectile failure from prior attempts at intercourse may lead to performance anxiety with attention focused on the ability to achieve and maintain an erection on subsequent attempts dissociated from the remainder of the sexual experience leading to anxiety and perpetuation of the erectile dysfunction. During sexual activity, particularly in midlife and later, the focus of a man's attention may drift away from the intimacy of sex and onto other stresses and concerns leading to a loss of the erection and difficulty in regaining the erection. This cognitive loss of awareness of the sensory and psychological impact of sexual desire and arousal is described as a loss of sensate focus. The effect of midlife and associated hormonal changes on sexual function has been discussed earlier.

Sexual dysfunction in men also correlates with their overall health. Chronic diseases that are associated with impaired sexual function include chronic musculoskeletal pain, arthritis, rheumatologic diseases; neurological conditions such as certain spinal cord injuries leading to erectile dysfunction, nerve damaging prostate cancer surgery, and multiple sclerosis; diabetes; atherosclerosis; pituitary gland tumors; chronic renal disease; hypertension, obesity, lipid disorders; and smoking. Unlike women, sexual dysfunction in men correlates with cardiovascular disease and erectile dysfunction may be an early manifestation of cardiovascular disease. Prescription and over-the-counter medications can affect the components of the male sexual response. These include medications that may affect brain neurotransmitters involved in the sexual response such as antidepressant medications and other psychoactive medications, medications that affect blood flow such as cardiovascular and blood pressure medications, medications that negatively affect nerve function involving erection, analgesic medications such as opioids that may reduce genital sexual sensitivity, alcohol, and other recreational drugs. Penile numbness and impotence are reported to develop in serious, competitive bicyclists related to nerve damage from bicycle seats.

In common to both men and women are issues related to the conduciveness of the environment and circumstance for sexual activity and the sexual dysfunction imposed by these factors. Another issue of sexual dysfunction shared by men and women is the issue of sexual dysfunction by proxy. This refers to sexual dysfunction imposed by the sexual dysfunction of a sex partner, the lack of an available partner for desired partnered sexual activity, or the sexual relationship disturbances due to psychological and social behavioral relationship issues.

These mechanisms of sexual dysfunction in the population are displayed in Table 13.2.

Causes of Sexual Dysfunction in Fibromyalgia Polypain

In polypain, sexual dysfunction occurs either from the general causes that affect any individual independent of polypain as well as sexual dysfunction that develops specifically because of factors related to polypain. Of the general causes of sexual dysfunction, midlife changes are particularly relevant as the average age of polypain patients is 52.9 years. In addition, the psychiatric, psychological, and psychosocial disturbances in polypain reviewed in Chapter 12 may adversely affect sexual function and are a significant source of sexual dysfunction given that 66% of polypain patients report reduced libido or reduced of sexual interest.

The polypain sources of pain consisting of primary generalized osteoarthritis predominantly involving the neck and back with associated degenerative disc disease and the variable combination of associated tendinitis, bursitis, and fasciitis not only cause pain that may interfere with sexual desire and arousal but may also cause mechanical difficulties in positioning for comfort to undertake sexual activity. Furthermore, the reduced pain thresholds from adverse pain processing generated by increased nociception amplifies pain and may cause sensitivity to non-painful contact. The sleep abnormalities contribute to the reduced pain thresholds. Psychiatric, psychological, and psychosocial disturbances identified in polypain as well as sleepiness and fatigue may impact sexual response. Fatigue limiting sexual activity may develop as a result of the pain, sleep disturbances, and medication. Finally, the antidepressants and opioids used to treat polypain may impair sexual function and opioids may reduce genital sensitivity to sexual stimulation. These polypain specific mechanisms of sexual dysfunction are displayed in Table 13.3.

Group	Category	Cause
Not Specific to Polypain	• See Table 13.2	
Specific to Polypain	• Psychiatric • Psychological • Psychosocial	• See Chapter 12
	• Primary Generalized Osteoarthritis, Bursitis, Tendinitis, Fasciitis	• Pain • Mechanical Positioning
	• Reduced Pain Thresholds	• Pain • Sensitivity to Non-painful Contact
	• Sleep Disturbances of Polypain	• See Chapter 11
	• Medications	• Antidepressants • Opioids
	• Fatigue	• Primary Generalized Osteoarthritis, Bursitis, Tendinitis, Fasciitis • Sleep Disturbances • Medications

Table 13.3: *Mechanisms of sexual dysfunction in men and women specific to polypain.*

The Interaction Between Sexual Function and Chronic Musculoskeletal Pain: Pain Is Bad For Sex, Sex Is Good For Pain

Sexual dysfunction in polypain may arise from factors independent of polypain or directly as a result of factors related to polypain. Regardless of how sexual dysfunction in polypain arises, it results in psychiatric, psychological, and psychosocial disturbances. These psychiatric, psychological, or psychosocial disturbances significantly influence pain suffering and pain behavior in chronic musculoskeletal pain. The adverse psychological contributors and consequences of sexual dysfunction in polypain ultimately lower pain thresholds and worsen the perception of pain. This leads to a progressive worsening spiral of increasing psychological and psychosocial disruption, poorer coping strategies, descending pain thresholds, and increasing perception of pain resulting in further impairments in sexual desire, arousal, and the normal sexual response. In essence, the psychiatric, psychological, and psychosocial aspects of sexual dysfunction in polypain beget further psychological and psychosocial disturbances, maladaptive pain suffering and pain behavior, maladaptive coping, increased pain, and worsened sexual dysfunction. Effective treatment strategies to improve sexual dysfunction improves psychological well-being and reverses this spiral to ultimately improve pain thresholds and reduce pain. Effective treatment strategies to reduce pain and raise pain thresholds improves sexual dysfunction imposed by the components driving polypain absent adverse sexual side effects of medication intervention. Thus, pain begets sexual dysfunction, good sex begets less pain, and less pain begets better sex.

The Fibromyalgia Polypain Wellness Core Sex Management Program: Returning Pleasure, Reducing Pain

The approach to the management of sexual dysfunction in polypain re-emphasizes the need for proper, thorough, and comprehensive assessment to determine the presence and nature of impairments in sexual desire, arousal, and the normal sexual response whether or not specifically related to polypain and to develop an appropriate understanding upon which to base treatment decisions. Only through such evaluation can the rheumatologist be sufficiently informed and knowledgeable as to be able to provide needed patient education in order that patients be able to fully participate in their own care and make truly informed decisions regarding treatment. As with managing any and all components of polypain, intensive follow-up regarding disturbances in sexual desire, arousal, and the normal sexual response with appropriate evaluation of progress to provide optimal benefit from a properly designed treatment program is of crucial importance.

The Polypain Wellness Core Sex Management Program forms part of the more comprehensive Polypain Wellness Core Program. In addition to their contributions to the symptoms and findings in polypain, the polypain sources of pain consisting of primary generalized osteoarthritis predominantly involving the neck and back with associated degenerative disc disease and the variable combination of associated tendinitis, bursitis, and fasciitis; the reduced pain thresholds from adverse pain processing generated by increased nociception; the sleep abnormalities; and the psychiatric, psychological, and psychosocial disturbances contribute to the sexual dysfunction identified in polypain. Thus, the fundamental and basic treatment for the disturbances of sexual desire, arousal, and the normal sexual response in polypain requires treatment with all the elements of the Polypain Wellness Core Program. Therefore, the Polypain Wellness Core Sex Management Program incorporates the pharmacologic intervention to control site specific pain symptoms, pain processing abnormalities, and psychological disturbances; biomechanical and postural intervention through exercises including the Integrated Daily Walking Program, orthotics, neuromuscular re-education, and weight control including the Rule of Thirds Polypain Weight Loss Program; ergonomic intervention through appropriate accommodation and modification; the Polypain Wellness Core Sleep Management Program; and the Polypain Wellness Core Psychological Management Program.

The specific sexual activity and behavior related interventions comprising the Polypain Wellness Core Sex Management Program component of the Polypain Wellness Core Program begins with the implementation of adaptive sexual cognitive coping behavior and appropriate sexual activity ergonomics. This is the foundation upon which the Polypain Wellness

Core Sex Management Program is built. The successful management of the disturbances of sexual desire, arousal, and the normal sexual response in polypain can only occur in the presence of appropriate adaptive sexual cognitive coping behavior and sexual activity ergonomics, biomechanics, and posture. Equally important is the need to incorporate appropriate joint and joint related alignment, posture, and biomechanics as detailed in the Polypain Wellness Core Program and specifically the components that relate to sleep biomechanics and posture in regard to the Polypain Wellness Core Sleep Management Program as well as the implementation of adaptive cognitive coping and pain behavior as described in the Polypain Wellness Core Psychological Management Program. Finally, these treatment elements must be appropriately considered before the consideration of adding medications to treat sexual dysfunction.

In the management of the disturbances of sexual desire, arousal, and the normal sexual response in polypain, medications are never enough. However, disturbances of sexual desire, arousal, and the normal sexual response in polypain may be adequately treated through the Polypain Wellness Core Program and all its components along with the adaptive sexual cognitive coping behavior and sexual activity ergonomics, biomechanics, and posture components of the Polypain Wellness Core Sex Management Program and sexual dysfunction specific medications may not be required.

Adaptive Sexual Cognitive Coping Self-Management and Sexual Activity Ergonomics, Biomechanics, Posture Program: Enhancing Sexual Outcomes, Lessening Pain

Sexual Activity Adaptive Cognitive Coping

1) The brain is the largest and most important sex organ.

2) It is crucial to incorporate all the elements of the Polypain Wellness Core Psychological Management Program. Psychiatric, psychological, and psychosocial well-being are vital for normal sexual responsiveness and function. The relationship aspects of this program are especially critical for established relationships with partnered sexual activity.

3) In a healthy, supportive, nurturing relationship, an orgasm is not always necessary to have satisfying sexual activity.

This is true more often for women than men. In particular, it is very important to have good sexual communication to determine if female orgasm is likely to occur during sexual intercourse in order to determine timing of the male orgasm, as the male orgasm will result in a loss of erection and loss of penile stimulation for the female.

4) An occasional or episodic lack of orgasm or ability to complete sex to orgasm in established healthy relationships should not be looked upon as failure or an illness requiring medical attention, but rather as foreplay for the next time around.

5) In sexual relationships, have sex.

As discussed in Chapter 12, sexual relationships require sexual contact to maintain not only that component of the relationship, but to maintain the relationship as a whole as sexual activity is a part of that relationship. Therefore, have sex as often as the relationship requires and ensure that it is as pleasant and satisfying as needed to satisfy the partners of the relationship. The more frequent the sexual activity, the greater the satisfaction with the sex life.

6) The more intimacy/pleasure/love/happiness/excitement/interest/trust you give in sex, the more you get. It is a true measure of the health and strength of a relationship.

7) If you are not having satisfying sex with your partner in a way that fulfills your partner's desires and needs, your partner may find someone else who will.

8) In the economy of sex in established relationships, men and women should be willing to give their partner what they want in order to get what they need.

What do men want from women?	What do women want from men?
Sex	Love
Sex in a variety of ways	Emotional Security
Sex in a variety of places	Relationship Security
Sex in the context of a secure loving relationship	Sex with someone who validates their contribution to the relationship
Sex with someone who validates their contribution to the relationship	Sex in the context of a secure loving relationship

Table 13.4: What men and women want from each other.

What women should be willing give to men to fulfill their own needs and wants.	What men should be willing give to women to fulfill their own needs and wants.
Sex	Love
Sex in a variety of ways	Emotional Security
Sex in a variety of places	Relationship Security
Sex in the context of a secure loving relationship	Sex with someone who validates their contribution to the relationship
Sex with someone who validates their contribution to the relationship	Sex in the context of a secure loving relationship

Table 13.5: What men and women should give one another to get what they want.

Sexual Activity Ergonomics, Biomechanics, and Posture

1) Make time and space for satisfying sexual activity.

2) In established healthy relationships in which there is also a sexual relationship, study and know your partner's sexual anatomy.

3) In established healthy relationships in which there is also a sexual relationship, study and know your partner's sexual responses. Sounds, posture, and motion distinguish pleasure from discomfort or tedium. Don't be shy or afraid to ask and tell. Be open, honest, willing to share, daring to explore, wise enough to learn, and courageous enough to try.

4) Learn how to touch and stimulate your partner's non-genital and genital sexual anatomy from your partner. Have your partner guide and show you if you do not know this.

5) Sex is a multisensory experience between you and your partner.

Sexual desire is the basis of normal sexual response. It is driven by sensory inputs based on touch, smell, taste, sound, sight, thoughts, fantasy, or hormonally driven drivers that stimulate sexual excitement. Initially, sexual desire is a cognitive experience coupled with a sensory experience. This sensory experience should, for the initial portion of the sex activity, be non-genital sex. This non-genital sex should involve pleasurable non-genital touching. The eyes are involved in seeing the surroundings and your partner in a sexually stimulating manner. The glare of bright lights or the television does not fall in this category. Look into your partner's eyes. Eye contact is very intimate. The sounds heard should be intimate and should be soothing, supportive, and stimulating such as words of affection or sounds of pleasure from you and your partner. This does not include the television, radio, or discussions about problems, politics, or the news. The smells should be stimulating and pleasant. Topical analgesic rubs do not fall in this category. Sex in established relationships must involve intimate passionate kissing, for a kiss represents an intimate bond that identifies a deep emotional bond and intimacy beyond the mere mechanics of genital sexual performance. However, be wary if the individual being kissed uses topical capsaicin. This does not wash off and lingers on the skin without odor for many hours. Kissing an area with active capsai-

Multisensory Non-Genital Sex

Fingers and feet

Eyes

Ears

Lips

Smell

Figure 13.1:
Multisensory non-genital
sex experience.

cin, genital contact with such an area, or contact with hands that have touched such an area to the genital area, lips, or eyes will produce intensely uncomfortable burning and basically destroy the mood and stop the activity. The multisensory experience of non-genital sex can be recalled by the acronym FEELS as shown in Figure 13.1.

Use your senses to express and receive pleasure. Non-genital sexual stimulation heightens the sexual tension and intensifies the sexual experience as a prelude to genital sexual activity. In addition, it affirms and enhances the relationship intimacy and strengthens the relationship bond beyond the sexual activity.

6) Get a genital lubricant for sexual activity.

If genital dryness or inadequate lubrication during arousal are issues in women, use a genital lubricant containing propylene glycol or butylene glycol, and glycerin with or without polyethylene glycol, hydroxycellulose, or other cellulose derivatives. Genital lubricants containing lactic acid provide a warming sensation and are described as warming formulas. These lubricants are highly effective in maintaining vaginal lubrication with penile thrusting and movement. They also work well on the penis for manual mechanical penile stimulation. The old water soluble jellies dry out very quickly, especially with friction from penile movement and are much less preferable.

7) Get a vibrator.

   Get an electric vibrator sufficient to provide clitoral and genital stimulation for the female partner. This is particularly important if female arousal and orgasm are difficult to achieve or require so much stimulation that the non-assisted sexual experience becomes tedious or unpleasant. However, even absent arousal and orgasmic difficulties, in the patient with polypain, the use of a vibrator facilitates female sexual arousal and orgasm and reduces the physical demands of the work and biomechanics of sexual intercourse and other sexual activity. Thus, the use of a vibrator during sexual activity improves sexual satisfaction and reduces adverse ergonomics, biomechanics, and posture regardless of whether the woman or man has polypain.

8) In partnered heterosexual sex, there are two positions for sexual intercourse that maximize intimacy while allowing for the individual affected by polypain to participate with minimal joint loading and optimal biomechanics and posture. Both positions involve facing each other.

   a) For the female with polypain: The woman should lie on her back with her hips and knees comfortably flexed and spread apart. Her partner should be kneeling in front of her, between her legs, on his knees, with his knees spread apart.

   b) For the male with polypain: The man should lie on his back with his partner straddling his thighs and pelvis on top.

   Both positions allow optimal neutral body posturing and avoid having the affected partner support excess weight. They readily allow easy genital positioning for intercourse, manual genital stimulation by either partner, the use of a vibrator for clitoral stimulation for the female coupled with penile entry, and the ability for penile thrusting while still using a vibrator. Both positions allow the affected individual to control the rate and degree of stimulation and depth of penile penetration.

   Both positions can provide significant penile and clitoral stimulation. As the woman's orgasm likely requires more time and stimulation than the man's, it is recommended that female stimulation take place orally, manually, or with a vibrator until closer to orgasm prior to penile entry in these positions.

Sexual Counseling

Sexual counseling is a form of psychological therapy directed towards the aspects of sexual function. The introduction of sexual counseling for the management of the impairments in sexual desire, arousal, and the normal sexual response in polypain should be considered: 1) only in the presence of a comprehensive polypain management program with implementation of at least the Polypain Wellness Core Program; 2) in the presence of the best possible implementation of the Polypain Wellness Core Psychological Management Program; 3) only in the presence of the best possible implementation of the Adaptive Sexual Cognitive Coping Self-Management and Sexual Activity Ergonomics, Biomechanics, Posture Program; 4) and in the presence of ongoing sexual dysfunction. In undertaking sexual counseling, it is critical for the psychotherapist to acknowledge and understand sexual dysfunction associated with life issues independent of polypain as well as the components of sexual dysfunction contributed to and driven by the polypain process itself.

Medication to Manage Sexual Dysfunction

The introduction of medications in the management of the impairments in sexual desire, arousal, and the normal sexual response associated with polypain should be considered: 1) only in the presence of a comprehensive polypain management program with implementation of at least the Polypain Wellness Core Program; 2) only in the presence of the best possible implementation of the Polypain Wellness Core Psychological Management Program; 3) and only in the presence of the best possible implementation of the Adaptive Sexual Cognitive Coping Self-Management and Sexual Activity Ergonomics, Biomechanics, Posture Program actively being managed by appropriate sexual counseling. While the discussion of specific medications for the management of sexual dysfunction is beyond the scope of this chapter, several crucial points about the use of such medications for these circumstances are notable.

Medications used to manage various health issues including polypain should be thoroughly reviewed as to their potential contribution to sexual dysfunction and appropriate adjustments should be undertaken. Medications to manage sexual dysfunction in polypain can be introduced at any time, independent of the use of NSAIDs, acetaminophen, and opioids. If antidepressant medication or other psycho-active medication is felt to appropriate in managing sexual dysfunction, these medications should be introduced as described in Chapter 12.

Thus, the Polypain Wellness Core Sex Management Program is a comprehensive subset of the Polpain Wellness Core Program that treats the sexual dysfunction impacting the symptoms of polypain. This sexual dysfunction has adverse effects on the pain of polypain and pain message processing. It results in maladaptive coping and adverse pain suffering and pain behavior. The psychiatric, psychological, and psychosocial disturbances related to sexual dysfunction beget pain; pain begets psychiatric, psychological, and psychosocial disturbances that may beget sexual dysfunction; sexual dysfunction begets adverse cognitive coping; adverse cognitive coping begets psychiatric, psychological, and psychosocial disturbances which in turn beget pain with further reductions in pain thresholds as well as further sexual dysfunction. The Polypain Wellness Core Sex Management Program incorporates adaptive sexual cognitive coping self-management, ergonomics, biomechanics, posture, and as appropriately indicated, sexual counseling and medications to manage sexual dysfunction to improve sexual dysfunction and the attendant psychiatric, psychological, and psychosocial disturbances. Consequently, pain thresholds are improved with concomitant reduction in pain symptoms and improvement in psychological well-being, pain suffering, pain behavior, and sexual response.

Chapter 14

Steps 8 and 9: Injections and Surgery May Sometimes Be Needed

"The only way to keep your health is to eat what you don't want, drink what you don't like, and do what you'd rather not." —Mark Twain

The Polypain Wellness Core – Step 8: Injections

In many patients, following a thorough and comprehensive analysis and patient education program, the introduction of appropriate medications, biomechanics, posture, and ergonomics through the Polypain Wellness Core Program may suffice to improve symptoms and control disease progression. In some patients, there may be one or several joint or periarticular sites that are significantly more involved with osteoarthritis or inflammation from tendinitis, bursitis, or fasciitis or are more resistant to the treatment program than the other sites despite the incorporation of pharmacologic intervention to control site specific pain symptoms, pain processing abnormalities, and psychological disturbances; biomechanical and postural intervention through exercises including the Integrated Daily Walking Program, orthotics, neuromuscular re-education and weight control including the Rule of Thirds Polypain Weight Loss Program; ergonomic intervention through appropriate accommodation and modification; the Polypain Wellness Core Sleep Management Program; and the Polypain Wellness Core Psychological Management Program.

In such situations, local injection with an anti-inflammatory glucocorticoid to the specific joint or joint related structure may be of benefit in bringing the site under control commensurate with the response seen at other sites. Similarly, the injection of very active or resistant trigger points, which are painful and tender taut muscle bands, with a local anesthetic, may be of similar benefit. Consideration to injection should be made with appropriate risk-benefit analysis. Injections should be performed by rheumatologists experienced in the management of polypain and in the injection procedures under consideration. Injections can be performed any time throughout the course of treatment as indicated.

The Polypain Wellness Core – Step 9: Surgery

This is rarely indicated, but is a consideration at localized joint sites demonstrating significant irreversible damage and intractable pain or refractory nerve related complications from which maximal non-surgical intervention has otherwise failed; injection of the joint site is not indicated or is not sufficient; and only in the presence of the optimal implementation of the Poylpain Wellness Core program including pharmacologic intervention to control site specific pain symptoms, pain processing abnormalities, and psychological disturbances; biomechanical and postural intervention through exercises including the Integrated Daily Walking Program, orthotics, neuromuscular re-education and weight control including the Rule of Thirds Polypain Weight Loss Program; ergonomic intervention through appropriate accommodation and modification; the Polypain Wellness Core Sleep Management Program; and the Polypain Wellness Core Psychological Management Program.

Part Five

A Unified Understanding of Fibromyalgia Pain

Chapter 15

The Fibromyalgia Polypain Network Paradigm Solves The Enigma of Fibromyalgia

"Who controls the past controls the future. Who controls the present controls the past." —George Orwell, *1984*

Polypain represents an integrated unified model that fully explains the development and evolution of fibromyalgia. It identifies the sources and cause of the widespread pain in fibromyalgia and the critical components that affect the modulation of pain by pain itself as well as the associated sleep disruptions and psychiatric, psychological, and psychosocial disturbances of fibromyalgia that lead to the presence of pain and painful fibromyalgia tender points. It explains how and why ergonomic and biomechanical factors; sleep disturbances; obesity; psychiatric, psychological, and psychosocial factors; cognitive coping factors; and sexual dysfunction affect the symptoms and behavioral responses in polypain. It shows how psychiatric, psychological, and psychosocial problems; sleep disturbances; weight; and sexual function difficulties independent of polypain and related to other life issues significantly affect the symptoms of pain and also influence behavioral responses related to the portions of pain affected by these components as well as behaviors driven by these elements independent of the pain. All patients with fibromyalgia have polypain. In individuals with chronic widespread musculoskeletal pain from any cause associated with widespread painful tenderness, the Polypain Model fully identifies the factors that modulate that pain and explains the development and evolution of the tenderness.

367

Connecting the Pieces: The Complete Fibromyalgia Polypain Network Linking The Source of Pain to What You Actually Feel

Fundamentally, polypain consists of two components: 1) the sources of pain generating nociception caused by primary generalized osteoarthritis predominantly involving the neck and back with associated degenerative disc disease and the variable combination of associated tendinitis, bursitis, and fasciitis influenced by ergonomic, biomechanical, and postural factors; 2) the reduced pain thresholds from adverse pain processing generated by increased nociception driven by the pain itself; the sleep abnormalities; and the psychiatric, psychological, and psychosocial disturbances including depression and anxiety which are modulated in the dorsal horn of the spinal cord and lead to tenderness and referred pain. Most importantly, there is an identified source of pain upon which the process develops. Without a pain source, there is no pain for the pain processing modulators to act on. In the presence of these pain generators in polypain, the modulated pain signal or pain message leads to intensified pain appreciation, increased tenderness with increased pain sensitivity, and a wider distribution of pain and tenderness identified as pain magnification and pain amplification. This processed pain results in pain suffering and pain behavior that leads to expressions of pain, impairment, activity limitation, and disability.

In polypain: 1) pain begets pain; 2) psychiatric, psychological, and psychosocial disturbances beget pain; 3) sleep abnormalities beget pain; 4) overweight and obesity beget pain; 5) sexual dysfunction begets pain; 6) sleep disturbances beget sleep disturbances; 7) psychiatric, psychological, and psychosocial disturbances beget psychiatric, psychological, and psychosocial disturbances; 8) sexual dysfunction begets sexual dysfunction; 9) pain begets psychiatric, psychological and psychosocial disturbances; 10) pain begets sleep disturbances; 11) pain begets overweight and obesity; 12) pain begets sexual dysfunction; 13) psychiatric, psychological, and psychosocial disturbances beget sexual dysfunction; 14) psychiatric, psychological and psychosocial disturbances beget sleep disturbances; 15) sexual dysfunction begets psychiatric, psychological, and psychosocial disturbances. These interactions are integrated into a biopsychosocial process that controls the expression of pain by the pain

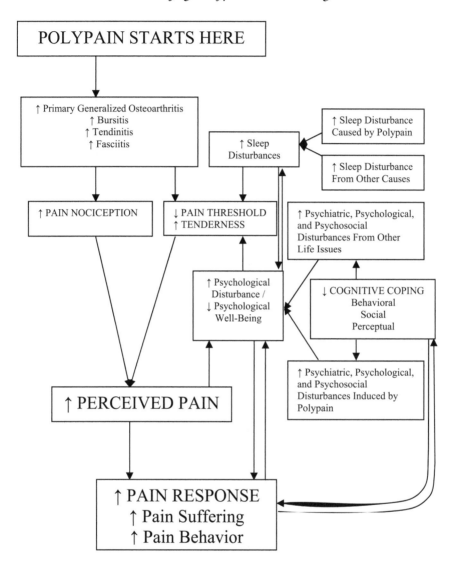

Figure 15.1: *The biopsychosocial network of polypain where increased pain appreciation is generated by the promotion of factors that increase pain and reduce pain thresholds with increased appreciation of pain and adverse pain suffering and behavior.*

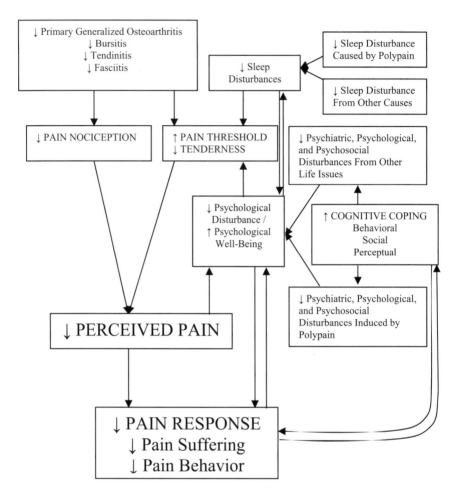

Figure 15.2: *The biopsychosocial network of polypain where treatment reduces the adverse effects on pain and pain processing with a concomitant reduction of pain appreciation and adverse pain suffering and behavior.*

generators and the modulation of pain messaging through altered pain thresholds. The biopsychosocial network of polypain is depicted in Figure 15.1 where increased pain appreciation is generated by the promotion of factors that increase pain and reduce pain thresholds with increased appreciation of pain and adverse pain suffering and behavior and Figure 15.2 where the treatment of these factors reduces their adverse effects on pain and pain processing with a concomitant reduction of pain appreciation and adverse pain suffering and behavior.

Integrated Well-Being and Polypain

In addition to addressing the biopsychosocial factors, polypain identifies the widespread impact of polypain at any point in time as well as over time. Polypain is a chronic disease process and changes over time. People and circumstances also change over time and this affects the presentation of polypain symptoms and related behavior. The chronicity of disease also requires chronic therapeutic intervention, to some degree, to treat unrecognized disease as well as obviously active disease in addition to preventing progression of the process. Thus, the context of polypain upon individuals and their specific life issues must be wholly considered to implement a beneficial and cost/risk effective management program.

Patient education and understanding are key to this. More importantly, the patient must be an actively involved participant in care and must understand the crucial importance of the self-management elements of treatment. Successful therapy hinges on the ability of the patient to understand the impact of medications, ergonomics, biomechanics, posture, behavioral coping, social coping, perceptual coping, weight, and sexual activity on pain, pain processing, pain suffering, and pain behavior. By this undertaking, the patient is able to make informed, free will choices regarding treatment and potential outcomes and readily comply to a long-term management program. Further, through this fully informed understanding, knowledge, and enlightenment, the patient can accept and incorporate the chronic issues of polypain and its management into a new definition of self in which self-concept is defined in consideration of polypain but not defined by polypain. The Polypain Wellness Core Program is ideally suited for these goals in that the program can be specifically individualized and accommodated to different circumstances and needs by the

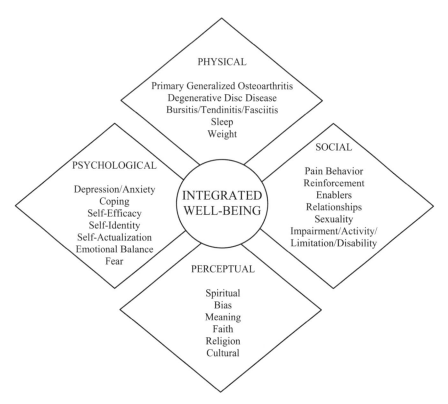

Figure 15.3: *The elements of integrated well-being in polypain.*

knowledgeable polypain patient at any point in time as well as over time. The Polypain Wellness Core Program addresses the components that lead to the integrated well-being of the polypain patient as shown in Figure 15.3.

Looking Ahead

In the past, the data regarding fibromyalgia had failed to identify the source of pain. The American College of Rheumatology widespread pain and tenderness criteria have wrongly diverted attention away from the musculoskeletal system. Based on the work published herein, polypain corrects these shortcomings by identifying the cause of pain in fibromyalgia arising from primary generalized osteoarthritis predominantly involving the neck and back with associated degenerative disc disease and the attendant association of a variable combination of tendinitis, bursitis, and fasciitis. Furthermore, polypain identifies how chronic widespread pain is modulated and ultimately perceived. Finally, it highlights the role of unrecognized, but detectable, musculoskeletal disease in the genesis of fibromyalgia and syndromes of chronic widespread pain. Future research in polypain must focus on a better understanding of how these disease processes develop in addition to increasing knowledge regarding pain message processing by the nervous system. This will provide the opportunity for even more targeted and directed treatment modalities.

References

Chapters 1 and 2

1. Aaron LA, Bradley LA, Alarcon GS et al. Perceived physical and emotional trauma as precipitating events in fibromyalgia. Associations with health care seeking and disability status but not pain severity. Arthritis Rheum 1997; 40: 453-460.

2. Aaron LA, Bradley LA, Alarcon GS et al. Psychiatric diagnoses in patients with fibromyalgia are related to health care-seeking behavior rather than to illness. Arthritis Rheum 1996; 39: 436-445.

3. Abraham GE, Flechas JD. Management of fibromyalgia: a rationale for the use of magnesium and malic acid. J Nutritional Med 1992; 3: 49-59.

4. Acasuso-Diaz M, Collantes-Estevez E. Joint hypermobility in patients with fibromyalgia syndrome. Arthritis Care Res 1998; 11: 39-42.

5. Adler GK, Kinsley BT, Hurwitz S et al. Reduced hypothalamic-pituitary and sympathoadrenal responses to hypoglycemia in women with fibromyalgia syndrome. Am J Med 1999; 106: 534-543.

6. Affleck G, Urrows S, Tennen H et al. Sequential daily relations of sleep, pain intensity, and attention to pain among women with fibromyalgia. Pain 1996; 68: 363-368.

7. Ahles TA, Yunus MB, Gaulier B et al. The use of contemporary MMPI norms in the study of chronic pain patients. Pain 1986; 24: 159-163.

8. Ahles TA, Yunus MB, Riley SD et al. Psychological factors associated with primary fibromyalgia syndrome. Arthritis Rheum 1984; 27: 1101-1106.

9. Airaksinen O, Vanninen E, Herno A et al. Decrease in regional cerebral perfusion in fibromyalgia. In: Abstracts of the 9th World Congress on Pain. Seattle: IASP Press; 1999: 43.

10. Alagiri M, Chottiner S, Ratner V et al. Interstitial cystitis: unexplained associations with other chronic disease and pain syndromes. Urology 1997; 49: 52-57.

11. Alberts KR, Bradley LA, Alarcon GS et al. Sertraline hydrochloride alters pain threshold, sensory discrimination ability, and functional brain activity in patients with fibromyalgia (FM): a randomized, controlled trial (RCT). Arthritis Rheum 1998; 41: S259.

12. Alfano AP, Taylor AG, Foresman PA et al. Static magnetic fields for treatment of fibromyalgia: a randomized controlled trial. J Altern Complement Med 2001; 7: 53-64.

13. Alnigenis MNY, Bradfley JD, Wallick J et al. Massage therapy in the management of fibromyalgia: a pilot study. J Musculoskel Pain 2001; 9: 55-67.

14. Ambrogio N, Cuttiford J, Lineker S et al. A comparison of three types of neck support in fibromyalgia patients. Arthritis Care Res 1998; 11: 405-410.

15. American Psychiatric Association. Diagnostic and Statistical Manual of Mental Disorders, Fourth Edition, Text Revision. Washington, DC: American Psychiatric Association; 2000.

16. Ammer K, Melnizky P. Medicinal baths for treatment of generalized fibromyalgia. Forsch Komplementarmed 1999; 6; 80-85.

17. And AKK, Schanberg L. Juvenile fibromyalgia syndrome. Curr Rheumatol Rep 2001; 3; 165-171

18. Anderberg UM, Marteinsdottir I, von Knorring L. Citalopram in patients with fibromyalgia – a randomized, double-blind, placebo-controlled study. Eur J Pain 2000; 4: 27-35.

19. Anonymous. Acupuncture. NIH Consensus Statement 1997; 15: 1-34.

20. Arnett FC, Edworthy SM, Bloch DA et al. The American Rheumatism Association 1987 revised criteria for the classification of rheumatoid arthritis 1988; 31: 315-324.

21. Arnold LM, Hess EV, Hudson JI et al. A randomized, placebo-controlled, double-blind, flexible-dose study of fluoxetine in the treatment of women with fibromyalgia. Am J Med 2002; 112: 191-197.

22. Arnold LM, Keck PE Jr, Welge JA. Antidepressant treatment of fibromyalgia. A meta-analysis and review. Psychosomatics 2000; 41: 104-113.

23. Arnold LM, Lu Y, Crofford LJ et al. A double-blind, multicenter trial comparing duloxetine with placebo in the treatment of fibromyalgia patients with or without major depressive disorder. Arthritis Rheum 2004; 50: 2974-84.

24. Arnold LM, Rosen A, Pritchett YL et al. A randomized, double-blind, placebo-controlled trial of duloxetine in the treatment of women with fibromyalgia with or without major depressive disorder. Pain. 2005;119:5-15.

25. Arroyo JF, Cohen ML. Abnormal responses to electrocutaneous stimulation in fibromyalgia. J Rheumatol 1993; 20: 1925-1931.

26. Azad KA, Alam MN, Haq SA et al. Vegetarian diet in the treatment of fibromyalgia. Bangladesh Med Res Counc Bull 2000; 26: 41-47.

27. Backman E, Bengtsson A, Bengtsson M et al. Skeletal muscle function in primary fibromyalgia. Effect of regional sympathetic blockade with guanethidine. Acta Neurol Scand 1988; 77: 187-191.

28. Bailey A, Starr L, Alderson M, Moreland J. A comparative evaluation of a fibromyalgia rehabilitation program. Arthritis Care Res 1999; 12: 336-340.

29. Balfour W. Observations, with cases illustrative of a new, simple and expeditious mode of curing rheumatism and sprains. J & C Muirhead, Edinburgh, 1816; 110.

30. Bannwarth B. Risk-benefit assessment of opioids in chronic non-cancer pain. Drug Saf 1999; 21: 283-296.

31. Barbour C. Use of complementary and alternative treatments by individuals with fibromyalgia syndrome. J Am Acad Nurse Pract 2000; 12: 311-316.

32. Bendtsen L, Norregaard J, Jensen R et al. Evidence of qualitatively altered nociception in patients with fibromyalgia. Arthritis Rheum 1997; 40: 98-102.

33. Bengtsson A, Henriksson KG, Jorfeldt L et al. Primary fibromyalgia. A clinical and laboratory study of 55 patients. Scand J Rheumatol 1986; 15: 340-347.

34. Bengtsson A, Henriksson KG, Larsson J. Reduced high-energy phosphate levels in the painful muscles of patients with primary fibromyalgia. Arthritis Rheum 1986; 29: 817-821.

35. Bennett R, DeGarmo P, Clark S. A 1 year double-blind, placebo-controlled study of guaifenesin in fibromyalgia. Arthritis Rheum 1996; 39: S212.

36. Bennett RM, Burckhardt CS, Clark SR et al. Group treatment of fibromyalgia: a 6 month outpatient program. J Rheumatol 1996; 23: 521-528.

37. Bennett RM, Clark SR, Campbell SM et al. Low levels of somatomedin C in patients with the fibromyalgia syndrome: a possible link between sleep and muscle pain. Arthritis Rheum 1992; 35: 1113-1116.

38. Bennett RM, Clark SR, Walczyk J. A randomized, double-blind, placebo-controlled study of growth hormone in the treatment of fibromyalgia. Am J Med 1998; 104: 227-231.

39. Bennett RM, Gatter RA, Campbell SM et al. A comparison of cyclobenzaprine and placebo in the management of fibrositis. A double-blind controlled study. Arthritis Rheum 1988; 31: 1535-1542.

40. Bennett RM. Confounding features of the fibromyalgia syndrome: a current perspective of differential diagnosis. J Rheumatol 1989; 16(suppl 19): 58-61.

41. Bennett RM. Emerging concepts in the neurobiology of chronic pain: evidence of abnormal sensory processing in fibromyalgia. Mayo Clin Proc 1999; 74: 385-398.

42. Bennett RM. Fibromyalgia and the disability dilemma. A new era in understanding a complex, multidimensional pain syndrome. Arthritis Rheum 1996; 39: 1627-1643.

43. Bennett RM. Fibrositis: misnomer for a common rheumatic disorder. West J Medicine 1981; 134: 405-413.

44. Bennett RM. Pharmacological treatment of fibromyalgia. J Functional Syndromes 2001; 1: 79-92.

45. Bennett RM. Physical fitness and muscle metabolism in the fibromyalgia syndrome: an overview. J Rheumatol 1989; 16(suppl 19): 28-29.

46. Bennett RM. The contribution of muscle to the generation of fibromyalgia symptomatology. J Musculoskeletal Pain 1996; 4: 35-39.

47. Bennett, RM. Fibromyalgia. In: Wall PD, Melzack R eds. Textbook of Pain. Fourth ed. Edinburgh: Churchill Livingston; 1999; 579-601.

48. Berg AM, Naides SJ, Simms RW. Established fibromyalgia and parvovirus B19 infection. J Rheumatol 1993; 20: 1941-1943.

49. Berman BM, Ezzo J, Hadhazy V et al. Is acupuncture effective in the treatment of fibromyalgia? J Fam Pract 1999; 48: 213-218.

50. Bessette L, Carette S, Fossel AH et al. A placebo controlled crossover trial of subcutaneous salmon calcitonin in the treatment of patients with fibromyalgia. Scand J Rheumatol 1998; 27: 112-116.

51. Biasi G, Manca S, Manganelli S et al. Tramadol in the fibromyalgia syndrome. Int J Clin Pharmacol Res 1998; 18: 13-19.

52. Blunt KL, Rajwani MH, Guerriero RC. The effectiveness of chiropractic management of fibromyalgia patients: a pilot study. J Manipulative Physiol Ther 1997; 20: 389-399.

53. Boisset-Pioro MH, Esdaile JM, Fitzcharles MA. Sexual and physical abuse in women with fibromyalgia syndrome. Arthritis Rheum 1995; 38: 235-241.

54. Bonafede RP, Downey DC, Bennett RM. An association of fibromyalgia with primary Sjogren's syndrome: A prospective study of 72 patients. J Rheumatol 1995; 22: 133-136.

55. Borenstein D. Prevalence and treatment outcome of primary and secondary fibromyalgia in patients with spinal pain. Spine 1995; 20: 796-800.

56. Bradley LA, Alarcon GS, Triana M et al. Health care seeking behavior in fibromyalgia: associations with pain thresholds, symptom severity, and psychiatric morbidity. J Musculoskel Pain 1994; 2: 79-87.

57. Bradley LA, Sotolongo A, Alberts KR et al. Abnormal regional cerebral blood flow in the caudate nucleus among fibromyalgia patients and non-patients is associated with insidious symptom onset. J Muscloskel Pain 1999; 7: 285-292.

58. Brattberg G. Connective tissue massage in the treatment of fibromyalgia. Eur J Pain 1999; 3: 235-244.

59. Buchwald D, Bombardier C. Disability and health care utilization in patients with chronic fatigue

and chronic fatigue syndrome. Med Care 1996; 34: 924-930.

60. Buckelew SP, Conway R, Parker J et al. Biofeedback/relaxation training and exercise interventions for fibromyalgia: a prospective trial. Arthritis Care Res 1998; 11: 196-209.

61. Burckhardt CS, Bjelle A. Education programmes for fibromyalgia patients: description and evaluation. Ballieres Best Pract Res Clin Rheumatol 1994; 8: 935-955.

62. Busch A, Schachter C, Peloso P et al. Exercise for treating fibromyalgia syndrome. The Cochrane Library. Oxford: Update Software, 2002.

63. Buskila D, Abu-Shakra M, Neumann L et al. Balneotherapy for fibromyalgia at the Dead Sea. Rheumatol Int 2001; 20: 105-108.

64. Buskila D, Neumann L, Alhoashie A et al. Fibromyalgia syndrome in men. Semin Arthritis Rheum 2000; 30: 47-51.

65. Buskila D, Neumann L, Hozanov I et al. Familial aggregation in the fibromyalgia syndrome. Semin Arthritis Rheum 1996; 26: 605-611.

66. Buskila D, Neumann L, Odes LR et al. The prevalence of musculoskeletal pain and fibromyalgia in patients hospitalized on internal medicine wards. Semin Arthritis Rheum 2001; 30: 411-417.

67. Buskila D, Neumann L. Fibromyalgia syndrome (FM) and nonarticular tenderness in relatives of patients with FM. J Rheumatol 1997; 24: 941-944.

68. Buskila D, Shnaider A, Newmann L et al. Musculoskeletal manifestations and autoantibody profile in 90 hepatitis C virus infected Israeli patients. Semin Arthritis Rheum 1998; 28: 107-113.

69. Cada DJ, Levien T, Baker DE. Pregabalin. Hospital Pharmacy 2006; 41: 157-172.

70. Campbell SM, Clark S, Tindall EA et al. Clinical characteristics of fibrositis. I. A "blinded" controlled study of symptoms and tender points. Arthritis Rheum 1983; 26: 817-824.

71. Carette S, Bell MJ, Reynolds WJ et al. Comparison of amitriptyline, cyclobenzaprine, and placebo in the treatment of fibromyalgia. A randomized, double-blind clinical trial. Arthritis Rheum 1994; 37: 32-40.

72. Carette S, McCain GA, Bell DA et al. Evaluation of amitriptyline in primary fibrositis: a double-blind, placebo-controlled study. Arthritis Rheum 1986; 29: 655-659.

73. Carli G, Suman AL, Biasi G et al. Reactivity to superficial and deep stimuli in patients with chronic musculoskeletal pain. Pain 2002; 100: 259-269.

74. Carmona L, Ballina J, Gabriel R et al. The burden of musculoskeletal diseases in the general population of Spain: results from a national study. Ann Rheum Dis 2001; 60: 1040-1045.

75. Chaiamnuay P, Darmawan J, Muirden KD et al. Epidemiology of rheumatic disease in rural Thailand: a WHO-ILAR COPCORD study. Community Oriented Programme for the control of Rheumatic Disease. J Rheumatol 1998; 25: 1382-1387.

76. Chambless DL, Baker MJ, Baucom DH et al. Update on empirically validated therapies, II. Clin Psychol 1998; 51: 3-16.

77. Chang L, Mayer EA, Johnson T et al. Differences in somatic perception in female patients with irritable bowel syndrome with and without fibromyalgia. Pain 2000; 84: 297-307.

78. Chun A, Desauteis S, Silvka A et al. Visceral algesia in irritable bowel syndrome, fibromyalgia, and sphincter of Oddi dysfunction, type III. Dig Dis Sci 1999; 44: 631-636.

79. Clark P, Burgos-Vargas R, Medina-Palma C et al. Prevalence of fibromyalgia in children: a clinical study of Mexican children. J Rheumatol 1998; 25: 2009-2014.

80. Clark S, Tindall E, Bennett RM. A double blind crossover trial of prednisone versus placebo in the treatment of fibrositis. J Rheumatol 1985; 12: 980-983.

81. Clauw DJ, Schmidt M, Radulovic D et al. The relationship between fibromyalgia and interstitial cystitis. J Psychiatr Res 1997; 31: 125-131.

82. Cohen H, Buskila D, Neumann L et al. Confirmation of an association between fibromyalgia and serotonin transporter promoter region (5-HTTLPR) polymorphism, and relationship to anxiety-related personality traits. Arthritis Rheum 2002; 46: 845-847.

83. Cohen H, Neumann L, Alhosshle A et al. Abnormal sympathovagal balance in men with fibromyalgia. J Rheumatol 2001; 28: 217-227.

84. Cohen H, Neumann L, Shore M et al. Autonomic dysfunction in patients with fibromyalgia: application of power spectral analysis of heart rate variability. Semin Arthritis Rheum 2000; 29: 217-227.

85. Cohen ML. Is fibromyalgia a distinct clinical entity? The disapproving rheumatologist's evidence. Baillieres Best Pract Res Clin Rheumatol 1999; 13: 421-425.

86. Colbert AP, Markov MS, Banerji M et al. Magnetic mattress pad use in patients with fibromyalgia: a randomized double-blind pilot study. J Back Musculoskeletal Rehabil 1999; 13: 19-31.

87. Cook DB, Lange G, Ciccone DS et al. Functional imaging of pain in patients with primary fibromyalgia. J Rheumatol 2004; 31: 364-378.

88. Cote KA, Moldofksy H. Sleep, daytime symptoms, cognitive performance in patients with fibromyalgia. J Rheumatol 1997; 24: 2014-2023.

89. Coward DM. Tizanidine: neuropharmacology and mechanism of action. Neurology 1994; 44: S6-10.

90. Crofford LJ, Appleton BE. Complementary and alternative therapies for fibromyalgia. Curr Rheumatol Rep 2001; 3: 147-156.

91. Crofford LJ, Pillemer SR, Kalogeras KT et al. Hypothalamic-pituitary-adrenal axis perturbations in patients with fibromyalgia. Arthritis Rheum 1994; 37: 1583-1592.

92. Crofford LJ, Rowbotham MC, Mease PJ et al. Pregabalin for the treatment of fibromyalgia syndrome: results of a randomized, double-blind, placebo-controlled trial. Arthritis Rheum 2005; 52: 1264-1273.

93. Crofford LJ, Simpson S, Young JP et al. A six-month, double-blind, placebo-controlled, durability of effect study of pregabalin for pain associated with fibromyalgia. Oasis-Online Abstract Submission and Invitation System 2005. 4 November 2006 <www.abstractsonline.com/viewer/SearchResults.asp>

94. Croft P, Burt J, Schollum J et al. More pain, more tender points: is fibromyalgia just one end of a continuous spectrum? Ann Rheum Dis 1996; 55: 482-485.

95. Croft P, Rigby AS, Boswell R et al. The prevalence of chronic widespread pain in the general population. J Rheumatol 1993; 20: 710-713.

96. Croft P, Schollum J, Silman A. Population study of tender point counts and pain as evidence of fibromyalgia. BMJ 1994; 309: 696-699.

97. Culclasure TF, Enzenauer RJ, West SG. Post-traumatic stress disorder presenting as fibromyalgia. Am J Med 1993; 94: 548-549.

98. Darmawan J, Valkenbug HA, Muirden KD et al. Epidemiology of rheumatic diseases in rural and urban populations in Indonesia: a World Health Organization International league against rheumatism COPCORD Study, Stage I, Phase 2. Ann Rheum Dis 1992; 51: 525-528.

99. De Stefano R, Selvi E, Villanova M et al. Image analysis quantification of substance P immunoreactivity in the trapezius muscle of patients with fibromyalgia and myofascial pain syndrome. J Rheumatol 2000; 27: 2906-2010.

100. DeBlecourt AC, Knipping AA, DeVoogd N et al. Weather conditions and complaints in fibromyalgia. J Rheumatol 1993; 20: 1932-1934

101. Deluze C, Bosia L, Zirbs A et al. Electroacupuncture in fibromyalgia: results of a controlled trial. Br Med J 1992; 305: 1249-1252.

102. Dessein PH, Shipton EA, Stanwix AE et al. Neuroendocrine deficiency-mediated development and persistence of pain in fibromyalgia: a promising paradigm? Pain 2000; 86: 213-215.

103. Deyo RA. Drug therapy for back pain. Which drugs help which patients? Spine 1996; 21: 2840-2849, discussion 2849-2850.

104. Di Piero V, Jones AKP, Iannotti F et al. Chronic pain: a PET study of the central effects of percutaneous high cervical cordotomy. Pain 1991; 46: 9-12.

105. Dinerman H, Goldenberg DL, Felson DT. A prospective evaluation of 118 patients with the fibromyalgia syndrome: prevalence of Raynaud's phenomenon, sicca symptoms, ANA, low complement, and Ig deposition at the dermal-epidermal junction. J Rheumatol 1986; 13: 368-373.

106. Dinerman H, Steere AC. Lyme disease associated with fibromyalgia. Ann Intern Med 1992; 117: 281-285.

107. Dohrenbusch R, Gruterich M, Genth E. Fibromyalgia and Sjogren syndrome – clinical and methodological aspects. J Rheumatol 1996; 55: 19-27

108. Donald F, Esdaile JM, Kimoff JR et al. Musculoskeletal complaints and fibromyalgia in patients attending a respiratory sleep disorders clinic. J Rheumatol 1996; 23: 1612-1616.

109. Drewes AM, Andreasen A, Jennum P et al. Zopiclone in the treatment of sleep abnormalities in fibromyalgia. Scand J Rheumatol 1991; 20: 288-293.

110. Drewes AM, Gade K, Nielson KD et al. Clustering of sleep electroencephalographic patterns in patients with the fibromyalgia syndrome. Br J Rheumatol 1995; 34: 1151-1156.

111. Dwight MD, Arnold LM, O'Brien H et al. An open clinical trial of venlafaxine treatment of fibromyalgia. Psychosomatics 1998; 39: 14-17.

112. Edwards AM, Blackburn L, Christie S et al. Food supplements in the treatment of primary fibromyalgia: a double-blind, crossover trial of anthocyanidins and placebo. J Nutr Environ Med 2000; 10: 189-199.

113. Edwards PW, Zeichner A, Kuczmierczyk AR et al. Familial pain models: the relationship between family history of pain and current pain experience. Pain 1985; 21: 379-384.

114. Elert J, Kendall SA, Jarsson B et al. Chronic pain and difficulty in relaxing postural muscles in patients with fibromyalgia and chronic whiplash associated disorders. J Rheumatol 2001; 28: 1361-1368.

115. Elert JE, Dahlqvist SR, Alamary B, Eismann M. Muscle endurance, muscle tension, and personality traits in patients with muscle of joint pain – a pilot study. J Rheumatol 1995; 20: 1550-1556.

116. Elert JE, Rantapaa-Dahlqvist SB, Henriksson-Larsen K et al. Muscle performance, electromyography and fibre type composition in fibromyalgia

and work-related myalgia. Scand J Rheumatol 1992; 21: 28-34.

117. Epstein SA, Kay G, Clauw D et al. Psychiatric disorders in patients with fibromyalgia. A multicenter investigation. Psychosomatics. 1999; 40: 57-63.

118. Farber L, Startz T, Bruckle W et al. Effiacacy and tolerability of tropisetron in primary fibromyalgia – a highly selective and competitive 5-HT$_3$ receptor antagonist. German Fibromyalgia Study Group. Scand J Rheumatol 2000; 113: 49-54.

119. Farber L, Startz TH, Bruckle W et al. Short-term treatment of primary fibromyalgia with the 5-HT$_3$-receptor antagonist tropisetron. Results of a randomized, double-blind, placebo-controlled multicenter trial in 418 patients. Int J Clin Pharmacol Res 2001; 21: 1-13.

120. Farooqi A, Gibson T. Prevalence of the major rheumatic disorders in the adult population of north Pakistan. Br J Rheumatol 1998; 37: 491-495.

121. Fassbender HG. Pathology of rheumatic disease. New York: Springer Verlag; 1975

122. Feldman D, Mariano E. Treatment of fibromyalgia with acupuncture: a randomized, placebo controlled trial of 16 weeks duration (abstract 91). American College of Rheumatology Meeting. November 2001.

123. Felson DT, Goldenberg DL. The natural history of fibromyalgia. Arthritis Rheum 1986; 29: 1522-1526.

124. Ferraccioli G, Ghirelli L, Scita F et al. EMG-biofeedback training in fibromyalgia syndrome. J Rheumatol 1987; 14: 820-825.

125. Fetrow CW, Avila JR. Efficacy of the dietary supplement S-adenosyl-L-methionine. Ann Pharmacother 2001; 35: 1414-1425.

126. Fisher P, Greenwood A, Juskisson EC et al. Effect of homeopathic treatment on fibrositis (primary fibromyalgia). Br Med J 1989; 299: 365-366.

127. Fitzcharles, MA. Is fibromyalgia a distinct clinical entity? The approving rheumatologist's evidence. Baillieres Best Pract Res Clin Rheumatol 1999; 13: 437-443.

128. Fors EA, Sexton H, Gotestam KG. The effect of guided imagery and amitriptyline on daily fibromyalgia pain: a prospective, randomized, controlled trial. J Psychiatr Res 2002; 36: 179-187.

129. Forseth KO, Gran JT, Husby G. A population study of the incidence of fibromyalgia among women aged 26-55 years. Br J Rheumatol 1997; 36: 1318-1323.

130. Forseth KO, Gran JT. The prevalence of fibromyalgia among women aged 20-49 years in Arendal, Norway. Scand J Rheumatol 1992; 21: 74-78.

131. Fryda-Kaurimsky Z, Muller-Fassbender H. Tizanidine (DS 103-282) in the treatment of acute paravertebral muscle spasm: a controlled trial comparing tizanidine and diazepam. J Int Med Res 1981; 9: 501-505.

132. Gallinaro AL, Feldman D, Natour J. An evaluation of the association between fibromyalgia and repetitive strain injuries in metalworkers on an industry in Guarulhos, Brazil. Joint Bone Spine 2001; 68: 59-64.

133. Gedalia A, Press J, Klein M et al. Joint hypermobility and fibromyalgia in schoolchildren. Ann Rheum Dis 1993; 52: 494-496.

134. Gendreau RM, Thorn MD, Gendreau JF et al. Efficacy of milnacipran in patients with fibromyalgia. J Rheumatol. 2005 32:1975-85.

135. Gibson JJ, Littlejohn GO, Gorman MM et al. Altered heat pain thresholds and cerebral event-related potential following painful CO_2 laser stimulation in subjects with fibromyalgia syndrome. Pain 1994; 58: 185-193.

136. Glass JM, Park DC. Cognitive dysfunction in fibromyalgia. Curr Rheumatol Rep 2001; 3: 123-127.

137. Goldberg RT, Pachas WN, Keith D. Relationship between traumatic events in childhood and chronic pain. Disability Rehab 1999; 21: 23-30.

138. Goldberg RT. Childhood abuse, depression, and chronic pain. Clin J Pain 1994; 10: 277-281.

139. Goldenberg DL, Felson DT, Dinerman H. A randomized, controlled trial of amitriptyline and naproxen in the treatment of patients with fibromyalgia. Arthritis Rheum 1986; 29: 1371-1377.

140. Goldenberg DL, Kaplan KH, Nadeau MG. A controlled study of stress-reduction, cognitive-behavioral treatment program in fibromyalgia. J Musculoskel Pain 1994; 2: 53-65.

141. Goldenberg DL, Mayskly M, Mossey CJ et al. A randomized double-blind crossover trial of fluoxetine and amitriptyline in the treatment of fibromyalgia. Arthritis Rheum 1996; 39: 1852-1859.

142. Goldenberg DL. Do infections trigger fibromyalgia? Arthritis Rheum 1993; 36: 1489-1492.

143. Goldenberg DL. Fibromyalgia syndrome a decade later: what have we learned? Arch Intern Med 1999; 1999: 777-785.

144. Goldenberg DL. Fibromyalgia syndrome. An emerging but controversial condition. JAMA 1987; 257: 2782-2787.

145. Goldenberg DL. Fibromyalgia: why such controversy? Ann Rheum Dis 1995; 54: 3-5.

146. Gonzalez VM, Goeppinger J, Lorig K. Four psychosocial theories and their application to patient education and clinical practice. Arthritis Care Res 1990; 3: 132-143.

147.Gowans SE, deHueck A, Voss S et al. A randomized, controlled trial of exercise and education
for individuals with fibromyalgia. Arthritis Care
Res 1999; 12: 120-128.

148.Gowers WR. Lumbago: its lessons and analogues.
BMJ 1904; 1:117-121.

149.Grace CM, Nielson WR, Hopkins M e al. Concentration and memory deficits in patients with
fibromyalgia syndrome. J Clin Exp Neuropsychol
1999; 21: 477-487.

150.Gracely RH, Petzke F, Wolf JM et al. Functional
magnetic resonance imaging evidence of aug-
mented pain processing in fibromyalgia. Arthritis
Rheum 2002; 46: 1333-1343.

151. Granges G, Littlejohn G. Pressure pain threshold
in pain-free subjects, in patients with chronic regional pain syndromes, and in patients with
fibromyalgia syndrome. Arthritis Rheum 1993; 36:
642-646.

152.Granges G, Littlejohn GO. A comparative study
of clinical signs in fibromyalgia/fibrositis syndrome, healthy and exercising subjects. J
Rheumatol 1993; 20: 344-351.

153. Granges G, Zilko P, Littlejohn GO. Fibromyalgia
syndrome: assessment of the severity of the condition 2 years after diagnosis. J Rheumatol 1997;
36: 1318-1323.

154.Graven-Nielsen T, Aspergren Kendall S,
Henriksson KG et al. Ketamine reduces muscle
pain, temporal summation, and referred pain in
fibromyalgia patients. Pain 2000; 85: 483-491.

155. Greenfield S, Fitzcharles MA, Esdaile JM. Reactive fibromyalgia syndrome. Arthritis Rheum 1992;
35: 678-681.

156.Griep EN, Boersma JW, deKloet ER. Altered reactivity of the hypothalamic-pituitary-adrenal axis
in the primary fibromyalgia syndrome. J Rheumatol
1993; 20: 469-474.

157.Guedj D, Weinberger A. Effect of weather conditions on rheumatic patients. Ann Rheum Dis 1990;
49: 158-159.

158.Haanen HCM, Hoenderdos HTW, van Romunde
LKJ et al. Controlled trial of hypnotherapy in the
treatment of refractory fibromyalgia. J Rheumatol
1991; 18: 72-75.

159. Hadhazy VA, Ezzo J, Creamer P et al. Mind-body
therapies for the treatment of fibromyalgia. A systematic review. J Rheumatol 2000; 27: 2911-2918.

160.Hagglund KJ, Deuser WE, Buckelew SP et al.
Weather, beliefs about weather, and disease se-
verity among patients with fibromyalgia. Arthritis
Care Res 1994; 7: 130-135.

161. Hanninen O, Kaariten K, Rauma A et al. Antioxi-
dants in vegan diet and rheumatic disorders. Toxi-
cology 2000; 155: 45-53.

162.Hannonen P, Malminiemi K, Yli-Kerttula U et al.
A randomized, double-blind, placebo-controlled
study of moclobemide and amitriptyline in the
treatment of fibromyalgia in females without psychiatric disorder. Br J Rheumatol 1998; 37: 1279-
1286.

163.Harvey CK. Fibromyalgia. Part II. Prevalence in
the podiatric patient population. Journal Am Podiatric Med Assoc 1993; 83: 416-417.

164.Haugen M, Kjeldsen-Kragh J, Nordvag BY et al.
Diet and disease symptoms in rheumatic diseases
– results of a questionnaire based study. Clin
Rheumatol 1991; 10: 401-407.

165.Hauri P, Hawkins DR. Alpha-delta sleep.
Electroencephalogr Clin Neurophysiol 1973; 34:
233-237.

166.Hawley DJ, Wolfe F, Cathey MA. Pain, functional
disability, and psychological status: a 12-month
study of severity in fibromyalgia. J Rheumatol
1988; 15: 1551-1556.

167.Hawley DJ, Wolfe F. Pain, disability, and pain/
disability relationships in seven rheumatic disorders: a study of 1,522 patients. J Rheumatol 1991;
10: 1552-1557.

168.Helleday U. Om myitis chronica (rheumatica). Ett
bidrag till dess diagnostic och behandling. Nord
Med Ark 1976; 8: 1-17.

169.Henriksson CM. Living with continuous muscular
pain – patient perspectives. Part I: Encounters
and consequences. Scand J Caring Sci 1995; 9:
67-76.

170.Henriksson CM. Longterm effects of fibromyalgia
on everyday life. A study of 56 patients. Scand J
Rheumatol 1994; 23: 36-41.

171. Henriksson KG. Is fibromyalgia a distinct clinical
entity? Pain mechanisms in fibromyalgia syndrome. A myologist's view. Baillieres Best Pract
Res Clin Rheumatol 1999; 13: 455-461.

172.Heymann RE, Helfenstein M, Feldman D. A
double-blinded, randomized, controlled study of
amitriptyline, nortriptyline and placebo in patients
with fibromyalgia. An analysis of outcome measures. Clin Exp Rheumatol 2001; 19: 697-702.

173.Ho M, Moreland J, Walker S et al. A comparison
randomized single-blind comparison of a supervised and unsupervised aerobic exercise regime
for patients with fibromyalgia. Br J Rheumatol
1998; 37: 27.

174.Hochberg MC. Updating the American College
of Rheumatology revised criteria for the classification of systemic lupus erythematosus [letter].
Arthritis Rheum 1997; 40: 1725.

175.Holdcraft LC, Assefi N, Buchwald D. Complementary and alternative medicine in fibromyalgia
and related syndromes. Best Pract Res Clin
Rheumatol 2003; 17: 667-683.

176.Hsu VM, Patella SJ, Sigal LH. 'Chronic Lyme disease' as the incorrect diagnosis in patients with fibromyalgia. Arthritis Rheum 1993; 36: 1493-1500.

177.Hudson JI, Goldenberg DL, Pope HG Jr et al. Comorbidity of fibromyalgia with medical and psychiatric disorders. Am J Med 1992; 92: 363-367.

178.Hudson JI, Pope HG Jr. Does childhood sexual abuse cause fibromyalgia? Arthritis Rheum 1995; 38: 161-163.

179.Hudson JI, Pope HG Jr. The relationship between fibromyalgia and major depressive disorder. Rheum Dis Clin N Am 1996; 22: 285-303.

180.Iadarola MJ, Max MD, Berman KF et al. Unilateral decrease in thalamic activity observed with position emission tomography in patients with chronic neuropathic pain. Pain 1995; 63: 55-64.

181.Jacobsen S, Danneskiold-Samsoe B, Andersen RB. Oral S-adenosylmethionine in primary fibromyalgia: a double-blind clinical evaluation. Scand J Rheumatol 1991; 20: 294-302.

182.Jacobsen S, Danneskiold-Samsoe B. Dynamic muscular endurance in primary fibromyalgia compared with chronic myofascial pain syndrome. Arch Phys Med Rehabil 1992; 73: 170-173.

183.Jacobsen S, Danneskiold-Samsoe B. Isometric and isokinetic muscle strength in patients with fibrositis syndrome. New characteristics for a difficult definable category of patients. Scand J Rheumatol 1987; 16: 61-65.

184.Jacobsen S, Jensen KE, Thomsen C et al. 31P magnetic resonance spectroscopy of skeletal muscle in patients with fibromyalgia. J Rheumatol 1992; 19; 1600-1603.

185.Jacobsen S, Jjensen KE, Thomsen C et al. [Magnetic resonance spectroscopy in fibromyalgia. A study of phosphate-31 spectra from skeletal muscles during rest and after exercise]. Ugeskr Laeger 1994; 156: 6841-6844.

186.Jacobsen S, Petersen IS, Danneskiold-Samsoe B. Clinical features in patients with chronic muscle pain – with special reference to fibromyalgia. Scand J Rheumatol 1993; 22: 69-76.

187.Jacobsen S, Wildschiodtz G, Danneskiold-Samsoe B. Isokinetic and isometric muscle strength combined with transcutaneous electrical muscle stimulation in primary fibromyalgia syndrome. J Rheumatol 1991; 18: 1390-1393.

188.Jacobsson L, Lindgarde F, Manthorpe R. The commonest rheumatic complaints of over six weeks' duration in a twelve-month period in a defined Swedish population. Prevalences and relationships. Scand J Rheumatol 1989; 18: 353-360.

189.Jaeschke R, Adachi J, Guyatt G, Keller J, Wong B. Clinical usefulness of amitriptyline in fibromyalgia: the results of 23 N-of-1 randomized controlled trials. J Rheumatol 1991; 18: 447-451.

190.Jentoft ES, Kvalvik AG, Mengshoel AM. Effects of pool-based and land-based aerobic exercise on women with fibromyalgia/chronic widespread muscle pain. Arthritis Rheum 2001; 45: 42-47.

191.Jubrias SA, Bennett RM, Klug GA. Increased incidence of a resonance in the phosphodiester region of 31P nuclear magnetic resonance spectra in the skeletal muscle of fibromyalgia patients. Arthritis Rheum 1994; 37: 801-807.

192.Kaartinen K, Lammi K, Hypen M et al. Vegan diet alleviates fibromyalgia symptoms. Scand J Rheumatol 2000; 29: 308-313.

193.Kameyama T, Nabeshma T, Matsuno K et al. Comparison of alpha-adrenoreceptor involvement in the antinociceptive action of tizanidine and clonidine in the mouse. Eur J Pharmacol 1986; 125: 257-264.

194.Kanner RM, Foley KM. Patterns of narcotic drug use in a cancer pain clinic. Ann N Y Acad Sci 1981; 362: 161-172.

195.Kaplan KH, Goldenberg DL, Galvin-Nadeau M. The impact of a meditation-based stress reduction program on fibromyalgia. Gen Hosp Psychiatry 1993; 15: 284-289.

196.Kazis LE, Meenan RF, Anderson JJ. Pain in the rheumatic diseases: investigations of a key health status component. Arthritis Rheum 1983; 26: 1017-1022.

197.Keel PJ, Bodoky C, Gerhard U et al. comparison of integrated group therapy and group relaxation training for fibromyalgia. Clin J Pain 1998; 14: 232-238.

198.Kellgren JH. Observations on referred pain arising from muscle. Clin Sci 1938; 3: 175-190.

199.Kemp P, Nielsen HV, Korsgard J et al. Blood flow in fibromyotic muscles. Scand J Rehabil Med 1982; 14: 81-86.

200.Kennedy M, Felson DT. A prospective long-term study of fibromyalgia syndrome. Arthritis Rheum 1996; 39: 682-685.

201.Kosek E Hansson P. Modulatory influence on somatosensory perception from vibration and heterotopic noxious conditioning stimulation (HNCS) in fibromyalgia patients and healthy subjects. Pain 1997; 70: 41-51.

202.Kosek E, Ekholm J, Hansson P. Increased pressure pain sensibility in fibromyalgia patients is located deep to skin but not restricted to muscle tissue. Pain 1995; 63: 335-339.

203.Kosek E, Ekholm J, Hansson P. Modulations of pressure pain thresholds during and following isometric contraction in patients with fibromyalgia and in healthy controls. Pain 1996a; 64: 415-423.

204.Kosek E, Ekholm J, Hansson P. Sensory dysfunction in fibromyalgia patients with implications for pathogenic mechanisms. Pain 1996; 68: 375-383.

205.Kurtze N, Gundersen KT, Svebak S. Quality of life, functional disability and lifestyle among sub-groups of fibromyalgia patients: the significance of anxiety and depression. Br J Med Psychol 1999; 72: 471-484.

206.Kurtze N, Gunderson KT, Svebak S. The role of anxiety and depression in fatigue and patterns of pain among subgroups of fibromyalgia patients. Br J Med Psychol 1998; 71: 185-194.

207.Kwiatek R, Barnden L, Rowe S. Pontine tegmental regional cerebral blood flow is reduced in fibromyalgia. Arthritis Rheum 1997; 40: S43.

208.Landis CA, Lentz MJ, Rothermel J et al. De-creased nocturnal levels of prolactin and growth hormone in women with fibromyalgia. J Clin Endocrinol Metab 2001; 86: 11-20.

209.Landro NI, Stiles TC, Sletvold H. Memory func-tioning in patients with primary fibromyalgia and major depression and healthy controls. J Psychosom Res 1997; 42: 297-306.

210.Larson AA, Glovengo SL, Russell U et al. Changes in the concentrations of amino acids in the cere-brospinal fluid that correlate with pain in patients with fibromyalgia: Implications for nitric oxide pathways. Pain 2000; 87: 201-211.

211. Lautenbacher S, Rollman GB, McCain GA. Multi-method assessment of experimental and clinical-pain in patients with fibromyalgia. Pain 1994; 59: 45-53.

212.Lautenbacher S, Rollman GB. Possible deficien-cies of pain modulation in fibromyalgia. Clin J Pain 1997; 13: 189-196.

213.Lautenschalager J, Bruckle W, Schorrenberger CC et al. Die Messung von Druckschmerzen im Bereichvon Sehen und Muskeln bei Gesuden und Patienten mit generalisierter Tendomyopathie (Fibromyalgie-Syndrom). Z Rheumatol 1988; 47: 397-404.

214.Le Bars D, Dickenson AH, Besson JM. Diffuse noxious inhibitory controls (DNIC). I. Effects on dorsal horn convergent neurons in the rat. Pain 1979; 6: 283-304.

215.Le Bars D, Dickenson AH, Besson JM. Diffuse noxious inhibitory controls (DNIC). II. Lack of effect on non-convergent neurons, supraspinal involvement and theoretical implications. Pain 1979; 6: 305-327.

216.Leal-Cerro A, Povedano J, Astorga R et al. the growth hormone (GH)- releasing hormone-GH-insulin-like growth factor-I axis in patients with fibromyalgia syndrome. J Clin Endocrinol Metab 1999; 84: 3378-3381.

217.Leavitt F, Katz RS. Is the MMPI invalid for as-sessing psychological disturbance in pain related organic conditions? J Rheumatol 1989; 16: 521-526.

218.Lentz MU, Landis CA, Rothermel J et al. Effects of selective slow wave sleep disruption on mus-culoskeletal pain and fatigue in middle aged women. J Rheumatol 1999; 26: 1586-1592.

219.Lester N, Lefebvre JC, Keefe FJ. Pain in young adults: I. Relationship to gender and family pain history. Clin J Pain 1994; 10: 282-289.

220.Lindell L, Bergman S, Petersson IF et al. Preva-lence of fibromyalgia and chronic widespread pain. Scand J Prim Health Care 2000; 18: 149-153.

221.Lindh MH, Johansson LG, Hedberg M et al. Stud-ies on maximal voluntary muscle contraction in patients with fibromyalgia. Arch Phys Med Rehabil 1994; 75: 1217-1222.

222.Lindman R, Eriksson A, Thornell LE. Fiber type composition of the human female trapezius muscle: enzyme-histochemical characteristics. Am J Anat 1991; 190: 385-392.

223.Lindman R, Hagberg M, Angqvist KA et al. Changes in muscle morphology in chronic trape-zius myalgia. Scand J Work Environ Health 1991; 17: 347-355.

224.Lindman R, Hagberg M, Bengtsson A et al. Cap-illary structure and mitochondrial volume density in the normal trapezius muscle and in chronic trapezius myalgia and in fibromyalgia. In: Chronic Trapezius Myalgia – a morphological study. PhD Thesis University of Umea, Sweden 1992.

225.Lindstrom I, Ohlund C, Eek C et al. The effect of graded activity on patients with subacute low back pain: a randomized prospective clinical study with an operant-conditioning behavioral approach. Phys Ther 1992; 72: 279-290.

226.Littlejohn GO. Fibrositis/fibromyalgia syndrome in the workplace. Rheum Dis Clin N Am 1989; 15: 45-60.

227.Lorenz J, Grasedyck K, Bromm B. Middle and long latency somatosensory evoked potentials after painful laser stimulations in patients with fibromyalgia syndrome. Electroencephalogr Clin Neurophysiol 1996; 100: 165-168.

228.Lund N, Bengtsson A, Thorborg P. Muscle tis-sue oxygen pressure in primary fibromyalgia. Scand J Rheumatol 1986; 15: 165-173.

229.Lydell C, Meyers OL. The prevalence of fibromyalgia in a South African community (ab-stract). Scand J Rheumatology 1992; 94 (supple-ment): 8. S143.

230.MacFarlane GJ, Thomas E, Papageorgiou AC et al. The natural history of chronic pain in the com-munity: a better prognosis than in the clinic? J Rheumatol 1996; 23: 1617-1620.

231.Makela M, Heliovaara M. Prevalence of primary fibromyalgia in the Finnish population. BMJ 1991; 303: 216-219.

232. Makela MO. Is fibromyalgia a distinct clinical entity? The epidemiologist's evidence. Baillieres Best Pract Res Clin Rheumatol 1999; 13: 415-419.

233. Mannerkorpi K, Nyberg B, Ahimen M et al. Pool exercise combined with an education program for patients with fibromyalgia syndrome. A prospective, randomized study. J Rheumatol 2000; 27: 2473-2481.

234. Marbach JJ. Medically unexplained chronic orofacial pain. Temporomandibular pain and dysfunction syndrome, orofacial phantom pain, burning mouth syndrome, and trigeminal neuralgia. Med Clin North Am 1999; 83: 691-710.

235. Martin L, Nutting A, MacIntosh BR et al. An exercise program in the treatment of fibromyalgia. J Rheumatol 1996; 23: 1050-1053.

236. Martinez-Lavin M, Hermosillo AG, Mendoza C et al. Orthostatic sympathetic derangement in subjects with fibromyalgia. J Rheumatol 1997; 24: 714-718.

237. Martinez-Lavin M, Hermosillo AG, Rasas M et al. Circadian studies of automatic nervous balance in patients with fibromyalgia: a heart rate variability analysis. Arthritis Rheum 1998; 41: 1966-1971.

238. Mathur AK, Gatter RA. Abnormal 31P-NMR spectroscopy of painful muscles of patients with fibromyalgia. Arthritis Rheum 1988; 31: S23

239. McBeth J, MacFarlane GJ, Benjamin J et al. The association between tender points, psychological distress, and adverse childhood experiences: a community-based study. Arthritis Rheum 1999; 42: 1397-1404.

240. McBeth J, Macfarlane GJ, Benjamin S et al. Features of somatization predict the onset of chronic widespread pain: results of a large population-based study. Arthritis Rheum 2001; 44: 940-946.

241. McBeth J, Silman AJ. The role of psychiatric disorders in fibromyalgia. Curr Rheumatol Rep 2001; 3: 157-164.

242. McCain GA, Bell DA, Mai FM et al. A controlled study of the effects of a supervised cardiovascular fitness training program on the manifestations of primary fibromyalgia. Arthritis Rheum 1988; 31: 1135-1141.

243. McCain GA, Tilbe KS. Diurnal hormone variation in fibromyalgia syndrome. A comparison with rheumatoid arthritis. J Rheumatol 1989; 16: 154-157.

244. McDermid AJ, Rollman GB, McCain GA. Generalized hypervigilance in fibromyalgia: evidence of perceptual amplification. Pain 1996; 66: 133-144.

245. Meiworm L, Jakob E, Walker UA et al. Patients with fibromyalgia benefit from aerobic endurance exercise. Clin Rheumatol 2000; 19: 253-257.

246. Melzack R. Prolonged relief of pain by brief, intense transcutaneous somatic stimulation. Pain 1975; 1: 357-373.

247. Mengshoel AM, Forre O, Komnaes HB. Muscle strength and aerobic capacity in primary fibromyalgia. Clin Exp Rheumatol 1990; 8: 475-479.

248. Mengshoel AM, Forre O. Physical fitness training in patients with fibromyalgia. J Musculoskel Pain 1993; 1: 267-272.

249. Mengshoel AM, Komnaes HB, Forre O. The effects of 20 weeks of physical fitness training in female patients with fibromyalgia. Clin Exp Rheumatol 1992; 10: 345-349.

250. Merchant RE, Andre C. A review of recent clinical trials of the nutritional supplement chlorella pyrenoidosa in the treatment of fibromyalgia, hypertension, and ulcerative colitis. Altern Ther Health Med 2001; 7: 79-91.

251. Middleton GD, McFarlin JE, Lipsky PE. The prevalence and clinical impact of fibromyalgia in systemic lupus erythematosus. Arthritis Rheum 1994; 37: 1181-1188.

252. Mikkelsson M, Latikka P, Kautiainen H et al. Muscle and bone pressure pain threshold and pain tolerance in fibromyalgia patients and controls. Arch Phys Med Rehabil 1992; 73: 814-818.

253. Mikkelsson M, Salminen JJ, Kautiainen H. Nonspecific musculoskeletal pain in preadolescents Prevalence and 1-year persistence. Pain 1997; 73: 29-35.

254. Miller LJ, Kubes KL. Serotonergic agents in the treatment of fibromyalgia syndrome. Ann Pharmacother 2002; 36: 707-712.

255. Moldofsky H, Lue FA, Mously C et al. The effect of zolpidem in patients with fibromyalgia: a dose ranging, double-blind, placebo controlled, modified crossover study. J Rheumatol 1996; 23: 529-533.

256. Moldofsky H, Scarisbrick P, England R et al. Musculoskeletal symptoms and non-REM sleep disturbance in patients with "fibrositis syndrome" and healthy subjects. Psychosom Med 1975; 37: 341-351.

257. Moldofsky H, Scarisbrick P. Induction of neurasthenic musculoskeletal pain syndrome by selective sleep stage deprivation. Psychosom Med 1976; 38: 35-44.

258. Moldofsky H. Chronobiological influences on fibromyalgia syndrome: theoretical and therapeutic implications. Ballieres Best Pract Res Clin Rheumatol 1994; 8: 801-810.

259. Moldofsky H. Sleep and fibrositis syndrome. Rheum Dis Clin North Am 1989; 15: 91-103.

260. Moore JE, McFall ME, Kivlahan DR et al. Risk of misinterpretation of MMPI Schizophrenia scale

elevations in chronic pain patients. Pain 1986; 32: 207-213.

261.Mountz JM, Bradley LA, Modell JG et al. Fibromyalgia in women. Abnormalities of regional cerebral blood flow in the thalamus and the caudate nucleus are associated with low pain threshold levels. Arthritis Rheum 1995; 38: 926-938.

262.Nabeshima T, Matsuno K, Sugimoto A et al. Antinociceptive activity induced by tizanidine and alpha 2-adrenoreceptors. Neuropharmacology 1987; 26: 1453-1455.

263.Neeck G, Riedel W. Thyroid function in patients with fibromyalgia syndrome. J Rheumatol 1992; 18: 1120-1122.

264.Ness TJ, San Pedro EC, Richards JS et al. A case of spinal cord injury-related pain with baseline rCBF brain SPECT imaging and beneficial response to gabapentin. Pain 1998; 78: 139-143.

265.Nicassio PM, Radojevic V, Weisman MH et al. A comparison of behavioral and educational interventions for fibromyalgia. J Rheumatol 1997; 24: 2000-2007.

266.Nichols DS, Glenn TM. Effects of aerobic exercise on pain perception, affects, and level of disability in individuals with fibromyalgia. PhysTher 1994; 74: 327-332.

267.Nielson WR, Merskey H. Psychosocial aspects of fibromyalgia. Curr Pain Headache Rep 2001; 5: 330-337.

268.Nielson WR, Walker C, McCain GA. Cognitive behavioral treatment of fibromyalgia syndrome: preliminary findings. J Rheumatol 1992; 19: 98-103.

269.Ninan PT. Use of venlafaxine in other psychiatric disorders. Depress Anxiety 2000; 12: 90-94.

270.Nordenskiold UM, Grimby G. Grip force in patients with rheumatoid arthritis and fibromyalgia and in healthy subjects. A study with the Grippit instrument. Scand J Rheumatol 1993; 22: 14-19

271.Norregaard J, Lykkegaard JJ, Mehlsen J et al. Exercise training in treatment of fibromyalgia. J Musculoskel Pain 1997; 5: 71-79.

272.Norregaard J, Volkmann H, Danneskiold-Samsoe B. A randomized controlled trial of citalopram in the treatment of fibromyalgia. Pain 1995; 61: 445-449.

273.O'Malley PG, Balden E, Tomkins G et al. Treatment of fibromyalgia with antidepressants: a meta-analysis. J Gen Intern Med 2000; 15: 659-666.

274.Offenbaecher M, Bondy B, de Johnge S et al. Possible association of fibromyalgia with a polymorphism in the serotonin transporter gene regulatory region. Arthritis Rheum 1999; 42: 2482-2488.

275.Okifuji A, Turk DC, Marcus DA. Comparison of generalized and localized hyperalgesia in patients

with recurrent headache and fibromyalgia. Psychosom Med 1999; 61: 771-180.

276.Okifuji A, Turk DC, Sherman JJ. Evaluation of the relationship between depression and fibromyalgia syndrome: why aren't all patients depressed? J Rheumatol 2000; 27: 212-219.

277.Olin R, Klein R, Berg PA. A randomized double-blind 16-week study of ritanserin in fibromyalgia syndrome: clinical outcome and analysis of autoantibodies to serotonin, gangliosides and phospholipids. Clin Rheumatol 1998; 17: 89-94.

278.Paira SO. Fibromyalgia associated with female urethral syndrome. Clin Rheumatol 1994; 13: 88-89.

279.Pappagallo M, Heinberg LJ. Ethical issues in the management of chronic non-malignant pain. Semin Neurol 1997; 17: 203-211.

280.Park JH, Phothimat P, Oates CT et al. Use of P-31 magnetic resonance spectroscopy to detect metabolic abnormalities in muscles of patients with fibromyalgia. Arthritis Rheum 1998; 41; 406-413.

281.Passik SD, Weinreb HJ. Managing chronic non-malignant pain: overcoming obstacles to the use of opioids. Adv Ther 2000; 17: 70-83.

282.Payne TC, Leavitt F, Garron DC et al. Fibrositis and psychologic disturbance. Arthritis Rheum 1982 ; 25 : 213-217.

283.Pellegrino MJ, Waylonis GW, Sommer A. Familial occurrence of primary fibromyalgia. Arch Phys Med Rehabil 1989; 70: 61-63.

284.Pillemer SR, Bradley LA, Crofford LJ et al. The neuroscience and endocrinology of fibromyalgia. Arthritis Rheum 1997; 40: 1928-1939.

285.Pincus T, Callahan LF, Bradley LA et al. Elevated MMPI scores for hypochondriasis, depression, and hysteria in patients with rheumatoid arthritis reflect disease rather than psychological status. Arthritis Rheum 1986; 29: 1456-1466.

286.Pioro-Boisset M, Esdaile JM & Fitzcharles MA. Alternative medicine use in fibromyalgia syndrome. Arthritis Care Res 1996; 9: 13-17

287.Portenoy RK. Opioid therapy for chronic non-malignant pain: a review of the critical issues. J Pain Symptom Manage 1996; 11: 203-217.

288.Porter J, Jick H. Addiction rare in patients treated with narcotics. N Engl J Med 1980; 302: 123.

289.Prescott E, Kjeller M, Jacobsen S et al. Fibromyalgia in the adult Danish Population: I. A prevalence study. Scand J Rheumatol 1993; 22: 233-237.

290.Quick DC. Joint pain and weather. A critical review of the literature. Minnesota Medicine 1997; 80: 25-29.

291.Quijada-Carrera J, Valenzuela-Castano A, Povedano-Gomez J et al. Comparison of tenoxicam and bromazepan in the treatment of fibromyalgia: a randomized, double blind, placebo-controlled trial. Pain 1996; 65: 221-225.

292. Quimby LG, Gratwick GM, Whitney CD et al. A randomized trial of cyclobenzaprine for the treatment of fibromyalgia. J Rheumatol 1989; 16: 140-143.

293. Ramos-Remus C, Salcedo-Rocha AL, Prieto-Parra RE, Galvan-Villegas F. How important is patient education? Baillieres Best Pract Res Clin Rheumatol 2000; 14: 689-703

294. Ramsay C, Moreland J, Ho M et al. an observer-blinded comparison of supervised and unsupervised aerobic exercise regimens in fibromyalgia. Rheumatology (Oxford) 2000; 39: 501-505.

295. Rao SG. The neuropharmacology of centrally-acting analgesic medications in fibromyalgia. Rheum Dis Clin North Am 2002; 28: 235-259.

296. Rau CL, Russell IJ. Is fibromyalgia a distinct clinical syndrome? Curr Rev Pain 2000; 4: 287-294.

297. Rea T, Russo J, Katon W et al. A prospective study of tender points and fibromyalgia during and after an acute viral infection. Arch Intern Med 1999; 159: 865-870.

298. Reilly PA, Littlejohn GO. Peripheral arthalgic presentation of fibrositis/fibromyalgia syndrome. J Rheumatol 1992; 19: 281-283.

299. Reynolds MD. The development of the concept of fibrositis. J Hist Med Allied Sci 1983; 38: 5-35.

300. Reynolds WJ, Moldofsky H, Saskin P et al. The effects of cyclobenzaprine on sleep physiology and symptoms in patients with fibromyalgia. J Rheumatol 1991; 18: 452-454.

301. Robinson RL, Birnbaum HG, Morley MA et al. Economic cost and epidemiological characteristics of patients with fibromyalgia claims. J Rheumatol 2003; 30: 1318-1325.

302. Roizenblatt S, Moldofsky H, Benedito-Silva AA et al. Alpha sleep characteristics in fibromyalgia. Arthritis Rheum 2001; 44: 222-230.

303. Rossy LA, Buckelew SP, Dorr N et al. A meta-analysis of fibromyalgia treatment interventions. Ann Behav Med 1999; 21: 180-191

304. Roy SH. Combined use of surface electromyography and 31P-NMR spectroscopy for the study of muscle disorders. Phys Ther 1993; 73: 892-901.

305. Russell IJ, Fletcher EM, Michalek JE et al. Treatment of primary fibrositis/fibromyalgia syndrome with ibuprofen and alprazolam : a double-blind, placebo-controlled study. Arthritis Rheum 1991; 34: 552-560.

306. Russell IJ, Kamin M, Bennett R et al. Efficacy of tramadol in treatment of pain in fibromyalgia. J Clin Rheumatol 2000; 6: 250-257.

307. Russell IJ, Kamin M, Sager D et al. Efficacy of Ultram™ [Tramadol HCL] treatment of fibromyalgia syndrome : preliminary analysis of a

multi-center, randomized, placebo-controlled study. Arthritis Rheum 1997; 40: S214.

308. Russell IJ, Michalek JE, Flechas JD et al. Treatment of fibromyalgia syndrome with Super Malic: a randomized, double-blind, placebo controlled, crossover pilot study. J Rheumatol 1995; 22: 953-958.

309. Russell IJ, Michalek JE, Vipario GA et al. Platelet ³H-imipramine uptake receptor density and serum serotonin levels in patients with fibromyalgia/fibrositis symptoms in the general population. J Rheumatol 1992; 19: 104-109.

310. Russell IJ, Michalek JE, Xiao Y et al. Therapy with a central alpha-2-adrenergic agonist [tizanidine] decreases cerebrospinal fluid substance P, and may reduce serum hyaluronic acid as it improves the clinical symptoms of the fibromyalgia syndrome. Arthritis Rheum 2002; 46: S614.

311. Russell IJ, Orr MD, Littman B et al. Elevated cerebrospinal fluid levels of substance P in patients with the fibromyalgia syndrome. Arthritis Rheum 1994; 37: 1593-1601.

312. Russell IJ, Vipraio GA, Morgan WW et al. Is there a metabolic basis for the fibrositis syndrome? Am J Med 1986; 81: 50-54.

313. Russell, IJ. Is fibromyalgia a distinct clinical entity? The clinical investigator's evidence. Baillieres Best Pract Res Clin Rheumatol 1999; 13: 445-454.

314. Scudds RA, McCain GA, Rollman GB et al. Improvements in pain responsiveness in patients with fibrositis after successful treatment with amitriptyline. J Rheumatol 1989; 16: 98-103.

315. Senna ER, De Barros AL, Silva EO et al. Prevalence of rheumatic diseases in Brazil: a study using the COPCORD approach. J Rheumatol 2004; 31: 594-597.

316. Shaver JL, Lentz M, Landis CA et al. Sleep, psychological distress, and stress arousal in women with fibromyalgia. Res Nurs Health 1997; 20: 247-257.

317. Siegel DM, Janeway D, Baum J. Fibromyalgia syndrome in children and adolescents: clinical features at presentation and status at follow-up. Pediatrics 1998; 101: 377-382.

318. Sietsema KE, Cooper DM, Caro X et al. Oxygen uptake during exercise in patients with primary fibromyalgia syndrome. J Rheumatol 1993; 20: 860-865.

319. Sigal LH. Persisting symptoms of Lyme disease – possible explanations and implications for treatment. J Rheumatol 1994; 21: 593-595.

320. Simms RW, Roy SH, Hrovat M et al. Lack of association between fibromyalgia syndrome and abnormalities in muscle energy metabolism. Arthritis Rheum 1994; 37: 794-800

321. Singh BB, Berman BM, Hadhazy VA et al. A pilot study of cognitive behavioral therapy in

fibromyalgia. Altern Ther Health Med 1998; 4: 67-70.

322.Sivri A, Cindas A, Dincer F et al. Bowel dysfunction and irritable bowel syndrome in fibromyalgia patients. Clin Rheumatol 1996; 15: 283-286.

323.Skootsky SA, Jaeger B, Dye RK. Prevalence of myofascial pain in general internal medicine practice. West J Med 1984; 151: 157-160.

324.Sletvold H, Stiles TC, Landro NI. Information processing in primary fibromyalgia, major depression and healthy controls. J Rheumatol 1995; 22: 137-142.

325.Slotkoff AT, Radulovic DA, Clauw DJ. The relationship between fibromyalgia and the multiple chemical sensitivity syndrome. Scand J Rheumatol 1997; 26: 364-367.

326.Smith HS, Barton AE. Tizanidine in the management of spasticity and musculoskeletal complaints in the palliative care population. Am J Hosp Palliat Care 2000; 17: 50-58.

327.Smythe HA, Moldofsky H. Two contributions to understanding the 'fibrositis syndrome'. Bull Rheum Dis 1978; 26: 928-931.

328.Smythe HA. Problems with the MMPI. J Rheumatol 1984; 11: 417-418.

329.Sorensen J, Bengtsson A, Ahlner J et al. Fibromyalgia – are there different mechanisms in the processing of pain? A double blind crossover comparison of analgesic drugs. J Rheumatol 1997; 24: 1615-1621.

330.Sorensen J, Bengtsson A, Backman E et al. Pain analysis in patients with fibromyalgia: effects of intravenous morphine, lidocaine and ketamine. Scand J Rheumatol 1995; 24: 360-365.

331.Sorensen J, Graven-Nielsen T, Henriksson KG et al. Hyperexcitability in fibromyalgia. J Rheumatol 1998; 25: 152-155.

332.Sperber AD, Atzmon Y, Neumann L et al. Fibromyalgia in the irritable bowel syndrome: studies of prevalence and clinical implications. Am J Gastroenterol 1999; 94: 3541-3456.

333.Staud R, Cannon RC, Mauderli AP et al. Temporal summation of pain from mechanical stimulation of muscle tissue in normal controls and subjects with fibromyalgia syndrome. Pain 2003; 102: 87-95.

334.Staud R, Robinson ME, Vierck CJ et al. Diffuse noxious inhibitory controls (DNIC) attenuate temporal summation of second pain in normal males but not in normal females or fibromyalgia patients. Pain 2003; 101: 167-174.

335.Staud R, Vierck CJ, Cannon RL et al. Abnormal sensitization and temporal summation of second pain (wind-up) in patients with fibromyalgia syndrome. Pain 2001; 91: 165-175.

336.Sternbach RA. Survey of pain in the United States: the

Nuprin Pain Report. Clin J Pain 1986; 2: 49-53.

337.Stratz T, Muller W. The use of 5-HT3 receptor antagonists in various rheumatic diseases – a clue to the mechanism of action of these agents in fibromyalgia? Scand J Rheumatol Suppl 2000; 113: 66-71.

338.Suhr JA. Neuropsychological impairment in fibromyalgia: relation to depression, fatigue, and pain. J Psychosom Res 2003; 55: 321-329.

339.Symons D. Epidemiologic concepts and rheumatology. In: Hochberg MC, Silman AJ, Smolen JS, Weinblatt ME, Weisman MH eds. Rheumatology, Third Edition. Edinburgh: Mosby; 2003: 13-20.

340.Tan EM, Cohen AS, Fries JF et al. The 1982 revised criteria for the classification of systemic lupus erythematosus (SLE) Arthritis Rheum 1982; 25: 1271-1277.

341.Tavoni A, Jeracitano G, Cirigliano G. Evaluation of S-adenosylmethionine in secondary fibromyalgia : a double-blind study. Clin Exp Rheumatol 1998; 16: 106-107.

342.Tavoni A, Vitali C, Bombardieri S et al. Evaluation of S-adenosylmethionine in primary fibromyalgia: a double-blind crossover study. Am J Med 1987; 83: 107-110.

343.Taylor ML, Trotter DR, Csuka ME. The prevalence of sexual abuse in women with fibromyalgia. Arthritis Rheum 1995; 38: 229-234.

344.Thieme K, Turk DC, Flor H. Comorbid depression and anxiety in fibromyalgia syndrome: relationship to somatic and psychosocial variables. Psychosom Med 2004; 66: 837-844.

345.Thorson, K. Is fibromyalgia a distinct clinical entity? The patient's evidence. Baillieres Best Pract Res Clin Rheumatol 1999; 13: 463-467.

346.Toomey TC, Seville JL, Mann JD et al. Relationship of sexual and physical abuse to pain description, coping, psychological distress, and healthcare utilization in a chronic pain sample. Clin J Pain 1995; 11: 307-315.

347.Torpy DJ, Papanicolaou DA, Lotsikas AJ et al. Responses of the sympathetic nervous system and the hypothalamic-pituitary-adrenal axis to interleukin-6: a pilot study in fibromyalgia. Arthritis Rheum 2000; 43: 872-880.

348.Travell J, Rinzler SH. The myofascial genesis of pain. Postgraduate Medicine 1952; 11: 425-434.

349.Travell JG, Simons DG. Myofascial Pain and Dysfunction: The Trigger Point Manual. Second ed. Baltimore: Williams & Wilkins; 1998.

350.Travell JG, Simons DG. Myofascial pain and Dysfunction: The Trigger Point Manual, Volume 2. Baltimore: Williams & Wilkins; 1992.

351.Tunks E, Crook J, Norman G et al. Tender points in fibromyalgia. Pain 1988; 34: 11-19.

352.Tunks E, McCain GA, Hart LE et al. The reliability of examination for tenderness in patients with myofascial pain, chronic fibromyalgia and controls. J Rheumatol 1995; 22: 944-962.

353.Turk DC, Flor H. The cognitive-behavioural approach to pain management. In: McMahon SB, Koltzenburg M eds. Wall and Melzack's Textbook of Pain, Fifth Edition. Edinburgh: Elsevier Churchill Livingstone; 2006: 339-348.

354.Turk DC, Okifuji A, Sinclair JD et al. Differential responses by psychosocial subgroups of fibromyalgia syndrome patients to an interdisciplinary treatment. Arthritis Care Res 1998; 11: 397-404.

355.Turk DC, Okifuji A, Sinclair JD et al. Interdisciplinary treatment for fibromyalgia syndrome; clinical and statistical significance. Arthritis Care Res 1998; 11: 186-195.

356.Vaeroy H, Helle R, Forre O et al. Cerebrospinal fluid levels of â-endorphin in patients with fibromyalgia (fibrositis syndrome). J Rheumatol 1988; 15: 1804-1806.

357.Vaeroy H, Helle R, Forre O et al. Elevated CSF levels of substance P and high incidence of Raynaud phenomenon in patients with fibromyalgia: new features for diagnosis. Pain 1988; 32: 21-26.

358.Vaeroy H, Nyberg F, Terenius L. No evidence for endorphin deficiency in fibromyalgia following investigation of cerebrospinal fluid (CSF) dynorphin A and Met-enkephalin-Arg6-Phe7. Pain 1991; 46: 139-143.

359.Vaeroy H, Sakurdda T, Foree O et al. Modulation of pain in fibromyalgia (fibrositis syndrome): cerebrospinal fluid (CSF) investigation of pain-related neuropeptides with special reference to calcitonin gene-related peptide (CGRP). J Rheumatol 1989; 19: 94-97.

360.van Santen M, Bolwijn P, Landewe R et al. High of low intensity aerobic fitness training in fibromyalgia: does it matter? J Rheumatol 2002; 29: 582-587.

361.van Santen M, Bolwijn P, Verstappen F et al. A randomized clinical trial comparing fitness and biofeedback training versus basic treatment in patients with fibromyalgia. J Rheumatol 1996; 25: 77-86.

362.Veale D, Kavanagh G, Fielding JF et al. Primary fibromyalgia and the irritable bowel syndrome: different expressions of a common pathogenetic process. Br J Rheumatol 1991; 30: 220-222.

363.Verstappen FTJ, van Santen-Hoeufft HMS, Bolwijn PH et al. Effects of a group activity program for fibromyalgia patients on physical fitness and well being. J Musculoskel Pain 1997; 5: 17-28.

364.Vierck CJ, Staud S, Price DD et al. The effect of maximal exercise on temporal summation of sec-

ond pain (windup) in patients with fibromyalgia syndrome. J Pain 2001; 6: 334-344.

365.Vlaeyen JW, Teeken-Gruben NJ, Goossens ME et al. Cognitive-educational treatment of fibromyalgia: a randomized clinical trial. I. Clinical effects. J Rheumatol 1996; 23: 1237-1245.

366.Volkmann H, Norregaard J, Jacobsen S et al. Double-blind, placebo-controlled cross-over study of intravenous S-adenosyl-L-methionine in patients with fibromyalgia. Scand J Rheumatol 1997; 26: 206-211.

367.Walker EA, Keegan D, Gardner G et al. Psychosocial factors in fibromyalgia compared with rheumatoid arthritis: I. Psychiatric diagnoses and functional disability. Psychosom Med 1997; 59: 565-571.

368.Wallace DJ. Genitourinary manifestations of fibrositis: an increased association with the female urethral syndrome. J Rheumatol 1990; 17: 238-239.

369.Waylonis GW, Perkins RH. Post-traumatic fibromyalgia. A long-term follow-up. Am J Phys Med Rehabil 1994; 73: 403-412.

370.Weigent DA, Bradley LA, Blalock JE et al. Current concepts in the pathophysiology of abnormal pain perception in fibromyalgia. Am J Med Sci 1998; 315: 405-412.

371.Weisman DE HJ. Opioid pseudo-addiction: an iatrogenic syndrome. Pain 1989; 36: 363-364.

372.Wessely S, Hotopf, M. Is fibromyalgia a distinct clinical entity? Historical and epidemiological evidence. Baillieres Best Pract Res Clin Rheumatol 1999; 13: 427-436.

373.White KP, Nielson WR, Harth M et al. Chronic widespread musculoskeletal pain with or without fibromyalgia: psychological distress in a representative community adult sample. J Rheumatol 2002; 29: 588-594.

374.White KP, Nielson WR. Cognitive behavioral treatment of fibromyalgia syndrome: a followup assessment. J Rheumatol 1995; 22: 717-721.

375.White KP, Speechley M, Harth M et al. Comparing self-reported function and work disability in 100 community cases of fibromyalgia syndrome versus controls in London, Ontario: the London Fibromyalgia Epidemiology Study. Arthritis Rheum 1999; 42: 76-83.

376.White KP, Speechley M, Harth M et al. Fibromyalgia in rheumatology practice: a survey of Canadian rheumatologists. J Rheumatol 1995; 22: 722-726.

377.White KP, Speechley M, Harth M et al. The London fibromyalgia epidemiology study: comparing the demographic and clinical characteristics in 100 random community cases of fibromyalgia versus controls. J Rheumatol 1999; 26: 1577-1585.

378.White KP, Speechley M, Harth M et al. The London fibromyalgia epidemiology study: the prevalence of fibromyalgia syndrome in London, Ontario. J Rheumatol 1999; 26: 1570-1576.

379.White KP, Speechley M, Harth M et al. The London fibromyalgia epidemiology study: direct health care cost of fibromyalgia syndrome in London, Canada. J Rheumatol 1999; 26: 885-889.

380.White KP, Thompson J. Fibromyalgia syndrome in an Amish community: a controlled study to determine disease and symptom prevalence. J Rheumatol 2003; 30: 1835-1840.

381.Wigers SH, Stiles TC, Vogel PA. Effects of aerobic exercise versus stress management treatment in fibromyalgia. A 4.5 year prospective study. Scand J Rheumatol 1996; 25: 77-86.

382.Wigers SH. Fibromyalgia outcome: the predictive values of symptom duration, physical activity, disability pension, and critical life events – a 4.5 year prospective study. J Psychosom Res 1996; 41: 235-243.

383.Williams DA, Cary MA, Groner KH et al. Improving physical functional status in patients with fibromyalgia: a brief cognitive behavioral intervention. J Rheumatol 2002; 29: 1280-1286.

384.Williams DA. Psychological and behavioral therapies in fibromyalgia and related syndromes. Best Pract Res Clin Rheumatol 2003; 17: 649-665.

385.Wittrup IH, Jensen B, Bliddal H et al. Comparison of viral antibodies in 2 groups of patients with fibromyalgia. J Rheumatol 2001; 28: 601-603.

386.Wolfe F, Anderson J, Harkness D et al. A prospective, longitudinal, multicenter study of service utilization and costs in fibromyalgia. Arthritis Rheum 1997; 40: 1560-1570.

387.Wolfe F, Anderson J, Harkness D et al. Health status and disease severity in fibromyalgia: results of a six-center longitudinal study. Arthritis Rheum 1997; 40: 1571-1579.

388.Wolfe F, Cathey MA, Hawley DJ. A double-blind placebo controlled trial of fluoxetine in fibromyalgia. Scand J Rheumatol 1994; 23: 255-259.

389.Wolfe F, Cathey MA, Kleinheksel SM et al. Psychological status in primary fibrositis and fibrositis associated with rheumatoid arthritis. J Rheumatol 1984; 11: 500-506.

390.Wolfe F, Michaud K. Severe rheumatoid arthritis (RA), worse outcomes, comorbid illness, and sociodemographic disadvantage characterize RA patients with fibromyalgia. J Rheumatol 2004; 31: 695-700.

391.Wolfe F, Ross K, Anderson J et al. The prevalence and characteristics of fibromyalgia in the general population. Arthritis Rheum 1995; 38: 19-28.

392.Wolfe F, Russell IJ, Vipario G et al. Serotonin levels, pain threshold, and fibromyalgia symptoms in the general population. J Rheumatol 1997; 24: 555-559.

393.Wolfe F, Simons DG, Fricton J et al. The fibromyalgia and myofascial pain syndromes: a preliminary study of tender points and trigger points in persons with fibromyalgia, myofascial pain syndrome and no disease. J Rheumatol 1992; 19: 944-951.

394.Wolfe F, Smythe HA, Yunus MB et al. The American College of Rheumatology 1990 criteria for the classification of fibromyalgia : Report of the Multicenter Criteria Committee. Arthritis Rheum 1990; 33: 160-172.

395.Wolfe F, Zhao S, Lane N. Preference for nonsteroidal anti-inflammatory drugs over acetaminophen by rheumatic disease patients: a survey of 1,799 patients with osteoarthritis, rheumatoid arthritis, and fibromyalgia. Arthritis Rheum 2000; 43: 378-385.

396.Wolfe F. Post-traumatic fibromyalgia: a case report narrated by the patient. Arthritis Care Res 1994; 7: 161-165.

397.Wolfe F. The Clinical syndrome of fibrositis. Am J Med 1986; 81: 7-14.

398.World Health Organization. Expert Committee on Drug Dependence, 16th report. Technical report series no. 407. Geneva: WHO; 1969.

399.Worrel LM, Krahn LE, Sletten CD et al. Treating fibromyalgia with a brief interdisciplinary program: initial outcomes and predictors of response. Mayo Clin Proc 2001; 76: 384-390.

400.Yunus M, Masi AT, Calabro JJ et al. Primary fibromyalgia (fibrositis): clinical study of 50 patients with matched normal controls. Semin Arthritis Rheum 1981; 11: 151-171.

401.Yunus MB, Aldag JC. Restless legs syndrome and leg cramps in fibromyalgia syndrome: a controlled study. BMJ 1996; 312: 1339.

402.Yunus MB, Dailey JW, Aldag JC et al. Plasma tryptophan and other amino acids in primary fibromyalgia: a controlled study. J Rheumatol 1992; 19: 90-94.

403.Yunus MB, Holt GS, Masi AT et al. Fibromyalgia syndrome among the elderly. Comparison with younger patients. J Am Geriatr Soc 1998; 36: 987-995.

404.Yunus MB, Inanici F, Aldag JC et al. Fibromyalgia in men: comparison of clinical features with women. J Rheumatol 2000; 27: 485-490.

405.Yunus MB, Masi AT, Aldag JC. A controlled study of primary fibromyalgia syndrome: clinical features and association with other functional syndromes. J Rheumatol 1989; 19: 62-71.

406.Yunus MB, Masi AT, Aldag JC. Short term effects of ibuprofen in primary fibromyalgia syndrome: a double-blind, placebo controlled trial.

J Rheumatol 1989; 16: 527-532.

407. Yunus MD, Kalyan-Raman UP, Masi AT et al. Electromicroscopic studies of muscle biopsy in primary fibromyalgia syndrome: a controlled and blinded study. J Rheumatol 1989; 16: 97-101.

408. Zijlstra TR, Barendregt PJ, van de Laar MA. Venlafaxine in fibromyalgia: results of a randomized, placebo-controlled, double-blind trial. Arthritis Rheum 2002; 46: S105.

References Chapter 3

1. Boivie J. Central Pain. In: McMahon SB, Koltzenburg M eds. Wall and Melzack's Textbook of Pain, Fifth Edition. Edinburgh: Elsevier Churchill Livingstone; 2006: 1057-1074.

2. Cohen ML. Is fibromyalgia a distinct clinical entity? The disapproving rheumatologist's evidence. Baillieres Best Pract Res Clin Rheumatol 1999; 13: 421-425.

3. Croft P, Burt J, Schollum J et al. More pain, more tender points: is fibromyalgia just one end of a continuous spectrum? Ann Rheum Dis 1996; 55: 482-485.

4. Croft P, Schollum J, Silman A. Population study of tender point counts and pain as evidence of fibromyalgia. Br Med J 1994; 309: 696-699.

5. Guyatt G, Rennie D. Users' Guide to the Medical Literature. Chicago: AMA Press; 2002.

6. Khostanteen I, Tunks ER, Goldsmith CH et al. Fibromyalgia: Can one distinguish it from simulation? An observer-blind controlled study. J Rheumatol 2000; 27: 2671-2676.

7. Landewe RBM, van der Heijde DMFM. Principles of assessment from a clinical perspective. Baillieres Best Pract Res Clin Rheumatol 2003; 17: 365-369.

8. National Center for Biotechnology Information. Pub Med. Il December 2007 <www.ncbi.nlm.nih.gov/sites/entrez>.

9. Sox HC, Blatt MA, Higgins MC et al. Medical Decision Making. Philadelphia: American College of Physicians; 2007.

10. Wolfe F, Smythe HA, Yunus MB et al. The American College of Rheumatology 1990 criteria for the classification of fibromyalgia : Report of the Multicenter Criteria Committee. Arthritis Rheum 1990; 33: 160-172.

References Chapter 4

1. American College of Rheumatology. Fibromyalgia. Il December 2007 <www.rheumatology.org/public/factsheets/fibromya_new.asp?aud=pat>.

2. Arthritis Foundation. Fibromyalgia. Il December 2007 <www.arthritis.org/disease-center.php?disease_id=10>.

3. Wolfe F, Smythe HA, Yunus MB et al. The American College of Rheumatology 1990 criteria for the classification of fibromyalgia : Report of the Multicenter Criteria Committee. Arthritis Rheum 1990; 33: 160-172.

References Chapter 5

1. Aaron LA, Bradley LA, Alarcon GS et al. Psychiatric diagnoses in patients with fibromyalgia are related to health care-seeking behavior rather than to illness. Arthritis Rheum 1996; 39: 436-445.

2. Affleck G, Urrows S, Tennen H et al. Sequential daily relations of sleep, pain intensity, and attention to pain among women with fibromyalgia. Pain 1996; 68: 363-368.

3. Akeson WH, Garfin S, Amiel D et al. Para-articular connective tissue in osteoarthritis. Semin Arthritis Rheum 1989; 18(suppl 2): 41-50.

4. Alagiri M, Chottiner S, Ratner V et al. Interstitial cystitis: unexplained associations with other chronic disease and pain syndromes. Urology 1997; 49: 52-57.

5. Altman RD, Asch E, Bloch D et al. Development of criteria for the classification and reporting of osteoarthritis: classification of osteoarthritis of the knee. Arthritis Rheum 1986; 29: 1039-1049.

6. Arnett FC, Edworthy SM, Bloch DA et al. The American Rheumatism Association 1987 revised criteria for the classification of theumatoid arthritis 1988; 31: 315-324.

7. Babul N, Darke AC. Reliability and accuracy for memory for acute pain. Pain 1994; 57: 131-132.

8. Badalamente MA, Cherney SB. Periosteal and vascular innervation of the human patella in degenerative joint disease. Semin Arthritis Rheum 1989; 18(suppl 2): 61-66.

9. Beck PW. Handwerker HO, Zimmerman M. Nervous outflow from the cat's foot during noxious radiant heat stimulation. Brain Res 1974; 67: 373-386.

10. Beitel RE, Dubner R. Response of unmyelinated (C) polymodal nociceptors to thermal stimuli applied to monkey's face. J Neurophysiol 1976; 39: 1160-1175.

11. Bellamy N, Sothern RB, Campbell J et al. Circadian and circaseptan variation in pain perception in osteoarthritis of the knee. J Rheumatol 1990; 17: 364-372.

12. Bengtsson A, Henriksson KG, Jorfeldt L et al. Primary fibromyalgia. A clinical and laboratory study of 55 patients. Scand J Rheumatol 1986; 15: 340-347.

13. Bennett GJ, Kajander KC, Sahara Y et al. Neurochemical and anatomical changes in the dorsal horn of rats with an experimental painful peripheral neuropathy. In: Cervero F, Bennett GJ, Headley PM eds. Processing of sensory information in the superficial dorsal horn of the spinal cord. Amsterdam: Plenum; 1989: 463-471.

14. Bennett RM. The contribution of muscle to the generation of fibromyalgia symptomatology. J Musculoskeletal Pain 1996; 4: 35-39.

15. Bessou P, Perl ER. Response of cutaneous sensory units with unmyelinated fibers to noxious stimuli. J Neurophysiol 1969; 32:1025-1043.

16. Brown GW, Harris T. Social Origins of Depression. London: Tavistock; 1978.

17. Bryant RA. Memory for pain and affect in chronic pain patients. Pain 1993; 54: 347-351.

18. Burckhardt CS, O'Reilly CA, Wiens AN et al. Assessing depression in fibromyalgia patients. Arthritis Care Res 1994; 7: 35-39.

19. Buskila D, Neumann L, Alhoashie A et al. Fibromyalgia syndrome in men. Semin Arthritis Rheum 2000; 30: 47-51.

20. Buskila D, Neumann L, Hozanov I et al. Familial aggregation in the fibromyalgia syndrome. Semin Arthritis Rheum 1996; 26: 605-611.

21. Buskila D, Neumann L. Fibromyalgia syndrome (FM) and nonarticular tenderness in relatives of patients with FM. J Rheumatol 1997; 24: 941-944.

22. Campbell SM, Clark S, Tindall EA et al. Clinical characteristics of fibrositis. I.A. 'blinded' controlled study of symptoms and tender points. Arthritis Rheum 1983; 26: 817-824.

23. Chang L, Mayer EA, Johnson T et al. Differences in somatic perception in female patients with irritable bowel syndrome with and without fibromyalgia. Pain 2000; 84: 297-307.

24. Chi S-I, Levine JD, Basbaum AI. Effects of injury discharge on the persistent expression of spinal cord fos-like immunoreactivity produced by sciatic nerve transaction in the rat. Brain Res 1993; 617: 220-224.

25. Chun A, Desauteis S, Silvka A et al. Visceral algesia in irritable bowel syndrome, fibromyalgia, and sphincter of Oddi dysfunction, type III. Dig Dis Sci 1999; 44: 631-636.

26. Clark DM, Teasdale JD. Constraints on effects of mood on memory. J Pers Soc Psychol 1985; 48: 1595-1608.

27. Clark DM, Teasdale JD. Diurnal variation in clinical depression and accessability of memories of positive and negative experiences. J Abnorm Psychol 1982; 91: 87-95.

28. Clark S, Campbell SM, Forehand ME et al. Clinical characteristics of fibrositis. II. A 'blinded', controlled study using standard psychological tests. Arthritis Rheum 1985; 28: 132-137.

29. Clauw DJ, Schmidt M, Radulovic D et al. The relationship between fibromyalgia and interstitial cystitis. J Psychiatr Res 1997; 31: 125-131.

30. Cook AJ, Woolf CJ, Wall PD et al. Dynamic receptive field plasticity in rat spinal cord dorsal horn following C primary afferent input. Nature 1987; 325: 151-153.

31. Cote KA, Moldofksy H. Sleep, daytime symptoms, cognitive performance in patients with fibromyalgia. J Rheumatol 1997; 24: 2014-2023.

32. Creamer P. Osteoarthritis. In: Wall PD, Melzack R eds. Textbook of Pain. Fourth ed. Edinburgh: Churchill Livingston; 1999: 493-504.

33. Crofford LJ, Pillemer SR, Kalogeras KT et al. Hypothalamic-pituitary-adrenal axis perturbations in patients with fibromyalgia. Arthritis Rheum 1994; 37: 1583-1592.

34. de Wied M, Verbaten MN. Affective pictures processing, attention and pain tolerance. Pain 2001; 90: 163-172.

35. Dickenson AH, Sullivan AF. Evidence for the role of the NMDA receptor in the frequency dependent potentiation of deep rat dorsal horn nociceptive neurons following C fiber stimulation. Neuropharmacology 1987; 26: 1235-1238.

36. Drewes AM. Pain and sleep disturbances with special reference to fibromyalgia and rheumatoid arthritis. Rheumatology (Oxford) 1999; 38: 1035-1038.

37. Dubner R, Ren K. Central mechanisms of thermal and mechanical hyperalgesia following tissue inflammation. In: Boivie J, Hansson P, Lindblom U eds. Touch, temperature, and pain in health and disease: mechanisms and assessments. Seattle: IASP Press; 1994: 267-277.

38. Eich E, Reeves JL, Jaeger B et al. Memory for pain: relation between past and present pain intensity. Pain 1985; 23: 375-379.

39. Eisenhower D, Mathiowetz NA, Morganstein D. Recall error: sources and bias reduction techniques. In: Beimer P, Groves R, Lyberg L et al eds. Measurement Errors in Surveys. New York: Wiley; 1991.

40. Erskine A, Morley S, Pearce S. Memory for pain: a review. Pain 1990; 41: 255-265.

41. Fields HL. Pain modulation: expectation, opioid analgesia and virtual pain. Prog Brain Res 2000; 122: 245-253.

42. Grigg P, Schaible H-G, Schmidt RF. Mechanical sensitivity of group III and IV afferents from posterior articular nerve in normal and inflamed cat knee. J Neurophysiol 1986; 55: 635-643.

43. Hochberg MC. Updating the American College of Rheumatology revised criteria for the classification of systemic lupus erythematosus [letter]. Arthritis Rheum 1997; 40: 1725.

44. Hoheisel U, Mense S. Long-term changes in discharge behaviour of cat dorsal horn neurones following noxious stimulation of deep tissues. Pain 1989; 36: 239-247.

45. Hu JW, Sessle BJ, Raboisson P et al. Stimulation of craniofacial muscle afferents induces prolonged facilitory effects in trigeminal nociceptive brainstem neurones. Pain 1992; 48: 53-60.

46. Hudson JI, Goldenberg DL, Pope HG Jr et al. Comorbidity of fibromyalgia with medical and psychiatric disorders. Am J Med 1992; 92: 363-367.

47. Hudson JI, Pope HG Jr. The relationship between fibromyalgia and major depressive disorder. Rheum Dis Clin N Am 1996; 22: 285-303.

48. Hunter M, Philips C, Rachman S. Memory for pain. Pain 1979; 6: 35-46.

49. Hylden JLK, Nahin RL, Traub RJ et al. Expansion of receptive fields of spinal lamina I projection neurons in rats with unilateral adjuvant-induced inflammation: the contribution of dorsal horn mechanisms. Pain 1989; 37: 239-243.

50. Jamison RN, Sbrocco T, Parris WCV. The influence of physical and psychosocial on accuracy of memory for pain in chronic pain patients. Pain 1989; 37: 289-294.

51. Kahneman D, Fredrickson BL, Schreiber CA et al. When more pain is preferred to less: adding a better end. Psychol Sci 1993; 4: 401-45.

52. Kantor TG. Concepts in pain control. Semin Arthritis Rheum1989; 18(suppl 2): 94-99.

53. Katz RS, Kravitz HM. Fibromyalgia, depression, and alcoholism: a family history study. J Rheumatol 1996; 23: 149-154.

54. Kazis LE, Meenan RF, Anderson JJ. Pain in the rheumatic diseases: investigations of a key health status component. Arthritis Rheum 1983; 26: 1017-1022.

55. Kiaer T, Gronlund J, Sorensen KH. Intraosseous pressure and partial pressures of oxygen and carbon dioxide in osteoarthritis. Semin Arthritis Rheum 1989; 18(suppl 2): 57-60.

56. Kidd B. Problems with pain – is the messenger to blame? Ann Rheum Dis 1996; 55: 276-283.

57. Kolasinski SL, Haines KA, Siegel EL et al. Neuropeptides and inflammation. A somatostatin analog as a selective antagonist of neutrophil activation by substance P. Arthritis Rheum 1992; 35: 369-375.

58. Kontinnen YT, Kemppinen P, Segerberg M et al. Peripheral and spinal neural mechanisms in arthritis with particular reference to treatment of inflammation and pain. Arthritis Rheum 1994; 37: 965-982.

59. Kosek E Hansson P. Modulatory influence on somatosensory perception from vibration and heterotopic noxious conditioning stimulation (HNCS) in fibromyalgia patients and healthy subjects. Pain 1997; 70: 41-51.

60. Kurtze N, Gundersen KT, Svebak S. Quality of life, functional disability and lifestyle among subgroups of fibromyalgia patients: the significance of anxiety and depression. Br J Med Psychol 1999; 72: 471-484.

61. Kurtze N, Gunderson KT, Svebak S. The role of anxiety and depression in fatigue and patterns of pain among subgroups of fibromyalgia patients. Br J Med Psychol 1998; 71: 185-194.

62. LaMotte RH, Thalhammer JG, Torebjork HE et al. Peripheral neural mechanisms of cutaneous hyperalgesia following mild injury by heat. J Neurosci 1982; 2: 765-781.

63. Lautenbacher S, Rollman GB. Possible deficiencies of pain modulation in fibromyalgia. Clin J Pain 1997; 13: 189-196.

64. Lentz MJ, Landis CA, Rothermel J et al. Effects of selective slow wave sleep disruption on musculoskeletal pain and fatigue in middle aged women. J Rheumatol 1999; 26: 1586-1592.

65. Lindblad S, Hedfors E. Arthroscopic and immunohistologic characterization of knee joint synovitis in osteoarthritis. Arthritis Rheum 1987; 30: 1081-1088.

66. Lindblad S, Hedfors E. Arthroscopic and synovial correlates of pain in osteoarthritis. Semin Arthritis Rheum 1989; 18(suppl 2): 91-93.

67. Linton SJ, Gotestam KG. A clinical comparison of two pain scales: correlation, remembering chronic pain, and a measure of compliance. Pain 1983; 17: 57-65.

68. Linton SJ, Melin L. The accuracy of remembering chronic pain. Pain 1982; 17: 57-65.

69. Linton SJ. Memory for chronic pain intensity: correlates of accuracy. Percept Mot Skills 1991; 72: 1091-1095.

70. Lund JP, Stohler CS, Widmer CG. The relationship between pain and muscle activity in fibromyalgia and similar conditions. In: Vaeroy H, Merskey H eds. Progress in fibromyalgia and myofascial pain. Amsterdam: Elsevier Science; 1993: 311-327.

71. Magni G, Caldieron C, Rigatti-Luchini S et al. Chronic musculoskeletal pain and depressive symptoms in the general population. An analysis of the 1st National Health and Nutrition Examination survey data. Pain 1990; 43: 299-307.

72. Matucci-Cerini M, Partsch G. The contribution of the peripheral nervous system and the neuropeptide network to the development of synovial inflammation. Clin Exp Rheumatol 1992; 10: 211-215.

73. McBeth J, Macfarlane GJ, Benjamin S et al. Fea-

tures of somatization predict the onset of chronic widespread pain: results of a large population-based study. Arthritis Rheum 2001; 44: 940-946.

74. McBeth J, Silman AJ. The role of psychiatric disorders in fibromyalgia. Curr Rheumatol Rep 2001; 3: 157-164.

75. McFarlane AC, Brooks PM. An analysis of the relationship between psychological morbidity and disease activity in rheumatoid arthritis. J Rheumatol 1988; 15: 926-931.

76. Mendel LM. Physiological properties of unmyelinated fiber projection to the spinal cord. Exp Neurol 1966; 16: 316-332.

77. Menon G, Yorkton EA. The use of memory and contextual cues in the formation of behavioral frequency judgments. In: Stone AA, Turkkan JS, Bachrach CA et al eds. The Science of Self Report: Implications for Research and Practice. New Jersey: Lawrence Earlbaum Associate; 2000.

78. Merskey H, Bogduk N, eds. Classification of chronic pain, 2nd ed. Seattle: IASP; 1994.

79. Meyer RA, Campbell JN. Myelinated nococeptive afferents account for the hyperalgesia that follows a burn to the hand. Science 1982; 213: 1527-1529.

80. Meyer RA, Campbell JN. Peripheral neural coding of pain sensation. Johns Hopkins APL Technical Digest 1981; 2: 164-171.

81. Moldofsky H, Scarisbrick P, England R et al. Musculoskeletal symptoms and non-REM sleep disturbance in patients with "fibrositis syndrome" and healthy subjects. Psychosom Med 1975; 37: 341-351.

82. Moldofsky H, Scarisbrick P. Induction of neurasthenic musculoskeletal pain syndrome by selective sleep stage deprivation. Psychosom Med 1976; 38: 35-44.

83. Moldofsky H. Sleep influences on regional and diffuse pain syndromes associated with osteoarthritis. Semin Arthritis Rheum 1989; 18(suppl 2): 18-21.

84. Neugebauer V, Schaible H-G. Evidence for a central component in the sensitization of spinal neurons with joint input during development of acute arthritis in cat's knee. J Neurophysiol 1990; 64: 299-311.

85. Nielson WR, Merskey H. Psychosocial aspects of fibromyalgia. Curr Pain Headache Rep 2001; 5: 330-337.

86. Okifuji A, Turk DC, Sherman JJ. Evaluation of the relationship between depression and fibromyalgia syndrome: why aren't all patients depressed? J Rheumatol 2000; 27: 212-219.

87. Paira SO. Fibromyalgia associated with female urethral syndrome. Clin Rheumatol 1994; 13: 88-89.

88. Pellegrino MJ, Waylonis GW, Sommer A. Familial occurrence of primary fibromyalgia. Arch Phys Med Rehabil 1989; 70: 61-63.

89. Pillemer SR, Bradley LA, Crofford LJ et al. The neuroscience and endocrinology of fibromyalgia. Arthritis Rheum 1997; 40: 1928-1939.

90. Price DD. Psychological and neural mechanisms of the affective dimension of pain. Science 2000; 288: 1769-1772.

91. Radanov BP, Sturzenegger M, Di Stefano G. Long-term outcome after whiplash injury. A 2-year follow-up considering features of injury mechanism and somatic, radiologic and psychosocial findings. Medicine (Baltimore) 1995; 74: 281-297.

92. Rainville P, Duncan GH, Price DD et al. Pain affect encoded in human anterior cingulated but not somatosensory cortex. Science 1997; 277: 968-971.

93. Rejeski WJ, Miller ME, Foy C et al. Self-efficacy and the progression of functional limitations and self-reported disability in older adults with knee pain. J Gerontol B Psychol Sci Soc Sci 2001; 56: S261-265.

94. Roizenblatt S, Moldofsky H, Benedito-Silva AA et al. Alpha sleep characteristics in fibromyalgia. Arthritis Rheum 2001; 44: 222-230.

95. Schaible H-G, Neugebauer V, Schmidt RF. Osteoarthritis and pain. Semin Arthritis Rheum 1989; 18: 30-34.

96. Schaible H-G, Schmidt RF. Effects of an experimental arthritis on the sensory properties of fine articular afferent units. J Neurophysiol 1985; 54: 1109-1122.

97. Schumacher HR. The role of inflammation and crystals in the pain of osteoarthritis. Semin Arthritis Rheum 1989; 18(suppl 2): 81-85.

98. Shiffman S, Hufford M, Hickox M et al. Remember that? A comparison of real-time versus retrospective recall of smoking lapses. J Consult Clin Psychol 1997; 65: 292-300.

99. Simone DA, Sorkin LS, Oh U et al. Neurogenic hyperalgesia: central neural correlates in responses of spinothalamic tract neurons. J Neurophysiol 1991; 66: 228-246.

100. Sivri A, Cindas A, Dincer F et al. Bowel dysfunction and irritable bowel syndrome in fibromyalgia patients. Clin Rheumatol 1996; 15: 283-286.

101. Sletvold H, Stiles TC, Landro NI. Information processing in primary fibromyalgia, major depression and healthy controls. J Rheumatol 1995; 22: 137-142.

102. Slotkoff AT, Radulovic DA, Clauw DJ. The relationship between fibromyalgia and the multiple chemical sensitivity syndrome. Scand J Rheumatol 1997; 26: 364-367.

103. Sorensen J, Graven-Nielsen T, Henriksson KG et

al. Hyperexcitability in fibromyalgia. J Rheumatol 1998; 25: 152-155.

104. Sperber AD, Atzmon Y, Neumann L et al. Fibromyalgia in the irritable bowel syndrome: studies of prevalence and clinical implications. Am J Gastroenterol 1999; 94: 3541-3456.

105. Staud R, Robinson ME, Vierck CJ et al. Diffuse noxious inhibitory controls (DNIC) attenuate temporal summation of second pain in normal males but not in normal females or fibromyalgia patients. Pain 2003; 101; 167-174.

106. Steultjens MP, Dekker J, Bijlsma JW. Coping, pain, and disability in osteoarthritis: a longitudinal study. J Rheumatol 2001; 28: 1068-1072.

107. Tan EM, Cohen AS, Fries JF et al. The 1982 revised criteria for the classification of systemic lupus erythematosus (SLE) Arthritis Rheum 1982; 25: 1271-1277.

108. Veale D, Kavanagh G, Fielding JF et al. Primary fibromyalgia and the irritable bowel syndrome: different expressions of a common pathogenetic process. Br J Rheumatol 1991; 30: 220-222.

109. Villemure C, Bushnell MC. Cognitive modulation of pain: how do attention and emotion influence pain processing? Pain 2002; 95: 195-199.

110. Villemure C, Slotnick BM, Bushnell MC. Effects of odors on pain perception: deciphering the roles of emotion and attention. Pain 2003; 106: 101-108.

111. Wallace DJ. Genitourinary manifestations of fibrositis: an increased assocatioin with the female urethral syndrome. J Rheumatol 1990; 17: 238-239.

112. Weiser S, Cedrashi C. Psychosocial issues in the prevention of chronic low back pain - a literature review. Ballieres Best Pract Res Clin Rheumatol 1992; 6: 657-684.

113. Wilcox GL. Excitatory neurotransmitters and pain. In: Bond MR, Charlton JE, Woolf CJ eds. Proceedings of the VIth World Congress on Pain. Amsterdam: Elsevier; 1991: 97-117.

114. Wilcox S, Brenes GA, Levine D et al. Factors related to sleep disturbance in older adults experiencing knee pain or knee pain with radiographic evidence of knee osteoarthritis. J Am Geriatr Soc 2000; 10: 1241-1251.

115. Wolfe F, Smythe HA, Yunus MB et al. The American College of Rheumatology 1990 criteria for the classification of fibromyalgia : Report of the Multicenter Criteria Committee. Arthritis Rheum 1990; 33: 160-172.

116. Woolf CJ, King AE. Dynamic alterations in the cutaneous mechanoreceptive fields of dorsal horn neurons in the rat spinal cord. J Neurosci 1990; 10: 2717-2726.

117. Woolf CJ, Shortland P, Coggeshall RE. Peripheral nerve injury triggers central sprouting of myelinated afferents. Nature 1992; 355: 75-78.

118. Woolf CJ, Thompson SWN. The induction and maintenance of central sensitization is dependent on N-methyl-D-aspartic acid receptor activation; implications for the treatment of post-injury pain hypersensitivity states. Pain 1991; 44: 293-299.

119. Woolf CJ. Evidence for a central component of post-injury pain hypersensitivity. Nature 1983; 306; 686-688.

120. Wyke B. The neurology of joints: a review of general principles. Clin Rheum Dis 1981; 7: 223-239.

121. Yunus M, Masi AT, Calabro JJ et al. Primary fibromyalgia (fibrositis) : clinical study of 50 patients with matched normal controls. Semin Arthritis Rheum 1981; 11: 151-171.

122. Yunus MB, Inanici F, Aldag JC et al. Fibromyalgia in men: comparison of clinical features with women. J Rheumatol 2000; 27: 485-490.

123. Yunus MB. Psychological aspects of fibromyalgia syndrome: a component of the dysfunctional spectrum syndrome. Ballieres Best Pract Res Clin Rheumatol 1994; 8: 811-837.

References Chapter 6

1. Akeson WH, Garfin S, Amiel D et al. Para-articular connective tissue in osteoarthritis. Semin Arthritis Rheum 1989; 18(suppl 2): 41-50.

2. Altman RD, Asch E, Bloch D et al. Development of criteria for the classification and reporting of osteoarthritis: classification of osteoarthritis of the knee. Arthritis Rheum 1986; 29: 1039-1049.

3. Altman RD, Fries JF, Bloch DA et al. Radiographic assessment of progression in osteoarthritis. Arthritis Rheum 1987; 30: 1214-1225.

4. Badalamente MA, Cherney SB. Periosteal and vascular innervation of the human patella in degenerative joint disease. Semin Arthritis Rheum 1989; 18(suppl 2): 61-66.

5. Baliunas AJ, Hurwitz DE, Ryals AB et al. Increased knee joint loads during walking are present in subjects with knee osteoarthritis. Osteoarthritis Cartilage 2002; 10: 573-579.

6. Bandler R, Shipley MT. Columnar organization in thje midbrain periaqueductal gray: modules for emotional expression? Trends Neurosci 1994; 17: 379-389.

7. Bellamy N, Sothern RB, Campbell J et al. Circadian and circaseptan variation in pain perception in osteoarthritis of the knee. J Rheumatol 1990; 17: 364-372.

8. Berry PH, Chapman CR, Covington EC et al. Pain: Current Understanding of Assessment, Management, and Treatments. Virginia: National Pharmaceutical Council, Inc.; 2001.

9. Boden SD, Davis DO, Dina TS et al. Abnormal magnetic resonance scans of the lumbar spine in asymptomatic subjects: a prospective investigation. J Bone Joint Surg 1990; 72A: 403-408.

10. Bogduk N. Cervical causes of headache and dizziness. In: Grieve G, ed. Modern manual therapy of the vertebral column. Edinburgh: Churchill Livingstone; 1986: 289-302.

11. Bogduk N. Innervation and pain patterns in the cervical spine. Clin Phys Ther 1988; 17: 1-13.

12. Bradley LA. Adherence with treatment regimens among adult rheumatoid arthritis patients: current status and future directions. Arthritis Care Res 1989; 2: 33-39.

13. Brandt KD. Animal models of osteoarthritis. Biorheology 2002; 39: 221-235.

14. Burke LE, Ockene IS, eds. Compliance in healthcare and research. New York: Futura; 2001.

15. Burr DB. The importance of subchondral bone in osteoarthrosis. Curr Opin Rheumatol 1998; 10: 256-262.

16. Chi S-I, Levine JD, Basbaum AI. Effects of injury discharge on the persistent expression of spinal cord fos-like immunoreactivity produced by sciatic nerve transaction in the rat. Brain Res 1993; 617: 220-224.

17. Class Complaints in Love. Corrected Fifth Amended Class Action Complaint. Welcome to HMO Settlements. 17 December 2007 <http://hmosettlements.com/settlements/class_action/CorrectedFifthAmendedClassActionComplaint.pdf>.

18. Classification of chronic pain: Descriptions of common pain syndromes and definition of pain terms. Prepared by the International Association for the Study of Pain, Subcommittee on Taxonomy. Pain Suppl 1986; 3: S1-S226.

19. Cloward RB. Cervical diskography: a contribution to the etiology and mechanism of neck, shoulder and arm pain. Ann Surg 1959; 150: 1052-1064.

20. Coderre TJ, Katz J, Vaccarino AL, Melzack R. Contribution of central neuroplasticity to pathologic pain: review of clinical and experimental evidence. Pain 1993; 52: 259-285.

21. Cooper C, Snow S, McAlindon TE et al. Risk factors for the incidence and progression of radiographic knee osteoarthritis. Arthritis Rheum 2000; 43: 995-1000.

22. Craig AD, Dostrovsky JO. Medulla to thalamus. In: Wall PD, Melzack R eds. Textbook of Pain. Fourth ed. Edinburgh: Churchill Livingstone; 1999: 183-214.

23. Creamer P. Osteoarthritis. In: Wall PD, Melzack R eds. Textbook of Pain. Fourth ed. Edinburgh: Churchill Livingstone; 1999: 493-504.

24. Daltroy LH. Doctor-patient communication in rheumatological disorders. Baillieres Clin Rheumatol 1993; 7: 221-239.

25. Danielsson LG. Incidence and prognosis of coxarthrosis Acta Orthop Scand 1964; 66(suppl): 1-87.

26. Deyo RA, McNeish LM, Cone RO III. Observer variability in the interpretation of lumbar spine radiographs. Arthritis Rheum 1985; 28: 1066-1070.

27. Deyo RA. Compliance with therapeutic regimens in arthritis: issues, current status, and a future agenda. Sem Arthritis Rheum 1982; 12: 233-244.

28. Dickenson AH, Sullivan AF. Evidence for a role of the NMDA receptor in the frequency dependent potentiation of deep rat dorsal horn nociceptive neurons following C fiber stimulation. Neuropharmacology 1987; 26: 1235-1238.

29. Dieppe P, Cushnaghan J, Tucker M et al. The Bristol OA500 Study: progression and impact of the disease after 8 years. Osteoarthritis Cartilage 2000; 8: 63-68.

30. Doubell TP, Mannion RJ, Woolf CJ. The dorsal horn state-dependent sensory processing, plasticity and the generation of pain. In: Wall PD, Melzack R eds. Textbook of Pain. Fourth ed. Edinburgh: Churchill Livingstone; 1999: 165-181.

31. Dougados M, Gueguen A, Nguyen M et al. Longitudinal radiologic evaluation of osteoarthritis of the knee. J Rheumatol 1992; 19: 378-383.

32. Dreyfuss P, Michaelsen M, Fletcher D. Atlanto-occipital and atlantoaxial joint pain patterns. Spine 1994; 19: 1125-1131.

33. Dwyer A, Aprill C, Bogduk N. Cervical zygapophyseal joint pain patterns. I: a study in normal volunteers. Spine 1990; 15: 453-457.

34. Eckstein F, Faber S, Muhlbauer R et al. Functional adaptation of human joints to mechanical stimuli. Osteoarthritis Cartilage 2002; 10: 44-50.

35. Edwards JCW, ed. Second International Meeting on Synovium; Cell Biology and Physiology. Ann Rheum Dis 1995; 54: 389-436.

36. Feinstein B, Langton NJK, Jameson RM, Schiller F. Experiments on pain referred from deep somatic tissues. J Bone Joint Surg 1954; 36A: 981-997.

37. Felson DT, Hannan MT, Naimark A et al. Occupational physical demands, knee bending, and knee osteoarthritis: results from the Framingham Study. J Rheumatol 1991; 18: 1587-1592.

38. Frankel VH, Burstein AH, Brooks DB. Biomechanics of internal derangement of the knee. Pathomedics as determined by analysis of the instant centers of motion. J Bone Joint Surg 1971; 53A: 945.

39. Grant JCB. Grant's Atlas of Anatomy, Fourth ed. Baltimore: The Williams and Wilkins Company; 1972.

40. Graven-Nielsen T, Mense S. The peripheral ap-

paratus of muscle pain: evidence from animal and human studies. Clin J Pain 2001; 17: 2-10.

41. Grigg P, Schaible H-G, Schmidt RF. Mechanical sensitivity of group III and IV afferents from posterior articular nerve in normal and inflamed cat knee. J Neurophysiol 1986; 55: 635-643.

42. Hakelius A, Hindmarsh J. The comparative reliability of preoperative diagnostic methods in lumbar disc surgery. Acta Orthop Scand 1972; 43: 234-238.

43. Harris PA, Hart DJ, Dacre JE et al. The progression of radiological hand osteoarthritis over 10 years: a clinical follow-up study. Osteoarthritis Cartilage 1994; 2: 247-252.

44. Hart DJ, Leedham-Green M, Spector TD. The prevalence of knee osteoarthritis in the general population using different clinical criteria: the Chingford Study. Br J Rheum 1991; 30: 72.

45. Hassan BS, Mockett S, Doherty M. Static postural sway, proprioception, and maximal voluntary quadriceps contraction in patients with knee osteoarthritis and normal control subjects. Ann Rheum Dis 2001; 60: 612-618.

46. Hasselbacher P. The biology of the joint. Clin Rheum Dis 1981; 7.

47. Hernborg JS, Nilsson BE. The natural course of untreated osteoarthritis of the knee. Clin Orthop 1977; 123: 130-137.

48. Holzer P 1998 Neurogenic vasodilatation and plasma leakage in the skin. General Pharmacology 30:5-11.

49. Hurwitz DE, Sumner DR, Block JA. Bone density, dynamic joint loading and joint degeneration. A review. Cells Tissues Organs 2001; 169: 201-209.

50. Janis I. The patient as decision-maker. In: Gentry WD, ed. Handbook of behavioral medicine. New York: Guilford Press; 1983: 326-368.

51. Jensen MC, Brant-Zawadzki MN, Obuchowski N et al. Magnetic resonance imaging of the lumbar spine in people without back pain. N Engl J Med 1994; 331: 69-73.

52. Jones AKP, Derbyshire SWG. Cerebral mechanisms operating in the presence and absence of inflammatory pain. Ann Rheum Dis 1996; 55: 411-420.

53. Kallman DA, Wigley FM, Scott WW et al. The longitudinal course of hand osteoarthritis in a male population. Arthritis Rheum 1990; 33: 1323-1332.

54. Kantor TG. Concepts in pain control. Semin Arthritis Rheum 1989; 18(suppl 2): 94-99.

55. Kazis LE, Meenan RF, Anderson JJ. Pain in the rheumatic diseases: investigations of a key health status component. Arthritis Rheum 1983; 26: 1017-1022.

56. Keefe FJ, Bonk V. Psychosocial assessment of pain in patients having rheumatic diseases. Rheum Dis Clin North Am 1999; 25: 81-103.

57. Kerin A, Patwari P, Kuettner K et al. Molecular basis of osteoarthritis: biomechanical aspects. Cell Mol Life Sci 2002; 59: 27-35.

58. Kiaer T, Gronlund J, Sorensen KH. Intraosseous pressure and partial pressures of oxygen and carbon dioxide in osteoarthritis. Semin Arthritis Rheum 1989; 18(suppl 2): 57-60.

59. Kidd B. Problems with pain – is the messenger to blame? Ann Rheum Dis 1996; 55: 276-283.

60. Kolasinski SL, Haines KA, Siegel EL et al. Neuropeptides and inflammation. A somatostatin analog as a selective antagonist of neutrophil activation by substance P. Arthritis Rheum 1992; 35: 369-375.

61. Kontinnen YT, Kemppinen P, Segerberg M et al. Peripheral and spinal neural mechanisms in arthritis with particular reference to treatment of inflammation and pain. Arthritis Rheum 1994; 37: 965-982.

62. Lane NE, Lin P, Christiansen L et al. Association of mild acetabular dysplasia with an increased risk of incident hip osteoarthritis in elderly white women: the study of osteoporotic fractures. Arthritis Rheum 2000; 43: 400-404.

63. Lawrence JS, Bremmer JM, Bier F. Osteo-arthrosis. Prevalence in the population and relationship between symptoms and x-ray changes. Ann Rheum Dis 1966; 25: 1-24.

64. Lawrence JS. Rheumatism in populations. London: William Heinemann; 1977.

65. Levine JD, Goetzl EJ, Basbaum AI. Contribution of the nervous system to the pathophysiology of rheumatoid arthritis and other polyarthritides. Rheum Dis Clin North Am 1987; 13: 369-383.

66. Ley P. Psychological studies of doctor-patient communication. In: Rachman S, ed. Contributions to medical psychology. Oxford: Pergamon Press; 1977: 9-42.

67. Lindblad S, Hedfors E. Arthroscopic and immunohistologic characterization of knee joint synovitis in osteoarthritis. Arthritis Rheum 1987; 30: 1081-1088.

68. Lindblad S, Hedfors E. Arthroscopic and synovial correlates of pain in osteoarthritis. Semin Arthritis Rheum 1989; 18(suppl 2): 91-93.

69. Little CB, Ghosh P. Variation in proteoglycan metabolism by articular chondrocytes in different joint regions is determined by post-natal mechanical loading. Osteoarthritis Cartilage 1997; 5: 49-62.

70. Loeser JD, Melzack R. Pain: an overview. Lancet 1999; 353: 1607-1609.

71. Loeser JD. Pain and suffering. Clin J Pain 2000;

16(2 suppl): S2-S6.

72. Loeser JD. What is chronic pain? Theor Med 1991; 12: 213-215.

73. Lynn B 1996 Efferent function of nociceptors. In: Belmonte C, Cervero F (eds) Neurobiology of nociceptors. Oxford University Press, Oxford, p 418-438.

74. Maggi C A, Meli A 1988 The sensory-efferent function of capsaicin-sensitive sensory neurons. General Pharmacology 19:1-43.

75. Matucci-Cerini M, Partsch G. The contribution of the peripheral nervous system and the neuropeptide network to the development of synovial inflammation. Clin Exp Rheumatol 1992; 10: 211-215.

76. McAlindon TE, Wilson PW, Aliabadi P et al. Level of physical activity and the risk of radiographic and symptomatic knee osteoarthritis in the elderly: the Framingham study. Am J Med 1999; 106: 151-157.

77. McFarlane AC, Brooks PM. An analysis of the relationship between psychological morbidity and disease activity in rheumatoid arthritis. J Rheumatol 1988; 15: 926-931.

78. Mendell LM. Physiological properties of unmyelinated fiber projection to the spinal cord. Exp Neurol 1966; 16: 316-332.

79. Moldofsky H. Sleep influences on regional and diffuse pain syndromes associated with osteoarthritis. Semin Arthritis Rheum 1989; 18(suppl 2): 18-21.

80. Mow VC, Ateshian GA, Spilker RL. Biomechanics of diarthrodial joints: a review of twenty years of progress. J Biomech Eng 1993; 115: 460-467.

81. Nachemson A. The lumbar spine: an orthopaedic challenge. Spine 1976; 1: 59-71.

82. Netter FH. Atlas of Human Anatomy, Fourth ed. Philadelphia: W.B. Saunders Company; 2006.

83. Nordin M, Frankel VH. Basic biomechanics of the musculoskeletal system, 3rd ed. Lippincott, Williams & Williams, Philadelphia; 2001.

84. O'Sullivan A, Sheffrin SM. Economics Principles and Tools. New Jersey: Prentice Hall; 1998.

85. Radanov BP, Sturzenegger M, Di Stefano G. Long-term outcome after whiplash injury. A 2-year follow-up considering features of injury mechanism and somatic, radiologic and psychosocial findings. Medicine (Baltimore) 1995; 74: 281-297.

86. Radin EL, Burr DB, Caterson B et al. Mechanical determinants of osteoarthrosis. Semin Arthritis Rheum 1991; 21(suppl 2): 12-21.9.

87. Raja SN, Meyer RA, Ringkamp M et al. Peripheral neural mechanisms of nociception. In: Wall PD, Melzack R eds. Textbook of Pain. Fourth ed. Edinburgh: Churchill Livingston; 1999: 11-57.

88. Rejeski WJ, Miller ME, Foy C et al. Self-efficacy and the progression of functional limitations and self-reported disability in older adults with knee pain. J Gerontol B Psychol Sci Soc Sci 2001; 56: S261-265.

89. Salter DM, Millward-Sadler SJ, Nuki G et al. Differential responses of chondrocytes from normal and osteoarthritic human articular cartilage to mechanical.

90. Samad TA, Sapirstein A, Woolf CJ. Prostanoids and pain: unraveling mechanisms and revealing therapeutic targets. Trends Mol Med 2002; 8: 390-396.

91. Saunders JB, Inman VT, Eberhardt HD. The major determinants in normal and pathological gait. J Bone Joint Surg 1953; 35A: 543-558.

92. Schaible H-G, Grubb BD. Afferent and spinal mechanisms of joint pain. Pain 1993; 55: 5-54.

93. Schaible H-G, Neugebauer V, Schmidt RF. Osteoarthritis and pain. Semin Arthritis Rheum 1989; 18: 30-34.

94. Schaible H-G, Schmidt RF. Effects of an experimental arthritis on the sensory properties of fine articular afferent units. J Neurophysiol 1985; 54: 1109-1122.

95. Schmelz M, Petersen L J 2001 Neurogenic inflammation in human and rodent skin. News in Physiological Sciences 16:33-37.

96. Schollmeier G, Uhthoff HK, Sarkar K, Fukuhara K. Effects of immobilization on the capsule of the canine glenohumeral joint. A structural functional study. Clin Orthop 1994; 304: 37-42.

97. Scholz J, Woolf CJ. Can we conquer pain? Nat Neurosci 2002; 5(suppl): 1062-1067.

98. Schumacher HR. The role of inflammation and crystals in the pain of osteoarthritis. Semin Arthritis Rheum 1989; 18(suppl 2): 81-85.

99. Seifert MH, Whiteside CG, Savage O. A five year follow up of 50 cases of idiopathic osteoarthritis of the hip (abstract). Ann Rheum Dis 1969; 28: 325-326.

100. Sewitch, MJ, Dobkin, PL, Bernatsky, S, et al. Medication non-adherence in women with fibromyalgia. Rheumatology (Oxford) 2004; 43:648.

101. Sharma L, Hurwitz DE, Thonar EJ et al. Knee adduction moment, serum hyaluronan level, and disease severity in medial tibiofemoral osteoarthritis. Arthritis Rheum 1998; 41: 1233-1240.

102. Sharma L, Pai YC. Impaired proprioception and osteoarthritis. Curr Opin Rheumatol 1997; 9: 253-258.

103. Sharma L, Song J, Felson DT et al. The role of knee alignment in disease progression and functional decline in knee osteoarthritis. JAMA 2001; 286: 188-195.

104. Slemenda C, Brandt KD, Heilman DK et al. Quadriceps weakness and osteoarthritis of the knee. Ann Intern Med 1997 15; 127: 97-104.

105. Sokoloff L. The joints and synovial fluid, vol 1. New York: Academic Press, 1978.

106. Sokoloff L. The joints and synovial fluid, vol 2. New York: Academic Press, 1980.

107. Spector TD, Dacre JE, Harris PA, Huskisson EC. The radiological progression of osteoarthritis: an eleven year follow up study of the knee. Ann Rheum Dis 1992; 51: 1107-1110.

108. Spector TD, Hart DJ, Doyle DV. Incidence and progression of osteoarthritis in women with unilateral knee disease in the general population: the effect of obesity. Ann Rheum Dis 1994; 53: 565-568.

109. Stadnik TW, Lee RR, Coen HL et al. Annular tears and disk herniation: prevalence and contrast enhancement on MR images in the absence of low back pain or sciatica. Radiology 1998; 206: 49-55.

110. Steig RL, Williams RC. Chronic pain as a biosociocultural phenomenon: implications for treatment. Semin Neurol 1983; 3: 370-376.

111. Steultjens MP, Dekker J, Bijlsma JW. Coping, pain, and disability in osteoarthritis: a longitudinal study. J Rheumatol 2001; 28: 1068-1072.

112. Van Saase JLCM. Osteoarthrosis in the general population: a follow up study of osteoarthrosis of the hip. PhD thesis, Leiden State University, The Netherlands; 1990.

113. Van Tulder MW, Assendelft WJJ, Koes BW et al. Spinal radiographic findings and nonspecific low back pain: a systematic review of observational studies. Spine 1997; 22: 427-434.

114. Vane JR. Inhibition of prostaglandin synthesis as a mechanism of action of aspirinlike drugs. Nature 1971; 231: 232-239.

115. Vuori IM. Dose-response of physical activity and low back pain, osteoarthritis, and osteoporosis. Med Sci Sports Exerc 2001; 33(suppl): S551-S586.

116. Weiser S, Cedrashi C. Psychosocial issues in the prevention of chronic low back pain - a literature review. Baillieres Clin Rheumatol 1992; 6: 657-684.

117. Weishaupt D, Zanetti M, Hodler J et al. MR imaging of the lumbar spine: prevalence of intervertebral disk extrusion and sequestration, nerve root compression, end plate abnormalities, and osteoarthritis of the facet joints in asymptomatic volunteers. Radiology 1998; 209: 661-666.

118. Wiesel SW, Tsourmas N, Feffer HL et al. A study of computer-assisted tomography. I. The incidence of positive CAT scans in an asymptomatic group of patients. Spine 1984; 9: 549-551.

119. Wilcox S, Brenes GA, Levine D et al. Factors related to sleep disturbance in older adults experiencing knee pain or knee pain with radiographic evidence of knee osteoarthritis. J Am Geriatr Soc 2000; 10: 1241-1251.

120. Witt I, Vestergaard A, Rosenklint A. A comparative analysis of X-ray findings of the lumbar spine in patients with and without lumbar pain. Spine 1984; 9: 298-300.

121. Woolf AD. History and physical examination. In: Hochberg, Silman AJ, Smolen JS, Weinblatt ME, Weisman MH eds. Rheumatology, Third Edition. Edinburgh: Mosby; 2003: 169-190.

122. Woolf CJ, Thompson SWN. The induction and maintenance of central sensitization is dependent on N-methyl-D-aspartic acid receptor activation; implications for the treatment of post-injury pain hypersensitivity states. Pain 1991; 44: 293-299.

123. Wyke B. The neurology of joints: a review of general principles. Clin Rheum Dis 1981; 7: 223-239.

References Chapter 7

1. Abramson SB, Weissmann G. The mechanisms of action of non-steroidal anti-inflammatory drugs. Arthritis Rheum 1989; 32: 1-9.

2. ACR Subcommittee on osteoarthritis guidelines. Recommendations for the medical management of osteoarthritis of the hip and knee: 2000 update. Arthritis Rheum 2000; 43: 1905-1915.

3. Akeson WH, Garfin S, Amiel D et al. Para-articular connective tissue in osteoarthritis. Semin Arthritis Rheum 1989; 18(suppl 2): 41-50.

4. Akil H, Owens C, Gutstein H et al. Endogenous opioids: overview and current issues. Drug Alcohol Depend 1998; 51: 127-140.

5. Alcoff J, Jones E, Rust P et al. Controlled trial of imipramine for chronic low back pain. J Fam Pract 1982; 14: 841-846.

6. Ali NM. Hyperalgesic response in a patient receiving high concentrations of spinal morphine. Anesthesiology 1986; 65: 449.

7. Aliberti J, Hieny S, Reis e Sousa C et al. Lipoxin-mediated inhibition of IL-12 production by DCs: a mechanism for regulation of microbial immunity. Nat Immunol 2002; 3: 76-82.

8. Altman R, Aven A, Holmburg C et al. Capsaicin cream 0.025% as monotherapy for osteoarthritis: a double blind study. Semin Arthritis Rheum 1994; 23(suppl): 25-33.

9. Altman RD, Asch E, Bloch D et al. Development of criteria for the classification and reporting of osteoarthritis: classification of osteoarthritis of the knee. Arthritis Rheum 1986; 29: 1039-1049.

10. Andersen G, Christrup L, Sjogren P. Relationships among morphine metabolism, pain and side effects during long-term treatment: an update. J Pain

Symptom Manage 2003; 25: 74-91.

11. Anderson GD, Hauser SD, McGarity KL et al. Selective inhibition of cyclooxygenase (COX)-2 reverses inflammation and expression of COX-2 and interleukin 6 in rat adjuvant arthritis. J Clin Invest 1996; 97: 2672-2679.

12. Ansari A. The efficacy of newer antidepressants in the treatment of chronic pain: a review of current literature. Harv Rev Psychiatry 2000; 7: 257-277.

13. Antal M, Petko M, Polgar E et al. Direct evidence of an extensive GABAergic innervation of the spinal dorsal horn by fibres descending from the rostral ventromedial medulla. Neuroscience 1996; 73: 509-518.

14. Arnold LM, Keck PE Jr, Welge JA. Antidepressant treatment of fibromyalgia. A meta-analysis and review. Psychosomatics 2000; 41: 104-113.

15. Arnold LM, Lu Y, Crofford LJ et al. A double-blind, multicenter trial comparing duloxetine with placebo in the treatment of fibromyalgia patients with or without major depressive disorder. Arthritis Rheum 2004; 50: 2974-2984.

16. Arnold LM, Rosen A, Pritchett YL et al. A randomized, double-blind, placebo-controlled trial of duloxetine in the treatment of women with fibromyalgia with or without major depressive disorder. Pain 2005; 119: 5-15.

17. Atkinson JH, Kremer EF, Risch SC et al. Basal and post-dexamethasone cortisol and prolactin concentrations in depressed and non-depressed patients with chronic pain syndromes. Pain 1986; 25: 23-24.

18. Atkinson JH, Slater MA, Wahlgren DR et al. Effects of noradrenergic and serotonergic antidepressants on chronic low back pain intensity. Pain 1999; 83: 137-145.

19. Attur MG, Dave M, Akamatsu M et al. Osteoarthritis or osteoarthrosis: the definition of inflammation becomes a semantic issue in the genomic era of molecular medicine. Osteoarthritis Cartilage 2002; 10: 1-4.

20. Badalamente MA, Cherney SB. Periosteal and vascular innervation of the human patella in degenerative joint disease. Semin Arthritis Rheum 1989; 18(suppl 2): 61-66.

21. Bajwa ZH, Warfield CA, Wooton RJ. Overview of the treatment of chronic pain. UpToDate Online 2005; 13.2: 1-17. 20 September 2005 <http://www.utdol.com>.

22. Bamigbade TA, Davidson C, Langford RM et al. Actions of tramadol, its enantiomers and principal metabolite, O-desmethyltramadol, on serotonin (5-HT) efflux and uptake in the rat dorsal raphe nucleus. Br J Anaesth 1997; 79: 352-356.

23. Bandler R, Shipley MT. Columnar organization in thje midbrain periaqueductal gray: modules for emotional expression? Trends Neurosci 1994; 17: 379-389.

24. Bannwarth B. Risk-benefit assessment of opioids in chronic non-cancer pain. Drug Saf 1999; 21: 283-96.

25. Bannwarth B, Demotes-Mainard F, Schaeverbeke T et al. Where are peripheral analgesics acting? Ann Rheum Dis 1993; 52: 1-4.

26. Barnes PJ, Brown MJ, Dollery CT et al. Histamine is released from skin by substance P but does not act as the final vasodilator in the axon reflex. Br J Pharmacol 1986; 88:741-745.

27. Barrett SL, O'Malley R. Plantar fasciitis and other causes of heel pain. Am Fam Physician 1999; 59: 2200-2206.

28. Beiche F, Klein T, Nusing R et al. Localization of cyclooxygenase-2 and prostaglandin E2 receptor EP3 in the rat lumbar spinal cord. J Neuroimmunol. 1998; 89: 26-34.

29. Bellamy N, Sothern RB, Campbell J et al. Circadian and circaseptan variation in pain perception in osteoarthritis of the knee. J Rheumatol 1990; 17: 364-372.

30. Benderdour M, Tardif G, Pelletier JP et al. Interleukin 17 (IL-17) induces collagenase-3 production in human osteoarthritic chondrocytes via AP-1 dependent activation: differential activation of AP-1 members by IL-17 and IL-1â. J Rheumatol 2002; 29: 1262-1272.

31. Bennett RM, Gatter RA, Campbell SM et al. A comparison of cyclobenzaprine and placebo in the management of fibrositis. A double-blind controlled study. Arthritis Rheum 1988; 31: 1535-1542.

32. Bennett RM. Pharmacological treatment of fibromyalgia. J Funct Syndr 2001; 1: 79-92.

33. Berry H, Bloom B, Hamilton EBD et al. Naproxen sodium, diflunisal, and placebo in the treatment of chronic back pain. Ann Rheum Dis 1982; 41: 129-132.

34. Besse D, Lombard MC, Zajac JM et al. Pre- and postsynaptic distribution of mu, delta and kappa opioid receptors in the superficial layers of the cervical dorsal horn of the rat spinal cord. Brain Res 1990; 521: 15-22.

35. Besse D, Lombard MC, Zajac JM et al. Pre- and postsynaptic location of mu, delta and kappa opioid receptors in the superficial layers of the dorsal horn of the rat spinal cord. Prog Clin Biol Res 1990; 328: 183-186.

36. Beydoun A, Backonja MM. Mechanistic stratification of antineuralgic agents. J Pain Symptom Manage 2003; 25(5 Suppl): S18-S30.

37. Birrell GJ, McQueen DS, Iggo A et al. PGI2-induced activation and sensitization of articular mechanonociceptors. Neurosci Lett 1991; 124: 5-8.

38. Blackshear JL, Napier JS, Davidman M et al. Renal complications of NSAIDs: Identification and monitoring of those at risk. Semin Arthritis Rheum 1985; 14: 163–175.

39. Blumer D, Zorick F, Heilbronn M et al. Biological markers for depression in chronic pain. J Nerv Ment Dis 1982; 170: 425-428.

40. Boardman PL, Burke MJ, Camp AV et al. Treatment of osteoarthritis with piroxicam. Eur J Rheumatol Inflamm 1983; 6: 73–83.

41. Bourgoin S, Pohl M, Mauborgne A et al. Monoaminergic control of the release of calcitonin gene-related peptide and substance P-like materials from rat spinal cord slices. Neuropharmacology 1993; 32: 633-640.

42. Bovill JG. Mechanisms of actions of opioids and non-steroidal anti-inflammatory drugs. Eur J Anaesthesiol 1997; 14(Suppl 15): 9–15.

43. Bradley JD, Brandt KD, Katz BP et al.. Comparison of an anti-inflammatory dose of ibuprofen, an analgesic dose of ibuprofen, and acetaminophen in the treatment of patients with osteoarthritis of the knee. N Engl J Med 1991; 325: 87–91.

44. Bradley JD, Brandt KT, Katz BP et al.. Treatment of knee osteoarthritis: Relationship of clinical features of joint inflammation to the response to a nonsteroidal anti-inflammatory drug or pure analgesic. J Rheumatol 1992; 19: 1950–1954.

45. Breshnihan B, Hughes G, Essigman WK. Diflunisal in the treatment of osteoarthritis: a double-blind study comparing diflunisal with ibuprofen. Curr Med Res Opin 1997; 5: 556–561.

46. Bridger S, Henderson K, Glucksman E et al. Deaths from low dose paracetamol poisoning. BMJ 1998; 316: 1724-1725.

47. Brooks PM, Day RO. Non-steroidal anti-inflammatory drugs differences and similarities. N Engl J Med 1991; 324: 1716-1725.

48. Brooks PM. Non-steroidal anti-inflammatory drugs. In: Hochberg MC, Silman AJ, Smolen JS, Weinblatt ME, Weisman MH eds. Rheumatology, Third Edition. Edinburgh: Mosby; 2003: 377-384.

49. Brune K, Zeilhofer HU. Antipyretic analgesics. In: Melzack R, Wall PD eds. Handbook of Pain Management. Edinburgh: Churchill Livingstone; 2003: 341-351.

50. Bryans JS, Wustrow DJ. 3-Substituted GABA analogs with central nervous system activity: a review. Med Res Rev 1999; 19: 149-177.

51. Cada DJ, Levien T, Baker DE. Pregabalin. Hospital Pharmacy 2006; 41: 157-172.

52. Cai Z, McCaslin PP. Amitriptyline, desipramine, cyproheptadine and carbamazepine, in concentrations used therapeutically, reduce kainate and N-methyl-D-aspartate-induced intracellular Ca2+ levels in neuronal culture. Eur J Pharmacol 1992; 219: 53-57.

53. Carette S, Bell MJ, Reynolds WJ et al. Comparison of amitriptyline, cyclobenzaprine, and placebo in the treatment of fibromyalgia. A randomized, double-blind clinical trial. Arthritis Rheum 1994; 37: 32-40.

54. Carette S, McCain GA, Bell DA et al. Evaluation of amitriptyline in primary fibrositis: a double-blind, placebo-controlled study. Arthritis Rheum 1986; 29: 655-659.

55. Caterina MJ, Schumacher MA, Tominaga M et al. The capsaicin receptor: a heat activated ion channel in the pain pathway. Nature 1997; 389: 816-824.

56. Celiker R, Cagavi Z. Comparison of amitriptyline and sertraline in the treatment of fibromyalgia syndrome. Poster presented at: 20th Annual Scientific Meeting of the American Pain Society; April 20, 2001.

57. Chandrasekharan NV, Dai H, Roos KL et al. COX-3, a cyclooxygenase-1 variant inhibited by acetaminophen and other analgesic/antipyretic drugs: cloning, structure, and expression. Proc Natl Acad Sci U S A 2002; 99: 13926-13931.

58. Chapman CR, Hill HF. Prolonged morphine self-administration and addiction liability. Cancer 1989; 63: 1636-1644.

59. Cherny NI. Opioid analgesics. Comparative features and prescribing guidelines. Drugs 1996; 51: 713–737.

60. Chi S-I, Levine JD, Basbaum AI. Effects of injury discharge on the persistent expression of spinal cord fos-like immunoreactivity produced by sciatic nerve transaction in the rat. Brain Res 1993; 617: 220-224.

61. Coderre TJ, Katz J, Vaccarino AL, Melzack R. Contribution of central neuroplasticity to pathologic pain: review of clinical and experimental evidence. Pain 1993; 52: 259-285.

62. Commissiong JW, Karoum F, Reiffenstein RJ et al. Cyclobenzaprine: a possible mechanism of action for its muscle relaxant effect. Can J Physiol Pharmacol 1981; 59: 37– 44.

63. Conrozier T, Chappuis-Cellier C, Richard M et al. Increased serum C-reactive protein levels by immunonephelometry in patients with rapidly destructive hip osteoarthritis. Rev Rhum Engl Ed 1998; 65: 759-765.

64. Corbett AD, Paterson SJ, Kosterlitz HW. Selectivity of ligands for opioid receptors. In: Herz A ed. Handbook of Experimental Pharmacology. Opioids I. Berlin: Springer-Verlag; 1993: 645-673.

65. Cornwall MW, McPoil TG. Plantar fasciitis: etiology and treatment. J Orthop Sports Phys Ther 1999; 29: 756-760.

66. Cotran RS, Kumar V, Collins T. Robbins pathologic basis of disease, 6th ed. Philadelphia, PA: WB Saunders; 1999.

67. Couch J R, Ziegler D K, Hassanein R. Amitriptyline in the prophylaxis of migraine. Effectiveness and relationship of antimigraine and antidepressant effects. Neurology 1976; 26: 121-127.

68. Craig AD, Dostrovsky JO. Medulla to thalamus. In: Wall PD, Melzack R eds. Textbook of Pain. Fourth ed. Edinburgh: Churchill Livingston; 1999: 183-214.

69. Creamer P. Osteoarthritis. In: Wall PD, Melzack R eds. Textbook of Pain. Fourth ed. Edinburgh: Churchill Livingston; 1999: 493-504.

70. Crofford LJ, Rowbotham MC, Mease PJ et al. Pregabalin for the treatment of fibromyalgia syndrome: results of a randomized, double-blind, placebo-controlled trial. Arthritis Rheum 2005; 52: 1264-1273.

71. Crofford LJ, Simpson S, Young JP Jr et al. A Six-month, Double-blind, Placebo-controlled, Durability of Effect Study of Pregabalin for Pain Associated With Fibromyalgia. Oasis-Online Abstract Submission and Invitation System 2005; 4 November 2006 <www.abstractsonline.com/viewer/SearchResults.asp>.

72. Crofford LJ, Wilder RL, Ristimaki AP et al. Cyclooxygenase-1 and -2 expression in rheumatoid synovial tissues. Effects of interleukin-1 beta, phorbol ester, and corticosteroids. J Clin Invest 1994; 93: 1095-1101.

73. Cush JJ, Jasin HE, Johnson R et al. Relationship between clinical efficacy and laboratory correlates of inflammatory and immunologic activity in rheumatoid arthritis patients treated with nonsteroidal anti-inflammatory drugs. Arthritis Rheum 1990; 33: 623–633.

74. Cush JJ, Lipsky PE, Postlethwaite AE et al. Correlation of serologic indicators of inflammation with effectiveness of nonsteroidal anti-inflammatory drug therapy in rheumatoid arthritis. Arthritis Rheum 1990; 33: 19–28.

75. Dalton SE. The shoulder. In: Hochberg MC, Silman AJ, Smolen JS, Weinblatt ME, Weisman MH eds. Rheumatology, Third Edition. Edinburgh: Mosby; 2003: 615-630.

76. Deal CL, Schnitzer TJ, Lipstein E et al. Treatment of arthritis with topical capsaicin: a double-blind trial. Clin Ther 1991; 13: 383-395.

77. Delmas PD. Non-steroidal anti-inflammatory drugs and renal function. Br J Rheumatol 1995; 34: 25-28.

78. Devchand PR, Arita M, Hong S et al. Human ALX receptor regulates neutrophil recruitment in transgenic mice: roles in inflammation and host defense. FASEB J 2003; 17: 652-659.

79. Deyo RA. Drug therapy for back pain. Which drugs help which patients? Spine 1996; 21: 2840–2849.

80. Diaz-Gonzalez F, Gonzalez-Alvaro I, Campenero MR et al. Prevention of in vitro neutrophil-endothelial attachment through shedding of l-selectin by nonsteroidal anti-inflammatory drugs. J Clin Invest 1995; 95: 1756–1765.

81. DiBona GF. Prostaglandins and nonsteroidal anti-inflammatory drugs. Effects on renal hemodynamics. Am J Med 1986; 80: 12–21.

82. Dickenson A. Where and how do opioids act? In: Gebhart G, Hammond D, Jensen T eds. Proceedings of the 7th World Congress on Pain. Progress in Pain Research and Management, Vol 2. Seattle: IASP Press; 1994: 525-552.

83. Dickenson AH, Kieffer B. Opiates: baisic mechanisms. In: McMahon SB, Koltzenburg M eds. Wall and Melzack's Textbook of Pain, Fifth Edition. Edinburgh: Elsevier Churchill Livingstone; 2006: 427-442.

84. Dickenson AH, Sullivan AF. Evidence for a role of the NMDA receptor in the frequency dependent potentiation of deep rat dorsal horn nociceptive neurons following C fiber stimulation. Neuropharmacology 1987; 26: 1235-1238.

85. Dooley DJ, Donovan CM, Pugsley TA. Stimulus-dependent modulation of [3H]-norepinephrine release from rat neocortical slices by gabapentin and pregabalin. J Pharmacol Exp Ther 2000; 295: 1086-1093.

86. Dooley DJ, Mieske CA, Borosky SA. Inhibition of K(+)-evoked glutamate release from rat neocortical and hippocampal slices by gabapentin. Neurosci Lett 2000; 280: 107-110.

87. Doubell TP, Mannion RJ, Woolf CJ. The dorsal horn state-dependent sensory processing, plasticity and the generation of pain. In: Wall PD, Melzack R eds. Textbook of Pain. Fourth ed. Edinburgh: Churchill Livingston; 1999: 165-181.

88. Dwight MM, Arnold LM, O'Brien H et al. An open clinical trial of venlafaxine treatment of fibromyalgia. Psychosomatics 1998; 39: 14-17.

89. Ebersberger A, Grubb BD, Willingale HL et al. The intraspinal release of prostaglandin E2 in a model of acute arthritis is accompanied by an up-regulation of cyclo-oxygenase-2 in the spinal cord. Neuroscience 1999; 93: 775-781.

90. Ebertz JM, Hirshman CA, Kettelkamp NS et al. Substance P-induced histamine release in human cutaneous mast cells. J Invest Dermatol 1987; 88: 682-685.

91. Eisenach JC, Gebhart GF. Intrathecal amitriptyline acts as an N-methyl-D-aspartate receptor antagonist in the presence of inflammatory hyperalgesia in rats. Anesthesiology 1995; 83: 1046-1054.

92. Escott KJ, Brain SD. Effect of a calcitonin gene-related peptide antagonist (CGRP8-37) on skin vasodilatation and oedema induced by stimulation of the rat saphenous nerve. Br J Pharmacol 1993; 110: 772-776.

93. Fabbri A, Cruccu G, Sperti P et al. Piroxicam-induced analgesia. Evidence for a central component which is not opioid-mediated. Experientia 1992; 48: 1139–1142.

94. Farrell GC. The hepatic side effects of drugs. Med J Aust 1986; 145: 600–604.

95. Feldman M. COX-2 inhibitors and gastroduodenal toxicity – major clinical trials. UpToDate Online 2005; 13.2: 1-6. 20 September 2005 <http://www.utdol.com>.

96. Feltner DE, Crockatt JG, Dubovsky SJ et al. A randomized, double-blind, placebo-controlled, fixed-dose, multicenter study of pregabalin in patients with generalized anxiety disorder. J Clin Psychopharmacol 2003; 23: 240-249.

97. Fields HL, Basbaum HI, Heinricher MM. Central nervous system mechanisms of pain modulation. In: McMahon SB, Koltzenburg M eds. Wall and Melzack's Textbook of Pain, Fifth Edition. Edinburgh: Elsevier Churchill Livingstone; 2006: 125-142.

98. Fields HL. Pain modulation: expectation, opioid analgesia and virtual pain. Prog Brain Res 2000; 122: 245-253.

99. Fierro IM, Kutok JL, Serhan CN. Novel lipid mediator regulators of endothelial cell proliferation and migration: aspirin-triggered-15R-lipoxin A(4) and lipoxin A(4). J Pharmacol Exp Ther 2002; 300: 385-392.

100.Furst DE. Are there differences among nonsteroidal anti-inflammatory drugs? Comparing acetylated salicylates, nonacetylated salicylates, and nonacetylated nonsteroidal anti-inflammatory drugs. Arthritis Rheum 1994; 37: 1–9.

101. Geba GP, Weaver AL, Polis AB et al. Efficacy of rofecoxib, celecoxib, and acetaminophen in osteoarthritis of the knee: a randomized trial. JAMA 2002; 287: 64-71.

102.Gelgor L, Cartmell S, Mitchell D. Intracerebroventricular micro-injections of non-steroidal anti-inflammatory drugs abolish reperfusion hyperalgesia in the rat's tail. Pain 1992; 50: 323–329.

103.Gendreau RM, Thorn MD, Gendreau JF et al. Efficacy of milnacipran in patients with fibromyalgia. J Rheumatol 2005; 32: 1975-1985.

104.Gibbon WW, Cassar-Pullicino VN. Heel pain. Ann Rheum Dis 1994; 53: 344-348.

105.Godson C, Mitchell S, Harvey K et al. Cutting edge: lipoxins rapidly stimulate nonphlogistic phagocytosis of apoptic neutrophils by monocyte-derived macrophages. J Immunol 2000; 164: 1663-1667.

106.Goldenberg DL, Felson DT, Dinerman H. A randomized, controlled trial of amitriptyline and naproxen in the treatment of patients with fibromyalgia. Arthritis Rheum 1986; 29: 1371-1377.

107.Goldenberg DL, Mayskly M, Mossey CJ et al. A randomized double-blind crossover trial of fluoxetine and amitriptyline in the treatment of fibromyalgia. Arthritis Rheum 1996; 39: 1852-1859.

108.Gonzalez E, de la Cruz C, de Nicolás R et al. Long-term effect of non-steroidal anti-inflammatory drugs on the production of cytokines and other inflammatory mediators by blood cells of patients with osteoarthritis. Agents Actions Suppl 1994; 41: 171–178.

109.Gottrup H, Hansen PO, Arendt-Nielsen L et al. Differential effects of systemically administered ketamine and lidocaine on dynamic and static hyperalgesia induced by intradermal capsaicin in humans. Br J Anaesth 2000; 84: 155-162.

110. Grigg P, Schaible H-G, Schmidt RF. Mechanical sensitivity of group III and IV afferents from posterior articular nerve in normal and inflamed cat knee. J Neurophysiol 1986; 55: 635-643.

111. Grond S, Radbruch L, Meuser T et al. High-dose tramadol in comparison to low-dose morphine for cancer pain relief. J Pain Symptom Manage 1999; 18: 174-179.

112. Guieu R, Blin O, Pouget J et al. Analgesic effect of indomethacin shown using the nociceptive flexion reflex in humans. Ann Rheum Dis 1992; 51: 391–393.

113. Hagermark O, Hokfelt T, Pernow B. Flare and itch induced by substance P in human skin. J Invest Dermatol 1978; 71: 233-235.

114. Hameroff SR, Weiss JL, Lerman JC et al. Doxepin effects on chronic pain and depression: a controlled study. J Clin Psychiatry 1984; 45: 45-52.

115. Hammond DL, Levy RA, Proudfit HK. Hypoalgesia following microinjection of noradrenergic antagonists in the nucleus raphe magnus. Pain 1980; 9: 85-101.

116. Hammond DL, Levy RA, Proudfit HK. Hypoalgesia induced by microinjection of a norepinephrine antagonist in the raphe magnus: reversal by intrathecal administration of a serotonin antagonist. Brain Res 1980; 201: 475-479.

117. Headley PM, Duggan AW, Griersmith BT. Selective reduction by noradrenaline and 5-hydroxytryptamine of nociceptive responses of cat dorsal horn neurones. Brain Res 1978; 145: 185-189.

118. Heinricher MM, Neubert MJ. Neural basis for the hyperalgesic action of cholecystokinin in the rostral ventromedial medulla. J Neurophysiol 2004; 92: 1982-1989.

119. Heinricher MM. Orphanin FQ/nociceptin: from neural circuitry to behavior. Life Sci 2003; 73: 813-822.

120.Helme RD, Koschorke GM, Zimmermann M. Immunoreactive substance P release from skin nerves in the rat by noxious thermal stimulation. Neurosci Lett 1986; 63: 295-299.

121. Hord AH, Denson DD, Stowe B et al. alpha-1 and alpha-2 adrenergic antagonists relieve thermal hyperalgesia in experimental mononeuropathy from chronic constriction injury. Anesth Analg 2001; 92: 1558-1562.

122. Hunt S, Mantyh P. The molecular dynamics of pain control. Nat Rev Neurosci 2001; 2: 83-91.

123. Huskisson EC, Woolf PC, Baume HW et al. Four new anti-inflammatory drugs - responses and variations. Br Med J 1974; 1: 1084-1089.

124. Ito S, Okuda-Ashitaka E, Minami T. Central and peripheral roles of prostaglandins in pain and their interactions with novel neuropeptides nociceptin and nocistatin. Neurosci Res. 2001; 41:299-332.

125. Jaeschke R, Adachi J, Guyatt G, Keller J, Wong B. Clinical usefulness of amitriptyline in fibromyalgia: the results of 23 N-of-1 randomized controlled trials. J Rheumatol 1991; 18: 447-451.

126. Janeso G, Kiraly E, Janeso-Gabor A et al. Direct evidence for an axonal site of action of capsaicin. Naunyn Schmiedebergs Arch Pharmacol 1993; 313: 91–94.

127. Janeso G, Kiraly E, Janeso-Gabor A. Pharmacologically induced selective degeneration of chemosensitive primary sensory neurons. Nature 1977; 270: 741–743.

128. Jenkins DG, Ebutt AF, Evans CD. Imipramine in the treatment of low back pain. J Int Med Res 1976; 4(Suppl 2): 28-40.

129. Jones AKP, Derbyshire SWG. Cerebral mechanisms operating in the presence and absence of inflammatory pain. Ann Rheum Dis 1996; 55: 411-420.

130. Joris J, Costello A, Dubner R et al. Opiates suppress carrageenan-induced edema and hyperthermia at doses that inhibit hyperalgesia. Pain 1990; 43: 95-103.

131. Jung AC, Staiger T, Sullivan M. The efficacy of selective serotonin reuptake inhibitors for the management of chronic pain [see comments]. J Gen Intern Med 1997; 12: 384-389.

132. Kalunian KC, Concoff AL, Brion PH et al. Pharmacologic and surgical therapy of osteoarthritis. UpToDate Online 2005; 13.2: 1-25. 4 August 2005 <http://www.utdol.com>.

133. Kantor TG. Concepts in pain control. Semin Arthritis Rheum1989; 18(suppl 2): 94-99.

134. Karr SD. Subcalcaneal heel pain. Orthop Clinic North Am 1994; 25: 161-175.

135. Kayser V, Chen YL, Guilbaud G. Behavioural evidence for a peripheral component in the enhanced antinociceptive effect of a low dose of systemic morphine in carrageenan-induced hyperalgesic rats. Brain Res 1991; 560: 237-244.

136. Kayser V, Guilbaud G. The analgesic effects of morphine, but not those of the enkephalinase inhibitor thiorphan, are enhanced in arthritic rats. Brain Res 1983; 267: 131-138.

137. Kiaer T, Gronlund J, Sorensen KH. Intraosseous pressure and partial pressures of oxygen and carbon dioxide in osteoarthritis. Semin Arthritis Rheum 1989; 18(suppl 2): 57-60.

138. Kidd B. Problems with pain – is the messenger to blame? Ann Rheum Dis 1996; 55: 276-283.

139. Kobayashi H, Hasegawa Y, Ono H. Cyclobenzaprine, a centrally acting muscle relaxant, acts on descending serotonergic systems. Eur J Pharmacol 1996; 311: 29-35.

140. Koes BW, Scholten RJPM, Mens JMA et al. Efficacy of nonsteroidal anti-inflammatory drugs for low back pain: a systematic review of randomized clinical trials. Ann Rheum Dis 1997; 56: 214-223.

141. Kolasinski SL, Haines KA, Siegel EL et al. Neuropeptides and inflammation. A somatostatin analog as a selective antagonist of neutrophil activation by substance P. Arthritis Rheum 1992; 35: 369-375.

142. Kontinnen YT, Kemppinen P, Segerberg M et al. Peripheral and spinal neural mechanisms in arthritis with particular reference to treatment of inflammation and pain. Arthritis Rheum 1994; 37: 965-982.

143. Krishnan KKR, France RD, Pelton S et al. Chronic pain and depression. I. Classification of depression in low back pain patients. Pain 1985; 22: 279-287.

144. Kuo CC. Imipramine inhibition of transient K+ current: an external open channel blocker preventing fast inactivation. Biophys J 1998; 75: 2845-2857.

145. Kuraishi Y, Hirota N, Sato Y et al. Noradrenergic inhibition of the release of substance P from the primary afferents in the rabbit spinal dorsal horn. Brain Res 1985; 359: 177-182.

146. Kuraishi Y, Hirota N, Satoh M et al. Antinociceptive effects of intrathecal opioids, noradrenaline and serotonin in rats: mechanical and thermal algesic tests. Brain Res 1985; 326: 168-171.

147. Lance JW, Curran DA. Treatment of chronic tension headache. Lancet 1964; 1: 1236-1239.

148. Langohr HD, Stohr M, Petruch F. An open end, double-blind, crossover study on the efficacy of clomipramine in patients with painful mono and polyneuropathies. Eur Neurol 1982; 21: 309-317.

149. Lascelles RG. Atypical facial pain and depression. Br J Psychiatry 1966; 122: 651-659.

150. Lauritsen K, Laursen LS, Kjeldsen J et al. Inhibition of eicosanoid synthesis and potential therapeutic benefits of 'dual pathway inhibition'. Pharmacol Toxicol 1994; 75: 9–13.

151. Lawlor PG, Turner KS, Hanson J et al. Dose ratio between morphine and methadone in patients with cancer pain: a retrospective study. Cancer 1998; 82: 1167-1173.

152. Lee YH, Ryu TG, Park SJ et al. Alphal-adrenoceptors involvement in painful diabetic neuropathy: a role in allodynia. Neuroreport 2000; 11: 1417-1420.

153. Lembeck F, Donnerer J, Tsuchiya M et al. The non-peptide tachykinin antagonist, CP-96,345, is a potent inhibitor of neurogenic inflammation. Br J Pharmacol 1992; 105: 527-530.

154. Levinson DJ, Rubinstein HM. Double-blind comparison of fenoprofen calcium and ibuprofen in osteoarthritis of large joints. Current Therapy Research 1983; 34: 280-284.

155. Levy BD, De Sanctis GT, Devchand PR et al. Multi-pronged inhibition of airway hyper-responsiveness and inflammation by lipoxin A(4). Nat Med 2002; 8: 1018-1023.

156. Lewis KS, Han NH. Tramadol: A new centrally acting analgesic. Am J Health Syst Pharm 1997; 54: 643-652.

157. Lindblad S, Hedfors E. Arthroscopic and immunohistologic characterization of knee joint synovitis in osteoarthritis. Arthritis Rheum 1987; 30: 1081-1088.

158. Lindblad S, Hedfors E. Arthroscopic and synovial correlates of pain in osteoarthritis. Semin Arthritis Rheum 1989; 18(suppl 2): 91-93.

159. Lloyd RS, Costello F, Eves MJ et al. The efficacy and tolerability of controlled-release dihydrocodeine tablets and combination dextropropoxyphene/paracetamol tablets in patients with severe osteoarthritis of the hips. Curr Med Res Opin 1992; 13: 37-48.

160. Lu X, Xie W, Reed D. Nonsteroidal anti-inflammatory drugs cause apoptosis and induce cyclooxygenases in chicken embryo fibroblasts. Proc Natl Acad Sci U S A 1995; 92: 7961-7965.

161. Lyrica [package insert]. New York, NY; Pfizer, Inc; 2005.

162. Machelska H, Binder W, Stein C. Opioid receptors in the periphery. In: Kalso E, McQuay H, Wiesenfeld-Hallin Z eds. Opioid Sensitivity of Chronic Noncancer Pain. Progress in Pain Research and Management, Vol 14. Seattle: IASP Press; 1999: 45-58.

163. Magni G, Rigatti-Luchini S, Fracca F et al. Suicidality in chronic abdominal pain: an analysis of the Hispanic Health and Nutrition Examination Survey (HHANES). Pain 1998; 76: 137-144.

164. Magni G, Marchetti M, Moreschi C et al.. Chronic musculoskeletal pain and depressive symptoms in the National Health and Nutrition Examination. I. Epidemiologic follow-up study. Pain 1993; 53: 163-168.

165. Magni G. The use of antidepressants in the treatment of chronic pain. A review of the evidence. Drugs 1991; 42: 730-748.

166. Malmberg AB, Yaksh TL. Antinociceptive actions of spinal nonsteroidal anti-inflammatory agents on the formalin test in the rat. J Pharmacol Exp Ther 1992; 263: 136-146.

167. Malmberg AB, Yaksh TL. Hyperalgesia mediated by spinal glutamate or substance P receptor blocked by spinal cyclooxygenase inhibition. Science 1992; 257: 1276-1279.

168. Maneuf YP, Hughes J, McKnight AT. Gabapentin inhibits the substance P-facilitated K(+)-evoked release of [(3)H]glutamate from rat caudal trigeminal nucleus slices. Pain 2001; 93: 191-196.

169. Marbach JJ. Medically unexplained chronic orofacial pain. Temporomandibular pain and dysfunction syndrome, orofacial phantom pain, burning mouth syndrome, and trigeminal neuralgia. Med Clin North Am 1999; 83: 691-710.

170. Max MB, Schafer SC, Culnane M et al. Amitriptyline but not lorazepam relieves postherpetic neuralgia. Neurology 1988; 38: 1427-1432.

171. McCarthy GM, McCarty DJ. Effect of topical capsaicin in the therapy of painful osteoarthritis of the hands. J Rheumatol 1992; 19: 604-607.

172. McCaslin PP, Yu XZ, Ho IK et al. Amitriptyline prevents N-methyl-D-aspartate (NMDA)-induced toxicity, does not prevent NMDA-induced elevations of extracellular glutamate, but augments kainate-induced elevations of glutamate. J Neurochem 1992; 59: 401-405.

173. McCormack K, Brune K. Dissociation between the antinociceptive and inflammatory effects of the nonsteroidal anti-inflammatory drugs. A survey of their analgesic efficacy. Drugs 1991; 41: 533-547.

174. McQuay HJ, Moore RA. An Evidence-based Resource for Pain Relief. Oxford: Oxford University Press; 1998.

175. Mendell LM. Physiological properties of unmyelinated fiber projection to the spinal cord. Exp Neurol 1966; 16: 316-332.

176. Millan MJ, Czlonkowski A, Pilcher CW et al. A model of chronic pain in the rat: functional correlates of alterations in the activity of opioid systems. J Neurosci 1987; 7: 77-87.

177. Minami T, Nakano H, Kobayashi T et al. Characterization of EP receptor subtypes responsible for prostaglandin E2-induced pain responses by use of EP1 and EP3 receptor knockout mice. Br J Pharmacol 2001; 133: 438-444.

178. Miyoshi HR, Leckband SG. Systemic opioid analgesics. In: Loeser JD, Butler SH, Chapman CR, Turk DC eds. Bonica's Management of Pain. Philadelphia: Lipincott, Williams ans Wilkins; 2001: 1682-1709.

179.Mizumura K, Sato J, Kumazawa T. Effects of prostaglandins and other putative chemical intermediaries on the activity of canine testicular polymodal receptors studied in vitro. Pflugers Arch 1987; 408: 565-572.

180.Moldofsky H. Sleep influences on regional and diffuse pain syndromes associated with osteoarthritis. Semin Arthritis Rheum 1989; 18(suppl 2): 18-21.

181.Moreland LW, St. Clair EW. The use of analgesics in the management of pain in the rheumatic diseases. Rheum Dis Clin North Am 1999; 25: 153-191.

182.Myers SL, Brandt KD, Ehlich JW et al. J Synovial inflammation in patients with early osteoarthritis of the knee. Rheumatol 1990; 17: 1662-1669.

183.Nakajima H, Hiyama Y, Tsukada W et al. Effects of interferon gamma on cultured synovial cells from patients with rheumatoid arthritis: inhibition of cell growth, prostaglandin E2, and collagenase release. Ann Rheum Dis 1990; 49: 312-316.

184.Nakazawa K, Inoue K, Ohno Y. Block and unblock by imipramine of cloned and mutated P2X2 receptor/channel expressed in Xenopus oocytes. Neurosci Lett 1999; 264: 93-96.

185.Neil A, Kayser V, Gacel G et al. Opioid receptor types and antinociceptive activity in chronic inflammation: both kappa- and mu-opiate agonistic effects are enhanced in arthritic rats. Eur J Pharmacol 1986; 130: 203-208.

186.North RA, Yoshimura M. The actions of noradrenaline on neurones of the rat substantia gelatinosa in vitro. J Physiol 1984; 349: 43-55.

187.O'Malley PG, Balden E, Tomkins G et al. Treatment of fibromyalgia with antidepressants: a meta-analysis. J Gen Intern Med 2000; 15: 659-666.

188.Onghena P, van Houdenhove B. Antidepressant-induced analgesia in chronic non-malignant pain: a meta-analysis of 39 placebo controlled studies. Pain 1992; 49: 205-219.

189.Pande AC, Crockatt JG, Feltner DE et al. Pregabalin in generalized anxiety disorder: a placebo-controlled trial. Am J Psychiatry 2003; 160: 533-540.

190.Paoli F, Darcourt G, Cossa P. Sur l'action de l'imipramine dans les etats douloureux. Congress of Psychiatry and Neurology, Lille. Paris: Masson; 1960.

191.Pappagallo M, Heinberg LJ. Ethical issues in the management of chronic nonmalignant pain. Semin Neurol 1997; 17: 203-211.

192.Park TJ, Shin SY, Suh BC et al. Differential inhibition of catecholamine secretion by amitriptyline through blockage of nicotinic receptors, sodium channels, and calcium channels in bovine adrenal chromaffin cells. Synapse 1998; 29: 248-256.

193.Passik SD, Weinreb HJ. Managing chronic nonmalignant pain: overcoming obstacles to the use of opioids. Adv Ther 2000; 17: 70-83.

194.Pelletier JP, Roughley PJ, DiBattista JA et al. Are cytokines involved in osteoarthritic pathophysiology? Semin Arthritis Rheum 1991; 20(suppl 2): 12-25.

195.Pilletta P, Porchet HC, Dayer P. Central analgesic effect of acetaminophen but not of aspirin. Clin Pharmacol Ther 1991; 49: 350-354.

196.Pincus T, Koch G, Lei H et al. Patient preference for placebo, acetaminophen (paracetamol) or celecoxib efficacy studies (PACES): two randomised, double blind, placebo controlled, crossover clinical trials in patients with knee or hip osteoarthritis. Ann Rheum Dis 2004; 63: 931-939.

197.Pincus T, Koch GG, Sokka T et al. A randomized, double-blind, crossover clinical trial of diclofenac plus misoprostol versus acetaminophen in patients with osteoarthritis of the hip or knee. Arthritis Rheum 2001; 44: 1587-1598.

198.Planells-Cases R, Garcia-Martinez C, Royo M et al. Small molecules targeting the vanilloid receptor complex as drugs for inflammatory pain. Drugs Future 2003; 28: 787-795.

199.Portenoy RK. Chronic opioid therapy in nonmalignant pain. J Pain Symptom Manage 1990; 5(1 suppl): S46-S62.

200.Prichasuk S, Subhadrabandhu T. The relationship of pes planus and calcaneal spur to plantar heel pain. Clin Orthop 1994; 306: 192-196.

201.Qiu FH, Devchand PR, Wada K et al. Aspirin-triggered lipoxin A4 and lipoxin A4 up-regulate transcriptional corepressor NAB1 in human neutrophils. FASEB J 2001; 15: 2736-2738.

202.Quimby LG, Gratwick GM, Whitney CD et al. A randomized trial of cylobenzaprine for the treatment of fibromyalgia. J Rheumatol 1989; 16: 140-143.

203.Rahman W, Dashwood MR, Fitzgerald M et al. Postnatal development of multiple opioid receptors in the spinal cord and development of spinal morphine analgesia. Brain Res Dev Brain Res 1998; 108: 239-254.

204.Rahman W, Suzuki R, Dickenson AH. Pains, brains and spinal gains: facilitatory mechanisms underlying altered pain states. J Palliat Med Palliat Care 2003; 2: 82-89.

205.Rajagopal A, Vassilopoulou-Sellin R, Palmer JL et al. Hypogonadism and sexual dysfunction in male cancer survivors receiving chronic opioid therapy. J Pain Symptom Manage 2003; 26: 1055-1061.

206.Rao SG. The neuropharmacology of centrally-acting analgesic medications in fibromyalgia. Rheum Dis Clin North Am 2002; 28: 235-259.

207.Reddy SV, Maderdrut JL, Yaksh TL. Spinal cord pharmacology of adrenergic agonist-mediated antinociception. J Pharmacol Exp Ther 1980; 213: 525-533.

208.Reddy SV, Yaksh TL. Spinal noradrenergic terminal system mediates antinociception. Brain Res 1980; 189: 391-401.

209.Rejeski WJ, Miller ME, Foy C et al. Self-efficacy and the progression of functional limitations and self-reported disability in older adults with knee pain. J Gerontol B Psychol Sci Soc Sci 2001; 56: S261-265.

210.Reynolds IJ, Miller RJ. Tricyclic antidepressants block N-methyl-D-aspartate receptors: similarities to the action of zinc. Br J Pharmacol 1988; 95: 95-102.

211. Reynolds WJ, Moldofsky H, Saskin P et al. The effects of cyclobenzaprine on sleep physiology and symptoms in patients with fibromyalgia. J Rheumatol 1991; 18: 452-454.

212.Robinson DR. Inflammation. In: Hochberg MC, Silman AJ, Smolen JS, Weinblatt ME, Weisman MH eds. Rheumatology, Third Edition. Edinburgh: Mosby; 2003: 147-158.

213.Roth S, Iwan T, Hou Y et al. Long term opioid administration: stable doses and pain control with reduction in side effects over time. In: Proceedings of the 8th World Congress on Pain of the International Association for the Study of Pain. Seattle: IASP Press; 1996: 53.

214.Sagen J, Proudfit HK. Evidence for pain modulation by pre- and postsynaptic noradrenergic receptors in the medulla oblongata. Brain Res 1985; 331: 285-293.

215.Salt TE, Hill RG. Transmitter candidates of somatosensory primary afferent fibres. Neuroscience 1983; 10: 1083-1103.

216.Samad TA, Moore KA, Sapirstein A et al. Interleukin-1beta-mediated induction of Cox-2 in the CNS contributes to inflammatory pain hypersensitivity. Nature 2001; 410: 471-475.

217.Samad TA, Saperstein A, Woolf CJ. Prostanoids and pain: unraveling mechanisms and revealing therapeutic targets. Trends Mol Med 2002; 8: 390-396.

218.Sanchez C, Hyttel J. Comparison of the effects of antidepressants and their metabolites on reuptake of biogenic amines and on receptor binding. Cell Mol Neurobiol 1999; 19: 467-489.

219.Sandrini G, Ruiz L, Capararo M et al. Central analgesic activity of ibuprofen. A neurophysiological study in humans. Int J Clin Pharmacol Res 1992; 12: 197-204.

220.Sang CN, Hayes KS. Anticonvulsant medications in neuropathic pain. In: McMahon SB, Koltzenburg M eds. Wall and Melzack's Textbook of Pain, Fifth Edition. Edinburgh: Elsevier Churchill Livingstone; 2006: 499-506.

221.Saria A. Substance P in sensory nerve fibres contributes to the development of oedema in the rat hind paw after thermal injury. Br J Pharmacol 1984; 82: 217-222.

222.Savage SR. Assessment for addiction in pain-treatment settings. Clin J Pain 2002; 18(4 suppl): S28-S38.

223.Savage SR. Opioid use in the management of chronic pain. Med Clin North Am 1999; 83: 761-86.

224.Schaible H-G, Neugebauer V, Schmidt RF. Osteoarthritis and pain. Semin Arthritis Rheum 1989; 18: 30-34.

225.Schaible H-G, Schmidt RF. Effects of an experimental arthritis on the sensory properties of fine articular afferent units. J Neurophysiol 1985; 54: 1109-1122.

226.Schaible H-G, Schmidt RF. Excitation and sensitization of fine articular afferents from cat's knee joint by prostaglandin E2. J Physiol 1988; 403: 91-104.

227.Schapira D, Nahir M, Scharf Y. Trochanteric bursitis: a common clinical problem. Arch Phys Med Rehabil 1986; 67: 815-817.

228.Schepsis AA, Leach RE, Gorzyca J. Plantar fasciitis: etiology, treatment, surgical results and review of the literature. Clin Orthop 1991; 266: 185-196.

229.Schlondorff D. Renal complications of non-steroidal anti-inflammatory drugs. Kidney Int 1993; 44: 643-653.

230.Schnitzer T, Morton C, Coker C et al. Effectiveness of reduced applications of topical capsaicin (0.025%) in osteoarthritis. Arthritis Rheum 1992; 35: S132.

231.Schug SA, Gandham N. Opioids: clinical use. In: McMahon SB, Koltzenburg M eds. Wall and Melzack's Textbook of Pain, Fifth Edition. Edinburgh: Elsevier Churchill Livingstone; 2006: 443-457.

232.Schug SA, Zech D, Grond S et al. A long-term survey of morphine in cancer pain patients. J Pain Symptom Manage 1992; 7: 259-266.

233.Schumacher HR. The role of inflammation and crystals in the pain of osteoarthritis. Semin Arthritis Rheum 1989; 18(suppl 2): 81-85.

234.Schumacher HR, Meng Z, Sieck M et al. Effect of a nonsteroidal anti-inflammatory drug on synovial fluid in osteoarthritis. J Rheumatol 1996; 23: 1774-1777.

235.Scott LJ, Perry CM. Tramadol: a review of its use in perioperative pain. Drugs 2000; 60: 139-176.

236.Scudds RA, McCain GA, Rollman GB et al. Improvements in pain responsiveness in patients with fibrositis after successful treatment with amitriptyline. J Rheumatol 1989; 16: 98-103.

237.Serhan CN. Eicosanoids and related compounds. In: Koopman WJ, Moreland LW eds. Arthritis and Allied Conditions, Fifteenth Edition. Philadelphia: Lippincott, Williams and Wilkins; 2005: 517-539.

238.Simmons DL, Botting RM, Robertson PM et al. Induction of an acetaminophen-sensitive cyclooxygenase with reduced sensitivity to nonsteroid antiinflammatory drugs. Proc Natl Acad Sci U S A 1999; 96: 3275-3280.

239.Simon LS. Hyperbole, innuendo, and fact.: the strange case of selective cox-2 inhibitors. J Rheumatol 2006; 33: 1-3.

240.Simon LS. NSAIDs: Mechanism of action. UpToDate Online 2005; 13.2: 1-13. 20 September 2005 <http://www.utdol.com>.

241.Simon LS. NSAIDs: Overview of adverse effects. UpToDate Online 2005; 13.2: 1-8. 20 September 2005 <http://www.utdol.com>.

242.Simon LS. NSAIDs: Therapeutic use and variability of response in adults. UpToDate Online 2005; 13.2: 1-8. 20 September 2005 <http://www.utdol.com>.

243.Simon LS. Biologic effects of nonsteroidal antiinflammatory drugs. Curr Opin Rheumatol 1997; 9: 178–182.

244.Sindrup SH, Jensen TS. Efficacy of pharmacological treatments of neuropathic pain: an update and effect related to mechanism of drug action. Pain 1999; 83: 389-400.

245.Sivilotti L, Woolf CJ. The contribution of GABA_A and glycine receptors to central sensitization: disinhibition and touch-evoked allodynia in the spinal cord. J Neurophysiol 1994; 72: 169-179.

246.Sjogren P, Jensen NH, Jensen TS. Disappearance of morphine-induced hyperalgesia after discontinuing or substituting morphine with other opioid agonists. Pain 1994; 59: 313-316.

247.Spector TD, Hart DJ, Nandra D et al. Low-level increases in serum C-reactive protein are present in early osteoarthritis of the knee and predict progressive disease. Arthritis Rheum 1997; 40: 723-727.

248.Stein C, Millan MJ, Yassouridis A et al. Antinociceptive effects of mu- and kappa-agonists in inflammation are enhanced by a peripheral opioid receptor-specific mechanism. Eur J Pharmacol 1988; 155: 255-264.

249.Stein D, Peri T, Edelstein E et al.. The efficacy of amitriptylin and acetaminophen in the management of acute low back pain. Psychosomatics 1996; 37: 63-70.

250.Steultjens MP, Dekker J, Bijlsma JW. Coping, pain,

and disability in osteoarthritis: a longitudinal study. J Rheumatol 2001; 28: 1068-1072.

251.Sukenik S, Henkin J, Zimlichman S et al. Serum and synovial fluid levels of serum amyloid A protein and C-reactive protein in inflammatory and noninflammatory arthritis. J Rheumatol 1988; 15: 942-945.

252.Sullivan MJL, Reesor K, Mikail S et al. The treatment of depression in chronic low back pain: review and recommendations. Pain 1992; 50: 5-13.

253.Sundy JS. Nonsteroidal anti-inflammatory drugs. Koopman WJ, Moreland LW eds. Arthritis and Allied Conditions, Fifteenth Edition. Philadelphia: Lippincott, Williams and Wilkins; 2005: 670-704.

254.Svensson CI, Yaksh TL. The spinal phospholipase-cyclooxygenase-prostanoid cascade in nociceptive processing. Annu Toxicol 2002; 42: 553-583.

255.Takagi H, Yamamoto K, Shiosaka S et al. Morphological study of noradrenaline innervation in the caudal raphe nuclei with special reference to fine structure. J Comp Neurol 1981; 203: 15-22.

256.Tannenbaum H, Bombardier C, Davis P et al. An evidence-based approach to prescribing nonsteroidal antiinflammatory drugs. Third Canadian Consensus Conference. J Rheumatol 2006; 33: 140-157.

257.Taylor F, Dickenson A. Nociceptin/orphanin FQ. A new opioid, a new analgesic? Neuroreport 1998; 9: R65-70.

258.Tilley SL, Coffman TM, Koller BH. Mixed messages: modulation of inflammation and immune responses by prostaglandins and thromboxanes. J Clin Invest 2001; 108: 15-23.

259.Todd AJ, Spike RC. The localization of classical transmitters and neuropeptides within neurons in laminae I-III of the mammalian spinal dorsal horn. Prog Neurobiol 1993; 41: 609-646.

260.Todd AJ, Sullivan AC. A light microscope study of the coexistence of GABA-like and glycine-like immunoreactivities in the spinal cord of the rat. J Comp Neurol 1990; 296: 496-505.

261.Todorovic SM, Meyenburg A, Jevtovic-Todorovic V. Redox modulation of peripheral T-type Ca^{2+} channels in vivo: alteration of nerve injury-induced thermal hyperalgesia. Pain 2004; 109: 328-339.

262.Torebjork HE, Lundberg LER, LaMotte RH. Central changes in processing of mechanoreceptor input in capsaicin-induced sensory hyperalgesia in humans. J Physiol 1992; 448: 765-780.

263.Towheed TE, Judd MJ, Hochberg MC et al. Acetaminophen for osteoarthritis. Cochrane Database Syst Rev 2003; (2): CD004257.

264.Twycross RG. Opioids. In: Wall PD, Melzack R eds. Textbook of Pain. Fourth ed. Edinburgh: Churchill Livingston; 1999; 1187-1214.

265.Urquhart E. Central analgesic activity of nonsteroidal anti-inflammatory drugs in animal and human pain models. Semin Arthritis Rheum 1993; 23: 198–205.

266.Vane JR, Botting RM. New insights into the mode of action of anti-inflammatory drugs. Inflamm Res 1995; 44: 1-10.

267.Vane JR. Inhbition of prostaglandin synthesis as a mechanism of action of aspirin-like drugs. Nature 1971; 231: 232-239.

268.Vane JR, Botting RM. Mechanisms of action of aspirin-like drugs. Semin Arthritis Rheum 1997; 26: 2–10.

269.Vane JR. Introduction: mechanism of action of NSAIDs. Br J Rheumatol 1996; 35: 1–3.

270.Videman T, Osterman K. Double-blind parallel study of piroxicam versus indomethacin in the treatment of low back pain. Ann Clin Res 1984; 16: 156-160.

271.Vlok GJ, van Vuren JP. Comparison of a standard ibuprofen treatment regimen with a new ibuprofen/paracetamol/codeine combination in chronic osteo-arthritis. S Afr Med J 1987; Suppl 1: 4-6.

272.Walker JS, Sheather-Reid RB, Carmody JJ et al. Nonsteroidal anti-inflammatory drugs in rheumatoid arthritis and osteoarthritis. Arthritis Rheum. 1997; 40: 1944–1954.

273.Watanabe Y, Saito H, Abe K. Tricyclic antidepressants block NMDA receptor-mediated synaptic responses and induction of long-term potentiation in rat hippocampal slices. Neuropharmacology 1993; 32: 479-486.

274.Watson CP, Evans RJ, Reed K et al. Amitriptyline versus placebo in postherpetic neuralgia. Neurology 1982; 32: 671-673.

275.Watson CPN, Chipman ML, Monks RC. Antidepessant analgesics: a systematic review and comparative study. In: McMahon SB, Koltzenburg M eds. Wall and Melzack's Textbook of Pain, Fifth Edition. Edinburgh: Elsevier Churchill Livingstone; 2006: 481-497.

276.Wegman A, van der Windt D, van Tulder M et al. Nonsteroidal antiinflammatory drugs or acetaminophen for osteoarthritis of the hip or knee? A systematic review of evidence and guidelines. J Rheumatol 2004; 31: 344-354.

277.Weissman DE, Haddox JD. Opioid pseudoaddiction-an iatrogenic syndrome. Pain 1989; 36: 363-366.

278.Wilcox S, Brenes GA, Levine D et al. Factors related to sleep disturbance in older adults experiencing knee pain or knee pain with radiographic evidence of knee osteoarthritis. J Am Geriatr Soc 2000; 10: 1241-1251.

279.Wilder-Smith C, Schimke J, Osterwalder B et al. Oral tramadol, a mu-opioid agonist and monoamine reuptake-blocker, and morphine for strong cancer-related pain. Ann Oncol 1994; 5: 141-146.

280.Wilder-Smith CH, Hill L, Osler W et al. Effect of tramadol and morphine on pain and gastrointestinal motor function in patients with chronic pancreatitis. Dig Dis Sci 1999; 44: 1107-1116.

281.Willer J-C, De Broucker T, Bussel B et al. Central analgesic effect of ketoprofen in humans: Electrophysiological evidence for a supraspinal mechanism in a double-blind and cross-over study. Pain 1989; 38: 1–7.

282.Willer J-C, Harrewyn J-M. Effet inhibiteur central du ketoprophene intravineux sur la reflexe nociceptif de flexion chez l'homme. Presse Med 1987; 16: 63–67.

283.Willer J-C. Comparative study of perceived pain and nociceptive flexion reflex in man. Pain 1977; 3: 69–80.

284.Willer J-C. Reactions nociceptives chez l'homme. Etude electrophysiologique et Pharmacologique. Nouv Presse Med 1982; 11: 2125–2129.

285.Williams HJ. Comparison of naproxen and acetaminophen in the treatment of osteoarthritis of the knees. Arthritis Rheum 1991; 34(Suppl 9): S84.

286.Willis WD, Westlund KN. Neuroanatomy of the pain system and of the pathways that modulate pain. J Clin Neurophysiol 1997; 14: 2-31.

287.Wolfe F, Zhao S, Lane N. Preference for nonsteroidal antiinflammatory drugs over acetaminophen by rheumatic disease patients: a survey of 1,799 patients with osteoarthritis, rheumatoid arthritis, and fibromyalgia. Arthritis Rheum 2000; 43: 378-385.

288.Wolfe F. The C-reactive protein but not erythrocyte sedimentation rate is associated with clinical severity in patients with osteoarthritis of the knee or hip. J Rheumatol 1997; 24: 1486-1488.

289.Wolfe MM, Lichtenstein DR, Singh G. Gastrointestinal toxicity of non steroidal anti-inflammatory drugs. N Engl J Med 1999; 340: 1888-1899.

290.Woolf CJ, Thompson SWN. The induction and maintenance of central sensitization is dependent on N-methyl-D-aspartic acid receptor activation; implications for the treatment of post-injury pain hypersensitivity states. Pain 1991; 44: 293-299.

291.World Health Organization. Cancer pain relief and palliative care. Geneva: WHO; 1996.

292.World Health Organization. Cancer pain relief. Geneva: WHO; 1986.

293.World Health Organization. Expert Committee on Drug Dependence, 16th report. Technical report series no. 407. Geneva: WHO; 1969.

294.Wyke B. The neurology of joints: a review of general principles. Clin Rheum Dis 1981; 7: 223-239.

295.Xie WL, Chipman JG, Robertson DL et al. Expression of a mitogen-responsive gene encoding prostaglandin synthetase is regulated by mRNA splicing. Proc Natl Acad Sci U S A 1991; 88: 2692-2696.

296.Yaksh T. Pharmacology and mechanisms of opioid analgesic activity. In: Yaksh T, Lynch C, Zapol W et al eds. Anesthesia: Biologic Foundations. Philadelphia: Lippincott-Raven; 1997: 921-934.

297.Yaksh TL, Noueihed R. The physiology and pharmacology of spinal opiates. Annu Rev Pharmacol Toxicol 1985; 25: 433-462.

298.Yaksh TL. Behavioral and autonomic correlates of the tactile evoked allodynia produced by spinal glycine inhibition: effects of modulatory receptor systems and excitatory amino acid antagonists. Pain 1989; 37: 111-123.

299.Yaksh TL. Pharmacology and mechanisms of opioid analgesic activity. Acta Anaesthesiol Scand 1997; 41: 94-111.

300.Yang LC, Marsala M, Yaksh TL. Characterization of time course of spinal amino acids citrulline and PGE2 release after carrageenan/kaolin-induced knee joint inflammation: a chronic microdialysis study. Pain 1996; 67: 345-354.

301.Young WS 3rd, Kuhar MJ. Noradrenergic alpha 1 and alpha 2 receptors: light microscopic autoradiographic localization. Proc Natl Acad Sci USA 1980; 77: 1696-1700.

302.Zhang WY, Li Wan Po A. The effectiveness of topically applied capsaicin. A meta-analysis. Eur J Clin Pharmacol 1994; 46: 517-522.

303.Zijlstra TR, Barendregt PJ, van de Laar MA. Venlafaxine in fibromyalgia: results of a randomized, placebocontrolled, double-blind trial. Arthritis Rheum 2002; 46(supplement 9): S105.

References Chapter 8

1. Brody DM. Running injuries. Clinical Symposia 1987; 39(3): 1-36.

2. Messier SP, Gutekunst DJ, Davis C et al. Weight loss reduces knee-joint loads in overweight and obese older adults with knee osteoarthritis. Arthritis Rheum 2005; 52: 2026-2032.

3. Nachemson A. Lumbar mechanics as revealed by lumbar intradiscal pressure measurements. In: Jayson MIV ed. The Lumbar Spin and Back Pain, Fourth Edition. Edinburgh: Churchill Livingstone; 1992: 157-171.

4. Peterson DM. Overview of the risks and benefits of exercise. UpToDate Online 2006; 14.1: 1-20. 22 May 2006 <http://www.utdol.com>.

5. Wolheim FA. Pathogenesis of osteoarthritis. In: Hochberg, Silman AJ, Smolen JS, Weinblatt ME, Weisman MH eds. Rheumatology, Third Edition. London: Mosby; 2003: 1801-1815.

References Chapter 9

1. Agurs-Collins TD, Kumanyika SK, Have TR et al. A randomized controlled trial of weight reduction and exercise for diabetes management in older African-American subjects. Diabetes Care 1997; 20: 1503-1511.

2. Albu J, Pi-Sunyer XF. Obesity and diabetes. In: Bray G ed. Handbook of Obesity. New York: Marcel Dekker; 1998: 697–707.

3. Allison DB, Mentore JL, Heo M et al. Antipsychotic-induced weight gain: a comprehensive research synthesis. Am J Psychiatry 1999; 156: 1686-1696.

4. Allison DB, Kaprio J, Korkeila M et al. The heritability of body mass index among an international sample of monozygotic twins reared apart. Int J Obes Relat Metab Disord 1996; 20: 501–506.

5. Andersen RE, Crespo CJ, Bartlett SJ et al. Relationship between body weight gain and significant knee, hip, and back pain in older Americans. Obes Res 2003; 11: 1159-1162.

6. Anderssen S, Holme I, Urdal P et al. Diet and exercise intervention have favourable effects on blood pressure in mild hypertensives: the Oslo Diet and Exercise Study (ODES). Blood Press 1995; 4: 343-349.

7. Arden N, Nevitt MC. Osteoarthritis: epidemiology. Best Pract Res Clin Rheumatol 2006; 20: 3-25.

8. Ashley FW, Kannel WB. Relation of weight change to changes in atherogenic traits: the Framingham Study. J Chronic Dis 1974; 27: 103–114.

9. Ballantyne D, Devine B, Fife R. Interrelation of age, obesity, cigarette smoking and blood pressure in hypertensive patients. BMJ. 1978;1:880-881.

10. Ballor D, Keesey R. A meta-analysis of the factors affecting exercise-induced changes in body mass, fat mass and fat-free mass in males and females. Int J Obes 1991; 15: 717-726.

11. Bassett DR, Schneider PL, Huntington GE. Physical activity in an Old Order Amish community. Med Sci Sports Exerc 2004; 36: 79-85.

12. Bostick RM, Potter JD, Kushi LH et al. Sugar, meat, and fat intake, and nondietary risk factors for colon cancer incidence in Iowa women (United States). Cancer Causes Control 1994; 5: 38-52.

13. Bouchard C, Perusse L, Leblanc C et al. Inheritance of the amount of distribution of human body fat. Int J Obes Relat Metab Disord 1988; 12: 205–215.

14. Bouchard C, Savard R, Despres JP et al.. Body composition in adopted and biological siblings. Hum Biol 1985; 57: 61-75.

15. Bray GA. Diet and the initiation of therapy for obesity. UpToDate Online 2005; 13.2: 1-12. 14 July 2005 <http://www.utdol.com>.

16. Bray GA. Role of physical activity and exercise in obesity. UpToDate Online 2006; 14.2: 1-12. 5 July 2006 <http://www.utdol.com>.

17. Bultman SJ, Michaud EJ, Woychik RP. Molecular characterization of the mouse agouti locus. Cell 1992; 71: 1195-1204.

18. Campfield LA, Smith FJ, Burn P. The OB protein (leptin) pathway — a link between adipose tissue mass and central neural networks. Horm Metab Res 1996; 28: 619-632.

19. Canning H, Mayer J. Obesity: its possible effect on college acceptance. N Eng J Med 1966; 275: 1172-1174.

20. Cardon LR, Carmelli D, Fabsitz RR et al. Genetic and environmental correlations between obesity and body fat distribution in adult male twins. Hum Biol 1994; 66: 465–479.

21. Carman WJ, Sowers M, Hawthorne VM et al. Obesity as a risk factor for osteoarthritis of the hand and wrist: a prospective study. Am J Epidemiol 1994; 139: 119–129.

22. Carriere G. Parent and child factors associated with youth obesity. Supplement to Health Reports; Statistics Canada Catalogue 82-003 2003: 29-39.

23. Champagne CM, Bray GA, Kurtz AA et al. Energy intake and energy expenditure: a controlled study comparing dietitians and non-dietitians. J Am Diet Assoc 2002; 102: 1428-1432.

24. Chan J, Rimm E, Colditz G et al. Obesity, fat distribution and weight gain as risk factors for clinical diabetes in men. Diabetes Care 1994; 17: 961–969.

25. Chu SY, Lee NC, Wingo PA et al. The relationship between body mass and breast cancer among women enrolled in the Cancer and Steroid Hormone Study. J Clin Epidemiol 1991; 44: 1197-1206.

26. Chute CG, Willett WC, Colditz GA et al. A prospective study of body mass, height, and smoking on the risk of colorectal cancer in women. Cancer Causes Control 1991; 2: 117-124.

27. Colditz G, Willett W, Rotnitzky A et al. Weight gain as a risk factor for clinical diabetes mellitus in women. Ann Intern Med 1995; 122: 481–486.

28. Cooper C, Inskip H, Croft P et al. Individual risk factors for hip osteoarthritis: obesity, hip injury, and physical activity. Am J Epidemiol 1998; 147: 516–522.

29. Cooper C, Snow S, McAlindon TE et al. Risk factors for the incidence and progression of radiographic knee osteoarthritis. Arthritis Rheum 2000; 43: 995–1000.

30. Croft PR, Brigg D, Smith S et al. How useful is weight reduction in the management of hypertension? J R Coll Gen Pract. 1986; 36: 445-448.

31. Dattilo AM, Kris-Etherton PM. Effects of weight reduction on blood lipids and lipoproteins: A meta-analysis. Am J Clin Nutr 1992; 56: 320–328.

32. Davis BR, Blaufox MD, Oberman A et al. Reduction in long-term antihypertensive medication requirements. Effects of weight reduction by dietary intervention in overweight persons with mild hypertension. Arch Intern Med 1993; 153: 1773-1782.

33. Denke MA, Sempos CT, Grundy SM. Excess body weight: An underrecognized contributor to high blood cholesterol levels in white American men. Arch Intern Med 1993; 153: 1093–1103.

34. Denke MA, Sempos CT, Grundy SM. Excess body weight: An underrecognized contributor to high blood cholesterol levels in white American women. Arch Intern Med 1994; 154: 401–410.

35. Epstein LH, Wing RR. Aerobic exercise and weight. Addict Behav 1980; 5: 371-388.

36. Ewing R, Schmid T, Killingsworth R et al. Relationship between urban sprawl and physical activity, obesity, and morbidity. Am J Health Promot 2003; 18: 47-57.

37. Faith M, Allison D. Assessment of psychological status among obese persons. In: Thompson J eds. Body Image, Eating Disorders and Obesity. Washington, DC: American Psychological Association; 1996: 365–388.

38. Fava M, Judge R, Hoog SL et al. Fluoxetine versus sertraline and paroxetine in major depressive disorder: changes in weight with long-term treatment. J Clin Psychiatry 2000; 61: 863-867.

39. Felson DT, Anderson JJ, Naimark A et al. Obesity and knee osteoarthritis. The Framingham Study. Ann Intern Med 1988; 109: 18–24.

40. Felson DT, Lawrence RC, Dieppe PA et al. Osteoarthritis: new insights. Part I: the disease and its risk factors. Ann Intern Med 2000; 133: 635–646.

41. Felson DT, Zhang Y, Anthony JM et al. Weight loss reduces the risk for symptomatic knee osteoarthritis in women. The Framingham Study. Ann Intern Med 1992; 116: 535–539.

42. Felson DT, Zhang Y, Hannan M et al. Risk factors for incident radiographic knee osteoarthritis in the elderly. Arthritis Rheum 1997; 40: 728–733.

43. Fernstrom MH. Drugs that cause weight gain. Obes Res 1995; 3 Suppl 4: 435S-439S.

44. Flegal KM, Graubard BI, Williamson DF et al. Excess deaths associated with underweight, overweight, and obesity. JAMA 2005; 293: 1861-1867.

45. Flegal KM, Troiano RP, Pamuk ER et al. The influence of smoking cessation on the prevalence of overweight in the United States. N Engl J Med 1995; 333: 1165-1170.

46. Foreyt JP, Goodrick GK. Factors common to successful therapy for the obese patient. Med Sci

Sports Exerc 1991; 23: 292-297.

47. Foster GD, Wadden TA, Vogt RA et al. What is a reasonable weight loss? Patients' expectations and evaluations of obesity treatment outcomes. J Consult Clin Psychol 1997; 65: 79-85.

48. Gardner RM, Tockerman YR. A computer-TV video methodology for investigating the influence of somatotype on perceived personality traits. J Soc Behav Pers 1994; 9: 555-563.

49. Garfinkel L. Overweight and mortality. Cancer 1986; 58: 1826-1829.

50. Garland C, Shekelle RB, Barrett-Connor E et al. Dietary vitamin D and calcium and risk of colorectal cancer: a 19-year prospective study in men. Lancet 1985; 1: 307-309.

51. Garrow, J, Summerbell, C. Meta-analysis: Effect of exercise, with or without dieting, on the body composition of overweight subjects. Eur J Clin Nutr 1995; 49:1.

52. Gelber AC, Hochberg MC, Mead LA et al. Body mass index in young men and the risk of subsequent knee and hip osteoarthritis. Am J Med 1999; 107: 542–548.

53. Gerace TA, Hollis J, Ockene JK et al. Smoking cessation and change in diastolic blood pressure, body weight, and plasma lipids. MRFIT Research Group. Prev Med 1991; 20: 602-620.

54. Giovannucci E, Ascherio A, Rimm EB et al. Physical activity, obesity, and risk for colon cancer and adenoma in men. Ann Intern Med 1995; 122: 327-334.

55. Giovannucci E, Colditz GA, Stampfer MJ, Willett WC. Physical activity, obesity, and risk of colorectal adenoma in women (United States). Cancer Causes Control 1996; 7: 253- 263.

56. Giovannucci E. Insulin and colon cancer. Cancer Causes Control 1995; 6: 164-179.

57. Goldstein DJ, Potvin JH. Long term weight loss — the effect of pharmacological agents. Am J Clin Nutr 1994; 60: 647-657.

58. Gortmaker SL, Must A, Perrin JM et al. Social and economic consequences of overweight in adolescence and young adulthood. N Engl J Med 1993; 329: 1008-1012.

59. Graham S, Marshall J, Haughey B et al. Dietary epidemiology of cancer of the colon in western New York. Am J Epidemiol 1988; 128: 490-503.

60. Grimm RH Jr, Cohen JD, Smith WM et al. Hypertension management in the Multiple Risk Factor Intervention Trial (MRFIT). 6-year intervention results for men in special intervention and usual care groups. Arch Intern Med 1985; 145: 1191-1199.

61. Hadjiolova I, Mintcheva L, Dunev S et al. Physical working capacity in obese women after an exercise program for body weight reduction. Int J Obes 1982; 6: 405-410.

62. Hall SM, Tunstall CD, Vila KL et al. Weight gain prevention and smoking cessation: cautionary findings. Am J Public Health 1992; 82: 799-803.

63. Hart DJ, Doyle DV, Spector TD. Association between metabolic factors and knee osteoarthritis in women: the Chingford study. J Rheumatol 1995; 22: 1118–1123.

64. Havlik R, Hubert H, Fabsitz R et al. Weight and hypertension. Ann Intern Med 1983; 98: 855–859.

65. Heller SR, Clarke P, Daly H et al. Group education for obese patients with type 2 diabetes: greater success at less cost. Diabet Med 1988;5:552-556.

66. Helmrich SP, Shapiro S, Rosenberg L et al. Risk factors for breast cancer. Am J Epidemiol 1983; 117: 35-45.

67. Herschopf RJ, Elahi D, Andres R et al. Longitudinal changes in serum cholesterol in man: An epidemiologic search for an etiology. J Chronic Dis 1982; 35: 101–114.

68. Heyden S. The workingman's diet. II. Effect of weight reduction in obese patients with hypertension, diabetes, hyperuricemia and hyperlipidemia. Nutr Metab 1978; 22: 141-159.

69. Hill JO, Wyatt HR, Melanson EL. Genetic and environmental contributions to obesity. Med Clin North Am 2000; 84: 333-346.

70. Hjermann I, Leren P, Norman N et al. Serum insulin response to oral glucose load during a dietary intervention trial in healthy coronary high risk men: the Oslo study. Scand J Clin Lab Invest 1980; 40: 89-94.

71. Hu FB, Li TY, Colditz GA et al. Television watching and other sedentary behaviors in relation to risk of obesity and type 2 diabetes mellitus in women. JAMA 2003; 289: 1785-1791.

72. Huang MH, Chen CH, Chen TW et al. The effects of weight reduction on the rehabilitation of patients with knee osteoarthritis and obesity. Arthritis Care Res 2000; 13: 398–405.

73. Huang Z, Hankinson SE, Colditz GA et al. Dual effects of weight and weight gain on breast cancer risk. JAMA 1997; 278: 1407-1411.

74. Hubert HB, Feinleib M, McNamara PM et al. Obesity as an independent risk factor for cardiovascular disease: A 26-year follow-up of participants in the Framingham Heart Study. Circulation 1983; 67: 968–977.

75. Hunter DJ, Willett WC. Diet, body size, and breast cancer. Epidemiol Rev 1993; 15: 110-132.

76. Jakicic JM, Marcus BH, Gallagher KI et al. Effect of exercise duration and intensity on weight loss in overweight, sedentary women: a randomized trial. JAMA 2003; 290: 1323-1330.

77. Jeffery RW, Wing RR, Thorson C et al. Strengthening behavioral interventions for weight loss: a

randomized trial of food provision and monetary incentives. J Consult Clin Psychol 1993; 61: 1038-1045.

78. Jousilahti P, Tuomilehto J, Vartiainen E et al. Body weight, cardiovascular risk factors, and coronary mortality. 15-year follow-up of middle-aged men and women in eastern Finland. Circulation 1996; 93: 1372-1379.

79. Karlson EW, Mandl LA, Aweh GN et al. Total hip replacement due to osteoarthritis: the importance of age, obesity, and other modifiable risk factors. Am J Med 2003; 114: 93–98.

80. Karris L. Prejudice against obese renters. J Soc Psych 1977; 101: 159-160.

81. Katzel LI, Bleecker ER, Colman EG et al.Effects of weight loss vs aerobic exercise training on risk factors for coronary disease in healthy, obese, middle-aged and older men. A randomized controlled trial. JAMA 1995; 274: 1915- 1921.

82. Kayman S, Bruvold W, Stern JS. Maintenance and relapse after weight-loss in women: Behavioral aspects. Am J Clin Nutr 1990; 52: 800-807.

83. Keppel KG, Taffel SM. Pregnancy-related weight gain and retention: implications of the 1990 Institute of Medicine guidelines. Am J Public Health 1993; 83: 1100-1103.

84. Keys A, Brozek J, Henschel A et al. The biology of human starvation, vols 1 and 2. Minneapolis: University of Minnesota University Press; 1950.

85. Kinsell, LW, Gunning, B, Michaels, GD, et al. Calories do count. Metabolism 1964; 13:195-204.

86. Klatsky AL, Armstrong MA, Friedman GD et al. The relations of alcoholic beverage use to colon and rectal cancer. Am J Epidemiol 1988; 128: 1007-1015.

87. Klesges RC, Meyers AW, Klesges LM et al. Smoking, body weight, and their effects on smoking behavior: a comprehensive review of the literature. Psychol Bull 1989; 106: 204-230.

88. Kromhout D. Changes in energy and macronutrients in 871 middle-aged men during 10 years of follow-up (the Zutphen Study). Am J Clin Nutr 1983; 37: 287-294.

89. Kumanyika SK, Bahnson J, Bottom J et al. Race and sex influences on the efficacy of non-pharmlogic step-down therapy in hypertensive older adults. Can J Cardiol 1997; 13 (Suppl B): 369B [abstract].

90. Laara E, Rantakallio L. Body size and mortality in women: A 29 year follow-up of 12,000 pregnant women in northern Finland. J Epidemiol Community Health 1996; 50: 408–414.

91. Langford HG, Blaufox MD, Oberman A et al. Dietary therapy slows the return of hypertension after stopping prolonged medication. JAMA 1985; 253: 657-664.

92. Langford HG, Davis BR, Blaufox D et al. Effect of drug and diet treatment of mild hypertension on diastolic blood pressure. The TAIM Research Group. Hypertension 1991; 17: 210-217.

93. Larkin JC, Pines HA. No fat persons need apply: experimental studies of the overweight stereotype and hiring preference. Sociol Work Occup 1979; 6: 312-327.

94. Le Marchand L, Wilkens LR, Mi MP. Obesity in youth and middle age and risk of colorectal cancer in men. Cancer Causes Control 1992; 3: 349-354.

95. Leboeuf-Y de C, Kyvik KO, Bruun NH. Low back pain and lifestyle. Part II - Obesity: information from a population-based sample of 29,424 twin subjects. Spine 1999; 24: 779-784.

96. Lee IM, Paffenbarger RS Jr. Quetelet's index and risk of colon cancer in college alumni. J Natl Cancer Inst 1992; 84: 1326- 1331.

97. Lee L, Kumar S, Leong L. The impact of five-month basic military training on the body weight and body fat of 197 moderately to severely obese Singaporean males aged 17-19 years. Int J Obes 1994; 18: 105-109.

98. Leibel RL, Rosenbaum M, Hirsch J. Changes in energy expenditure resulting from altered body weight. N Engl J Med 1995; 332: 621-628. Erratum in: N Engl J Med 1995; 333: 399.

99. Leslie WS, Hankey CR, Lean ME. Weight gain as an adverse effect of some commonly prescribed drugs: a systematic review. QJM 2007; 100:395-404.

100.Lew EA, Garfinkel L. Variations in mortality by weight among 750,000 men and women. J Chronic Dis 1979; 32: 563-576.

101.Li Z, Maglione M, Tu W et al. Meta-analysis: pharmacologic treatment of obesity. Ann Intern Med 2005; 142: 532-546.

102.Lichtman SW, Pisarska K, Berman ER et al. Discrepancy between self-reported and actual caloric intake and exercise in obese subjects. N Engl J Med 1992; 327: 1893-1898.

103.Lievense AM, Bierma-Zeinstra SM, Verhagen AP et al. Influence of obesity on the development of osteoarthritis of the hip: a systematic review. Rheumatology (Oxford) 2002; 41: 1155-1162.

104.Lin PH, Proschan MA, Bray GA et al. Estimation of energy requirements in a controlled feeding trial. Am J Clin Nutr 2003; 77: 639-645.

105.Luo W, Morrison H, de Groh M et al. The burden of adult obesity in Canada. Chronic Dis Can 2007; 27: 135-144.

106.MacMahon S, Cutler J, Brittain E et al. Obesity and hypertension: epidemiological and clinical issues. Eur Heart J 1987; 8 (Suppl B): 57-70.

107.MacMahon SW, Macdonald GJ, Bernstein L et

al. A randomized controlled trial of weight reduction and metoprolol in the treatment of hypertension in young overweight patients. Clin Exp Pharmacol Physiol 1985; 12: 267-271.

108.Maggard MA, Shugarman LR, Suttorp M et al. Meta-analysis: surgical treatment of obesity. Ann Intern Med 2005; 142: 547-559.

109.Martinez ME, Giovannucci E, Spiegelman D et al. Physical activity, body size, and colorectal cancer in women. Am J Epidemiol 1996:146; S73.

110.Messier SP, Gutekunst DJ, Davis C et al. Weight loss reduces knee-joint loads in overweight and obese older adults with knee osteoarthritis. Arthritis Rheum 2005; 52: 2026-2032.

111. Messier SP, Loeser RF, Miller GD et al. Exercise and dietary weight loss in overweight and obese older adults with knee osteoarthritis: the Arthritis, Diet, and Activity Promotion Trial. Arthritis Rheum 2004; 50: 1501–1510.

112. Meyer JM, Stunkard AJ. Twin studies of human obesity. In: Bouchard C ed. The Genetics of Obesity. Boca Raton: CRC Press; 1994: 63–78.

113. Miller WC, Koceja DM, Hamilton EJ. A meta-analysis of the past 25 years of weight loss research using diet, exercise or diet plus exercise intervention. Int J Obes 1997; 21: 941-947.

114.Mokdad AH, Serdula MK, Dietz WH et al. The spread of the obesity epidemic in the United States, 1991-1998. JAMA 1999; 282: 1519-1522.

115. Must A, Jacques PF, Dallal GE et al. Long-term morbidity and mortality of overweight adolescents. A followup of the Harvard Growth Study of 1922 to 1935. N Engl J Med 1992; 327: 1350- 1355.

116. National Center for Health Statistics. Health, United States, 2005 with Chartbook on Trends in the Health of Americans. Maryland: U.S. Government Printing Office; 2005.

117. National Health and Nutrition Examination Survey. Anthropometric reference data, United States, 1988-1994. Center for Disease Control, National Center for Health Statistics. 3 June 2006 <www.cdc.gov/nchs/about/major/nhanes/Anthropometric%20Measures.htm>.

118. National Institute of Health, National Heart, Lung and Blood Institute. Clinical Guidelines on the Identification, Evaluation and Treatment of Overweight and Obesity in Adults: The Evidence Report. Washington, D.C.: NIH Publication No.: 98-4083; 1998.

119. National Institutes of Health, National Heart, Lung, Blood Institute and the North American Association for the study of Obesity. The Practical Guide. Identification, Evaluation and Treatment of Overweight and Obesity in Adults. Wahington, D.C.: Publication no. 00-4084; 2000.

120.Nilsson PM, Lindholm LH, Schersten BF. Lifestyle changes improve insulin resistance in hyperinsulinaemic subjects: a 1-year intervention study of hypertensives and normotensives in Dalby. J Hypertens 1992; 10: 1071-1078.

121. Ogden CL, Fryar CD, Carroll MD et al. Mean body weight, height, and body mass index, United States 1960-2002. Advance Data from Vital and Health Statistics. National Center for Health Statistics 2004; 347: 1-20.

122.Oliveria SA, Felson DT, Cirillo PA et al. Body weight, body mass index, and incident symptomatic osteoarthritis of the hand, hip, and knee. Epidemiology 1999; 10: 161-166.

123.Olshansky SJ, Passaro DJ, Hershow RC et al. A potential decline in life expectancy in the United States in the 21st century. N Engl J Med 2005; 352: 1138-1145.

124.Pan XR, Li GW, Hu YH et al. Effects of diet and exercise in preventing NIDDM in people with impaired glucose tolerance. The Da Qing IGT and Diabetes Study. Diabetes Care 1997; 20: 537-544.

125.Pavlou KN, Krey S, Steffee WP. Exercise as an adjunct to weight loss and maintenance in moderately obese subjects. Am J Clin Nutr 1989; 49: 1115-1123.

126.Pelleymounter MA, Cullen MJ, Baker MB et al. Effects of the obese gene product on body weight regulation in ob/ob mice. Science 1995; 269: 540-543.

127.Peltonen M, Lindroos AK, Torgerson JS. Musculoskeletal pain in the obese: a comparison with a general population and long-term changes after conventional and surgical obesity treatment. Pain 2003; 104: 549-557.

128.Perri MG, Nezu AM, Patti ET et al. Effect of length of treatment on weight loss. J Consult Clin Psychol 1989; 57: 450-452.

129.Phillips RL, Snowdon DA. Dietary relationships with fatal colorectal cancer among Seventh-Day Adventists. J Natl Cancer Inst 1985; 74: 307-317.

130.Pingitore R, Dugoni BL, Tindale RS et al. Bias against overweight job applicants in a simulated employment interview. J Appl Psychol 1994; 79: 909-917.

131. Pirie PL, McBride CM, Hellerstedt W et al. Smoking cessation in women concerned about weight. Am J Public Health 1992; 82: 1238-1243.

132.Pi-Sunyer XF. Clinical guidelines on the identification, evaluation and treatment of overweight and obesity in adults—the evidence report. Obes Res 1998; 6: 51S-210S.

133.Prather RC, Williamson DA. Psychopathology associated with bulimia, binge eating, and obesity. Int J Eat Disord 1988; 7: 177-184.

134. Prentice AM, Jebb SA. Obesity in Britain: Gluttony or sloth? BMJ 1995; 311: 437-439.

135. Ramsay LE, Ramsay MH, Hettiarachchi J et al. Weight reduction in a blood pressure clinic. BMJ 1978; 2: 244-245.

136. Ravussin E, Lillioja S, Knowler WC et al. Reduced rate of energy expenditure as a risk factor for body-weight gain. N Engl J Med 1988; 318: 467-472.

137. Reisin E, Abel R, Modan M et al. Effect of weight loss without salt restriction on the reduction of blood pressure in overweight hypertensive patients. N Engl J Med 1978; 298: 1-6.

138. Rejeski WJ, Focht BC, Messier SP et al. Obese, older adults with knee osteoarthritis: weight loss, exercise, and quality of life. Health Psychol 2002; 21: 419–426.

139. Report of a Joint FAO/WHO/UNU Expert Consultation. Energy and protein requirements. World Health Orgnization Technical Report Series 724, 1985.

140. Rexrode KM, Hennekens CH, Willett WC, et al. A prospective study of body mass index, weight change, and risk of stroke in women. JAMA. 1997;277:1539- 1545.

141. Richman R, Elliot L, Burns C et al.. The prevalence of obstructive sleep apnea in an obese female population. Int J Obes Relat Metab Disord 1994; 18: 173–177.

142. Roe DA, Eickwort KR. Relationships between obesity and associated health factors with unemployment among low income women. J Am Med Womens Assoc 1976; 31: 193-194, 198-199, 203-204.

143. Rosenberg L, Palmer JR, Miller DR et al. A case-control study of alcoholic beverage consumption and breast cancer. Am J Epidemiol 1990; 131: 6-14.

144. Ross R, Dagnone, D, Jones PJ et al. Reduction in obesity and related comorbid conditions after diet-induced weight loss or exercise-induced weight loss in men. A randomized, controlled trial. Ann Intern Med 2000; 133: 92-103.

145. Rubinstein S, Caballero B. Is Miss America an undernourished role model? JAMA 2000; 283: 1569.

146. Savage MP, Krolewski AS, Kenien GG et al.. Acute myocardial infarction in diabetes mellitus and significance of congestive heart failure as a prognostic factor. Am J Cardiol 1998; 62: 665–669.

147. Schoeller DA, Shay K, Kushner RF. How much physical activity is needed to minimize weight gain in previously obese women? Am J Clin Nutr 1997; 66: 551-556.

148. Schottenfeld D, Fraumeni JF. Cancer Epidemiology and Prevention. New York: Oxford University Press; 1996.

149. Schouten JS, van den Ouweland FA, Valkenburg HA. A 12 year follow up study in the general population on prognostic factors of cartilage loss in osteoarthritis of the knee. Ann Rheum Dis 1992; 51: 932–937.

150. Segal K, Dunaif A, Gutin B et al. Body composition, not body weight is related to cardiovascular disease risk factors and sex hormone levels in men. J Clin Invest 1987; 80: 1050–1055.

151. Sempos CT, Durazo-Arvizu R, McGee DL et al.. The influence of cigarette smoking on the association between body weight and mortality: The Framingham Heart Study revisited. Ann Epidemiol 1998; 8: 286–288.

152. Shaper AG, Wannamethee SG, Walker M. Body weight: implications for the prevention of coronary heart disease, stroke, and diabetes mellitus in a cohort study of middle aged men. BMJ 1997; 314: 1311-1317.

153. Shepard J. Hypertension, cardiac arrhythmias, myocardial infarction and stroke in relation to obstructive sleep apnea. Clin Chest Med 1992; 13: 437–458.

154. Simkin-Silverman L, Wing RR, Hansen DH et al. Prevention of cardiovascular risk factor elevations in healthy premenopausal women. Prev Med 1995; 24: 509-517.

155. Sjöström CD, Lissner L, Sjöström L. Relationships between changes in body composition and changes in cardiovascular risk factors: the SOS Intervention Study. Swedish Obese Subjects. Obes Res 1997; 5: 519-530.

156. Slentz CA, Duscha BD, Johnson JL et al. Effects of the amount of exercise on body weight, body composition, and measures of central obesity: STRRIDE—a randomized controlled study. Arch Intern Med 2004; 164: 31-39.

157. Smith DE, Lewis CE, Caveny JL et al. Longitudinal changes in adiposity associated with pregnancy. The CARDIA Study. Coronary Artery Risk Development in Young Adults Study. JAMA 1994; 271: 1747-1751.

158. Snow V, Barry P, Fitterman N et al. Pharmacologic and surgical management of obesity in primary care: a clinical practice guideline from the American College of Physicians. Ann Intern Med 2005; 142: 525-531

159. Sorensen TI, Holst C, Stunkard AJ et al. Correlations of body mass index of adult adoptees and their biological and adoptive relatives. Int J Obes Relat Metab Disord 1992; 16: 227–236.

160. Sorensen TI. The genetics of obesity. Metabolism 1995; 44: 4–6.

161. Sowers M, Jannausch ML, Stein E et al. C-reactive protein as a biomarker of emergent osteoarthritis. Osteoarthritis Cartilage 2002; 10: 595–601.

162.Spector TD, Hart DJ, Doyle DV. Incidence and progression of osteoarthritis in women with unilateral knee disease in the general population: the effect of obesity. Ann Rheum Dis 1994; 53: 565–568.

163.Spector TD, Hart DJ, Nandra D et al. Low-level increases in serum creative protein are present in early osteoarthritis of the knee and predict progressive disease. Arthritis Rheum 1997; 40: 723–727.

164.Spiegel K, Tasali E, Penev P et al. Brief communication: Sleep curtailment in healthy young men is associated with decreased leptin levels, elevated ghrelin levels, and increased hunger and appetite. Ann Intern Med 2004; 141: 846-850.

165.Spiegelman D, Israel R, Bouchard C et al. Absolute fat mass, percent body fat and body fat distribution: Which is the real determinant of blood pressure and serum glucose?. Am J Clin Nutr 1992; 55: 1033–1044.

166.Stamler R, Stamler J, Grimm R et al. Nutritional therapy for high blood pressure. Final report of a 4-year randomized controlled trial—the Hypertension Control Program. JAMA 1987; 257: 1484-1491.

167.Stampfer MJ, Maclure KM, Colditz GA et al.. Risk of symptomatic gallstones in women with severe obesity. Am J Clin Nutr 1992; 55: 652–658.

168.Stevens J, Cal J, Pamuk ER et al. The effect of age on the association between body-mass index and mortality. N Engl J Med 1998; 338: 1–7.

169.Stunkard AJ, Harris JR, Pedersen NL et al. The body-mass index of twins who have been reared apart. N Engl J Med 1990; 322: 1483-1487.

170.Stunkard AJ, Foch TT, Hrubec Z. A twin study of human obesity. JAMA 1986; 256: 51–54.

171. Stunkard AJ, Sorensen TI, Hanis C et al.. An adoption study of human obesity. N Engl J Med 1986; 314: 193–198.

172.Tambs K, Mourn T, Eaves L. Genetic and environmental contributions to the variance of body mass index in a Norwegian sample of first and second degree relatives. Am J Hum Biol 1991; 3: 257–267.

173.Thomas, PR ed. Weighing the Options: Criteria for evaluating Weight-Management Programs. Wasington: National Academy Press; 1995.

174.Toda Y, Toda T, Takemura S et al. Change in body fat, but not body weight or metabolic correlates of obesity, is related to symptomatic relief of obese patients with knee osteoarthritis after a weight control program. J Rheumatol 1998; 25: 2181–2186.

175. Toda Y. The effect of energy restriction, walking, and exercise on lower extremity lean body mass in obese women with osteoarthritis of the knee. J Orthop Sci 2001; 6: 148–154.

176.Tokunaga K, Matsuzawa Y, Kotani K et al. Ideal body weight estimated from the body mass index with the lowest morbidity. Int J Obes. 1991; 15: 1-5.

177.Tremblay A, Despres J, Maheux J et al. Normalization of the metabolic profile in obese women by exercise and a low fat diet. Med Sci Sports Exerc 1991; 23: 1326-1331.

178.United Kingdom Prospective Diabetes Study Group. United Kingdom prospective diabetes study group (UKPDS) 13: Relative efficacy of randomly allocated diet, sulphonylureas, insulin, or metformin in patients with newly diagnosed non-insulin-dependent diabetes followed for three years. BMJ 1995; 310: 83-88.

179.Vingard E, Alfredsson L, Malchau H. Lifestyle factors and hip arthrosis. A case reference study of body mass index, smoking and hormone therapy in 503 Swedish women. Acta Orthop Scand 1997; 68: 216–220.

180.Vogler GP, Sorensen TI, Stunkard AJ et al. Influences of genes and shared family environment on adult body mass index assessed in an adoption study by a comprehensive path model. Int J Obes Relat Metab Disord 1995; 19: 40-45.

181.Voracek M, Fisher ML. Shapely centrefolds? Temporal change in body measures: trend analysis. BMJ 2002; 325: 1447-1448.

182.Waaler HT. Height, weight, and mortality: The Norwegian experience. Acta Med Scand 1984; 679(suppl): 1–51.

183.Wadden TA, Berkowitz RI, Vogt RA et al. Lifestyle modification in the pharmacologic treatment of obesity: a pilot investigation of a potential primary care approach. Obes Res 1997; 5: 218-226.

184.Wadden TA, Foster GD, Wang J et al. Clinical correlates of short- and long-term weight loss. Am J Clin Nutr 1992; 56: 271S-274S.

185.Wadden TA, Kuehnel RH, Wilk J et al. Exercise in the treatment of obesity: Effects of four interventions on body composition, resting energy expenditure, appetite and mood. J Consult Clin Psychol 1997; 65: 269-277.

186.Wadden TA, Stunkard AJ. Controlled trial of very low calorie diet, behavior therapy, and their combination in the treatment of obesity. J Consult Clin Psychol 1986; 54: 482-488.

187.Wadden TA, Sternberg JA, Letizia KA et al.. Treatment of obesity by very low calorie diet, behavior therapy, and their combination: A five-year perspective. Int J Obes Relat Metab Disord 1989; 13: 39–46.

188.Wadden TA. New goals of obesity treatment: A healthier weight and other ideals. Prim Psychiatry 1998; 5: 45–54.

189.Walker SP, Rimm EB, Ascherio A et al. Body size

and fat distribution as predictors of stroke among US men. Am J Epidemiol 1996; 144: 1143-1150.

190. Wassertheil-Smoller S, Langford HG, Blaufox MD et al. Effective dietary intervention in hypertensives: sodium restriction and weight reduction. J Am Diet Assoc 1985; 85: 423- 430.

191. Webb R, Brammah T, Lunt M et al. Prevalence and predictors of intense, chronic, and disabling neck and back pain in the UK general population. Spine 2003; 28: 1195-1202.

192. Weight gain associated with intensive therapy in the diabetes control and complications trial. The DCCT Research Group. Diabetes Care 1988; 11:567-573.

193. Whelton PK, Applegate WB, Ettiger WH et al. Efficacy of weight loss and reduced sodium intake in the Trial of Nonpharmacologic Interventions in the Elderly (TONE). Circulation 1996; 94 (Suppl I): 1-178 [abstract].

194. Willett WC, Browne ML, Bain C et al. Relative weight and risk of breast cancer among premenopausal women. Am J Epidemiol 1985; 122: 731-740.

195. Willett WC, Manson JE, Stampfer MJ et al. Weight, weight change, and coronary heart disease in women. Risk within the 'normal' weight range. JAMA 1995; 273: 461-465.

196. Williamson DF, Madans J, Anda RF et al. Recreational physical activity and ten-year weight change in a US national cohort. Int J Obes Relat Metab Disord 1993; 17: 279-286.

197. Williamson DF, Madans J, Anda RF et al. Smoking cessation and severity of weight gain in a national cohort. N Engl J Med 1991; 324: 739-745.

198. Williamson DF, Madans J, Pamuk E et al. A prospective study of childbearing and 10-year weight gain in US white women 25 to 45 years of age. Int J Obes Relat Metab Disord 1994; 18: 561-569.

199. Williamson DF, Pamuk E, Thun M et al. Prospective study of intentional weight loss and mortality in overweight white men aged 40-64 years. Am J Epidemiol 1999; 149: 491-503.

200. Wright JD, Kennedy-Stephenson J, Wang CY et al. Trends in intake of energy and macronutrients – United States, 1971-2000. MMWR Weekly 2004; 53: 80-82.

201. Young T, Palt M, Dempsey J et al.. Occurrence of sleep disordered breathing among middle-aged adults. N Engl J Med 1993; 328: 1230–1273.

References Chapter 10

1. Klippel JH ed. Primer on the Rheumatic Diseases. Edition 12. Atlanta: Arthritis Foundation; 2001.

References Chapter 11

1. Aaron LA, Bradley LA, Alarcon GS et al. Psychiatric diagnoses in patients with fibromyalgia are related to health care-seeking behavior rather than to illness. Arthritis Rheum 1996; 39: 436-445.

2. Adam K, Oswald I. Sleep is for tissue restoration. J R Coll Physicians Lond 1977; 11: 376-388.

3. Affleck G, Urrows S, Tennen H et al. Sequential daily relations of sleep, pain intensity, and attention to pain among women with fibromyalgia. Pain 1996; 68: 363-368.

4. Akerstedt T, Palmblad J, de la Torre B et al. Adrenocortical and gonadal steroids during sleep deprivation. Sleep 1980; 3: 23-30.

5. Aldrich MS. Insomnia in neurological diseases. J Psychosomatic Res 1993; 37 Suppl I: 3-11.

6. Allan JS, Czeisler CA. Persistence of the circadian thyrotropin rhythm under constant conditions and after light-induced shifts of circadian phase. J Clin Endocrinol Metab 1994; 79: 508-512.

7. Alluisi EA, Coates GD, Morgan BBJ. Effects of temporal stressors on vigilance and information processing. In Mackie RR ed. Vigilance: Theory, Operational Performance, and Physiological Correlates. New York: Plenum Press; 1977: 361-421.

8. Althuis MD, Fredman L, Langenberg PW et al. The relationship between insomnia and mortality among community-dwelling older women. J Am Geriatr Soc 1998; 46: 1270-1273.

9. American Academy of Sleep Medicine. International Classification of Sleep Disorders: Diagnostic and Coding Manual, Second Edition. Westchester: American Academy of Sleep Medicine; 2005.

10. American Psychiatric Association. Diagnostic and Statistical Manual of Mental Disorders, Fourth Edition, Text Revision. Washington, DC: American Psychiatric Association; 2000.

11. American Sleep Disorders Association. International Classification of Sleep Disorders-Revised. Rochester: American Sleep Disorders Association; 1997.

12. Ancoli-Israel S, Schnierow B, Kelsoe J et al. A pedigree of one family with delayed sleep phase syndrome. Chronobiol Int 2001; 18: 831–841.

13. Appels A, de Vos Y, van Diest R et al. Are sleep complaints predictive of future myocardial infarction? Act Nerv Super (Praha) 1987; 29: 147-151.

14. Ashton H, Young AH. GABA-ergic drugs: Exit stage left, enter stage right. J Psychopharmacol 2003; 17: 174-178.

15. Atkinson JH, Ancoli-Israel S, Slater MA et al. Subjective sleep disturbance in chronic back pain. Clin J Pain 1988; 4: 225-232.

16. Ayas NT, White DP, Manson JE et al. A prospective study of sleep duration and coronary heart disease in women. Arch Intern Med 2003; 163: 205-209.

17. Beaumont M, Batejat D, Pierard C et al. Slow release caffeine and prolonged (64-h) continuous wakefulness: Effects on vigilance and cognitive performance. J Sleep Res 2001; 10: 265-276.

18. Belenky G, Wesensten NJ, Thorne DR et al. Patterns of performance degradation and restoration during sleep restriction and subsequent recovery: A sleep dose-response study. J Sleep Res 2003; 12: 1-12.

19. Benca RM, Obermeyer WH, Thisted RA et al. Sleep and psychiatric disorders: A meta-analysis. Arch Gen Psychiatry 1992; 49: 651-668.

20. Bengtsson A, Henriksson KG, Jorfeldt L et al. Primary fibromyalgia. A clinical and laboratory study of 55 patients. Scand J Rheumatol 1986; 15: 340-347.

21. Bennett RM, Gatter RA, Campbell SM et al. A comparison of cyclobenzaprine and placebo in the management of fibrositis. A double-blind controlled study. Arthritis Rheum 1988; 31: 1535-1542.

22. Bertrand B, Jamart J, Arendt C. Cetirizine and pseudoephedrine retard alone and in combination in the treatment of perennial allergic rhinitis: A double-blind multicentre study. Rhinology 1996: 34: 91-96.

23. Billiard M, Dolenc L, Aldaz C et al. Hypersomnia associated with mood disorders: A new perspective. J Psychosom Res 1994; 38(Suppl 1): 41-47.

24. Bixler, EO, Kales, A, Soldatos, CR, et al. Prevalence of sleep disorders in the Los Angeles metropolitan area. Am J Psychiatry 1979; 136: 1257-1262.

25. Bjerner B, Holm A, Swensson A. Diurnal variation in mental performance: A study of three-shift workers. Br J Ind Med 1955; 12: 103-110.

26. Bliwise DL. Sleep in normal aging and dementia: Review. Sleep 1993; 16:40-81.

27. Bonnet MH, Arand DL. 24-Hour metabolic rate in insomniacs and matched normal sleepers. Sleep 1995; 18: 581-588.

28. Bonnet MH, Arand DL. We are chronically sleep deprived. Sleep 1995; 18: 908-911.

29. Bonnet MH, Arand DL. Caffeine use as a model of acute and chronic insomnia. Sleep 1992; 15: 526-536.

30. Bonnet MH, Arand DL. The consequences of a week of insomnia. Sleep 1996; 19: 453-461.

31. Borbely AA, Tobler I, Loepfe M et al. All-night spectral analysis of the sleep EEG in untreated depressives and normal controls. Psychiatry Res 1984; 12: 27-33.

32. Borkovec TD, Lane TW, Van Oot PH. Short re-

port: Phenomenology of sleep among insomniacs and good sleepers: Wakefulness experience when cortically asleep. J Abnorm Psychol 1981; 90: 607-609.

33. Bradley TD, McNicholas WT Rutherford R et al. Clinical and physiological heterogeneity of the central sleep apnea syndrome. Am Rev Respir Dis 1986; 134: 217-221.

34. Branco J, Atalaia A, Paiva T. Sleep cycles and alpha-delta sleep in fibromyalgia syndrome. J Rheumatol 1994; 21: 1113-1117.

35. Breslau N, Roth T, Rosenthal L et al. Sleep disturbance and psychiatric disorders: a longitudinal epidemiological study of young adults. Biol Psychiatry 1996; 39: 411-418.

36. Brock S, Wiesel B. The narcoleptic-cataplectic syndrome-and excessive and dissociated reaction of the sleep mechanism-accompanying mental states. J Nerv Ment Dis 1941; 94: 700-712.

37. Broughton R, Ghanem Q, Hishikawa Y et al. Life effects of narcolepsy in 180 patients from North America, Asia and Europe compared to matched controls. Can J Neurol Sci 1981; 8: 299-304.

38. Burckhardt CS, O'Reilly CA, Wiens AN et al. Assessing depression in fibromyalgia patients. Arthritis Care Res 1994; 7: 35-39.

39. Bursztyn M, Ginsberg G, Stessman J. The siesta and mortality in the elderly: Effect of rest without sleep and daytime sleep duration. Sleep 2002; 25: 187-191.

40. Buysse DJ, Reynolds CF, Hoch CC et al. Longitudinal effects of nortriptyline on EEG sleep and the likelihood of recurrence in elderly depressed patients. Neuropsychopharmacology 1996; 14: 243-252.

41. Buysse DJ, Schweitzer PK, Moul DE. Clinical pharmacology of other drugs used as hypnotics. In: Kryger MH, Roth T, Dement WC eds. Principles and Practice of Sleep Medicine, Fourth Edition. Philadelphia: Elsevier Saunders; 2005: 452-467.

42. Buysse DJ, Reynolds CF, Kupfer DJ et al. Clinical diagnoses in 216 insomnia patients using the International Classification of Sleep Disorders (ICSD), DSM-IV and ICD-10 categories: a report from the APA/NIMH DSM-IV Field Trial. Sleep 1994; 17: 630-637.

43. Cajochen C. TAK-375 Takeda. Curr Opin Investig Drugs 2005; 6: 114-121.

44. Caldwell J, Rapoport R, Davis J et al. Efficacy and safety of a once-daily morphine formulation in chronic, moderate-to-severe osteoarthritis pain: Results from a randomized placebo-controlled, double-blind trial and an open-label extension trial. J Pain Symptom Manage 2002; 23: 278-291.

45. Campbell SM, Clark S, Tindall EA et al. Clinical

characteristics of fibrositis. I.A. 'blinded' controlled study of symptoms and tender points. Arthritis Rheum 1983; 26: 817-824.

46. Campos H, Siles X. Siesta and the risk of coronary heart disease: results from a population-based, case-control study in Costa Rica. Int J Epidemiol 2000; 29: 429-437.

47. Carette S, Bell MJ, Reynolds WJ et al. Comparison of amitriptyline, cyclobenzaprine, and placebo in the treatment of fibromyalgia. A randomized, double-blind clinical trial. Arthritis Rheum 1994; 37: 32-40.

48. Carette S, McCain GA, Bell DA et al. Evaluation of amitriptyline in primary fibrositis: a double-blind, placebo-controlled study. Arthritis Rheum 1986; 29: 655-659.

49. Carskadon MA, Brown ED, Dement WC. Sleep fragmentation in the elderly: Relationship to daytime sleep tendency. Neurobiol Aging 1982; 3: 321-327.

50. Carskadon MA, Dement WC, Mitler MM et al. Self-reports versus sleep laboratory findings in 122 drug-free subjects with complaints of chronic insomnia. Am J Psychiatry 1976; 133: 1382-1388.

51. Carskadon MA, Dement WC. Cumulative effects of sleep restriction on daytime sleepiness. Psychophysiology 1981; 18: 107-113.

52. Carskadon MA, Dement WC. Normal sleep: an overview. In: Kryger MH, Roth T, Dement WC eds. Principles and Practice of Sleep Medicine, Fourth Edition. Philadelphia: Elsevier Saunders; 2005: 13-23.

53. Casey DE. The relationship of pharmacology to side effects. J Clin Psychiatry 1997; 58(Suppl 10): 55-62.

54. Chang PP, Ford DE, Mead LA et al. Insomnia in young men and subsequent depression. The Johns Hopkins Precursors Study. Am J Epidemiol 1997; 146: 105-114.

55. Chen H, Tank Y. Sleep loss impairs inspiratory muscle endurance. Am Rev Respir Dis 1989; 140: 907-909.

56. Chesson A Jr, Hartse K, Anderson WM et al. Practice parameters for the evaluation of chronic insomnia. An American Academy of Sleep Medicine report. Standards of Practice Committee of the American Academy of Sleep Medicine. Sleep 2000; 23: 237-241.

57. Ciechanowski P, Katon W. Overview of generalized anxiety disorder. UpToDate Online 2006; 14.2: 1-10. 10 August 2006 <http://www.utdol.com>.

58. Claghorn JL, Mathew RJ, Weinman ML et al. Daytime sleepiness in depression. J Clin Psychiatry 1981; 42: 342-343.

59. Clark S, Campbell SM, Forehand ME et al. Clinical characteristics of fibrositis. II. A 'blinded', controlled study using standard psychological tests. Arthritis Rheum 1985; 28: 132-137.

60. Clauw D, Blank C, Hiltz R et al. Polysomnography in fibromyalgia patients (abstract). Arthritis Rheum 1994; 37(Suppl 9): S348.

61. Clemons M, Regnard C, Appleton T. Alertness, cognition and morphine in patients with advanced cancer. Cancer Treat Rev 1996; 122: 451-468.

62. Cohen M, Menefee LA, Doghramji K et al. Sleep in chronic pain: Problems and treatments. Int Rev Psychiatry 2000; 12: 115-126.

63. Coleman R, Roffwarg H, Kennedy S et al. Sleep-wake disorders based on a polysomnographic diagnosis: a national cooperative study. JAMA 1982; 247: 997-1003.

64. Conway J, Greenwood DT, Middlemiss DN. Central nervous actions of beta-adrenoreceptor antagonists. Clin Sci Mol Med 1978; 54: 119-124.

65. Cooper JA, Sagar HJ, Doherty SM et al. Different effects of dopaminergic and anticholinergics therapies on cognitive and motor function in Parkinson's disease. A follow-up study of untreated patients. Brain 1992; 115: 1701–1725.

66. Cote KA, Moldofsky H. Sleep, daytime symptoms, and cognitive performance in patients with fibromyalgia. J Rheumatol 1997; 24: 2014-2023.

67. Cousins MS, Roberts DCS, de Wit H. GABA$_B$ receptor agonists for the treatment of drug addiction: A review of recent findings. Drug Alcohol Depend 2002; 65: 209-220.

68. Cronin A, Keifer J, Davies M et al. Postoperative sleep disturbance: Influences of opioids and pain in humans. Sleep 2001; 24: 39-44.

69. Cumming JL. Behavioral complications of drug treatment of Parkinson's disease. J Am Geriatr Soc 1991; 39: 708–716.

70. Czeisler CA, Zimmerman JC, Ronda JM et al. Timing of REM sleep is coupled to the circadian rhythm of body temperature in man. Sleep 1980; 2: 329-346.

71. Daly D, Yoss R. Narcolepsy. In Magnus O, Lorentz de Haas A eds. The Epilepsies, vol 15, Handbook of Clinical Neurology. Amsterdam: North Holland Publishing; 1974: 836-852.

72. Daly DD, Yoss RE. The treatment of narcolepsy with methyl phenylpiperidylacetate: A preliminary report. Proc Staff Meet Mayo Clin 1956; 31: 620-625.

73. Dao TTT, Lavigne GJ, Charbonneau A et al. The efficacy of oral splints in the treatment of myofascial pain of the jaw muscles: A controlled clinical trial. Pain 1994; 56: 85-94.

74. Dauvilliers Y, Touchon J. Le sommeil du fibromyalgique: Revue des données cliniques et polygraphiques. Neurophysiol Clin 2001; 31: 18-33.

75. Dement WC, Vaughan C: The Promise of Sleep. New York: Dell; 1999.

76. Diagnostic classification of sleep and arousal disorders. 1979 first edition. Association of Sleep Disorders Centers and the Association for the Psychophysiological Study of Sleep. Sleep 1979; 2:1-154.

77. Diagnostic Classification Steering Committee. The International Classification of Sleep Disorders, Revised: Diagnostic and Coding Manual. Rochester: American Sleep Disorders Association; 1997.

78. Dinges DF, Pack F, Williams K et al. Cumulative sleepiness, mood disturbance, and psychomotor vigilance performance decrements during a week of sleep restricted to 4-5 hours per night. Sleep 1997; 20: 267-277.

79. Dinges DF. Nap patterns and effects in human adults. In Dinges DF, Broughton RJ eds. Sleep and Alertness: Chronobiological, Behavioral, and Medical Aspects of Napping. New York: Raven Press; 1989: 171-204.

80. Donnell JM. Performance decrement as a function of total sleep loss and task duration. Percept Mot Skills 1969; 29: 711-714.

81. Drewes AM, Gade J, Nielsen KD et al. Clustering of sleep electro-encaphalopathic patterns in patients with the fibromyalgia syndrome. Br J Rheumatol 1995; 34: 1151-1140.

82. Drewes AM, Nielsen KD, Taagholt SJ et al. Sleep intensity in fibromyalgia: Focus on the microstructure of the sleep process. Br J Rheumatol 1995; 34: 629-635.

83. Drewes AM. Pain and sleep disturbances with special reference to fibromyalgia and rheumatoid arthritis. Rheumatology (Oxford) 1999; 38: 1035-1038.

84. Drugs and insomnia. NIH Consensus Development Conference. Consensus development conference summary. Vol 4, No 10, National Institutes of Health, Bethesda, MD, 1984.

85. Dunleavy DLF, Brezinova V, Oswald I et al. Changes during weeks in effects of tricyclic drugs on the human sleep brain. Br J Psychiatry 1972; 120: 663-672.

86. Eaker ED, Pinsky J, Castelli WP. Myocardial infarction and coronary death among women: Psychosocial predictors from a 20-year follow-up of women in the Framingham Study. Am J Epidemiol 1992; 135: 854-864.

87. Eaton LM. Treatment of narcolepsy with desoxyephedrine hydrochloride. Staff Meet Mayo Clin 1943; 7: 262-264.

88. Edgar DM, Seidel WF: Modafinil induces wakefulness without intensifying motor activity or subsequent rebound hypersomnolence in the rat. J Pharmacol Exp Ther 1997; 283: 757-769.

89. Edinger JD, Fins AI, Glenn DM et al. Insomnia and the eye of the beholder: Are there clinical markers of objective sleep disturbances among adults with and without insomnia complaints? J Consult Clin Psychol 2000; 68: 586-593.

90. Edinger JD, Means MK. Overview of insomnia: definitions, epidemiology, differential diagnosis, and assessment. In: Kryger MH, Roth T, Dement WC eds. Principles and Practice of Sleep Medicine, Fourth Edition. Philadelphia: Elsevier Saunders; 2005: 702-713.

91. Eisen J, MacFarlane J, Shapiro CM. Psychotropic drugs and sleep: ABC of sleep disorders. BMJ 1993; 306: 1331-1334.

92. Ewing SB, Balachandran DD, LeBeau L et al. Subjective and objective indices of sleep loss: Effects of chronic partial sleep restriction. Sleep 2002; 25: A448.

93. Fenn KM, Nusbaum HC, Margoliash D. Consolidation during sleep of perceptual learning of spoken language. Nature 2003; 425: 614-616.

94. Feuillade P, Pringuey D, Belugou JL et al. Trimipramine: acute and lasting effects on sleep in healthy and major depressive subjects. J Affect Disord 1992; 24: 135-145.

95. Ford DE, Kamerow DB. Epidemiologic study of sleep disturbances and psychiatric disorders: An opportunity for prevention? JAMA 1989; 262: 1479-1484.

96. Fosse R, Stickgold R, Hobson JA. Brain-mind states: reciprocal variation in thoughts and hallucinations. Psychol Sci 2001; 12: 30-36.

97. Frazer A. Pharmacology of antidepressants. J Clin Psychopharmacol 1997; 17(Suppl 1) :2S-18S.

98. Gallup Organization. Sleep in America: A National Survey of US Adults. National Sleep Foundation, Princeton, NJ, 1991.

99. Gary KA, Winokur A, Douglas SD et al. Total sleep deprivation and the thyroid axis: Effects of sleep and waking activity. Aviat Space Environ Med 1996; 67: 513-519.

100. Gerlach J, Peacock L. New antipsychotics: The present status. Int Clin Psychopharmacol 1995; 10(Suppl 3): 39-48.

101. Goldenberg DL, Felson DT, Dinerman H. A randomized, controlled trial of amitriptyline and naproxen in the treatment of patients with fibromyalgia. Arthritis Rheum 1986; 29: 1371-1377.

102. Guilleminault C, Eldridge FL, Dement WC. Insomnia with sleep apnea: A new syndrome. Science 1973; 181: 856-858.

103. Guilleminault C, Pool P, Motta J et al. Sinus arrest during REM sleep in young adults. N Engl J Med 1984; 311: 1006-1010.

104. Guilleminault C, Powell NB, Martinez S et al. Preliminary observations on the effects of sleep

time in a sleep restriction paradigm. Sleep Med 2003; 4: 177-184.

105. Guilleminault C, Robinson A. Central sleep apnea. Neurol Clin 1996; 14: 611-628.

106. Gursky JT, Krahn LE. The effects of antidepressants on sleep: A review. Harv Rev Psychiatry 2000; 8: 298-306.

107. Hajak G, Rodenbeck A, Adler L et al. Nocturnal melatonin secretion and sleep after doxepin administration in chronic primary insomnia. Pharmacopsychiatry 1996; 29: 187-192.

108. Hajak G, Rodenbeck A, Voderholzer U et al. Doxepin in the treatment of primary insomnia: A placebo-controlled, double-blind, polysomnographic study. J Clin Psychiatry 2001; 62: 453-463.

109. Harding SM. Sleep in fibromyalgia patients: subjective and objective findings. Am J Med Sci 1998; 315: 367-376.

110. Hartmann E, Cravens J. The effects of long term administration of psychotropic drugs on human sleep: III. The effects of amitriptyline. Psychopharmacology (Berl) 1973; 33: 185-202.

111. Harvey AG. Identifying safety behaviors in insomnia. J Nerv Ment Dis 2002; 190: 16-21.

112. Hauri P, Hawkins DR. Alpha-delta sleep. Electroencephalogr Clin Neurophysiol 1973; 34: 233-237.

113. Hays JC, Blazer DG, Foley DJ. Risk of napping: Excessive daytime sleepiness and mortality in an older community population. J Am Geriatr Soc 1996; 44: 693-698.

114. Hendricks JC, Finn SM, Panckeri KA et al. Rest in Drosophila is a sleep-like state. Neuron 2000; 25: 129-138.

115. Hirshkowitz M. Normal human sleep: an overview. Med Clin North Am 2004; 88: 551-565

116. Hohagen F, Montero RF, Weiss E et al. Treatment of primary insomnia with trimipramine: An alternative to benzodiazepine hypnotics? Eur Arch Psychiatry Clin Neurosci 1994; 244: 65-72.

117. Hohagen F. Nonpharmacological treatment of insomnia. Sleep 1996; 19:S50.

118. Horne J, Percival J, Traynor J. Aspirin and human sleep. Electroencephalogr Clin Neurophysiol 1980; 49: 409-413.

119. Horne J. Why We Sleep. Oxford: Oxford University Press; 1988.

120. Horne JA, Baulk SD. Awareness of sleepiness when driving. Psychophysiology 2004; 41: 161-165.

121. Horne JA, Shackell BS. Alpha-like EEG activity in non-REM sleep and the fibromyalgia (fibrositis) syndrome. Electroencephalogr Clin Neurophysiol 1991; 79: 271-276.

122. Hornyak M, Cejnar M, Elam M et al. Sympathetic muscle nerve activity during sleep in man. Brain 1991; 114: 1281-1295.

123. Hudson JI, Goldenberg DL, Pope HG Jr et al. Comorbidity of fibromyalgia with medical and psychiatric disorders. Am J Med 1992; 92: 363-367.

124. Hudson JI, Pope HG Jr. The relationship between fibromyalgia and major depressive disorder. Rheum Dis Clin N Am 1996; 22: 285-303.

125. Idzikowski C, Shapiro C. Non psychotropic drugs and sleep: ABC of sleep disorders. BMJ 1993; 306: 1118-1121.

126. Inturrisi C. Clinical pharmacology of opioids for pain. Clin J Pain 2002; 18: S3-S13.

127. Irwin M, Mascovich A, Gillin JC et al. Partial sleep deprivation reduces natural killer cell activity in humans. Psychosom Med 1994; 56: 493-498.

128. Irwin M, McClintick J, Costlow C et al. Partial night sleep deprivation reduces natural killer and cellular immune responses in humans. FASEB J 1996; 10: 643-653.

129. Jaeschke R, Adachi J, Guyatt G, Keller J, Wong B. Clinical usefulness of amitriptyline in fibromyalgia: the results of 23 N-of-1 randomized controlled trials. J Rheumatol 1991; 18: 447-451.

130. Janson C, Lindberg E, Gislason T et al. Insomnia in men: A 10-year prospective population based study. Sleep 2001; 24: 425-430.

131. Johnson LC, MacLeod WL. Sleep and awake behavior during gradual sleep reduction. Percept Mot Skills 1973; 36: 87-97.

132. Johnson MP, Duffy JF, Dijk DJ et al. Short-term memory, alertness and performance: A reappraisal of their relationship to body temperature. J Sleep Res 1992; 1: 24-29.

133. Jones BE. Basic mechanisms of sleep-wake states. In: Kryger MH, Roth T, Dement WC eds. Principles and Practice of Sleep Medicine, Fourth Edition. Philadelphia: Elsevier Saunders; 2005: 136-153.

134. Jones CR, Campbell SS, Zone SE et al. Familial advanced sleep-phase syndrome: a short-period circadian rhythm variant in humans. Nat Med 1999; 5: 1062-1065.

135. Karacan I, Aslan C, Hirshkowitz M. Erectile mechanisms in man. Science 1983; 220: 1080-1082.

136. Karacan I, Goodenough DR, Shapiro A et al. Erection cycle during sleep in relation to dream anxiety. Arch Gen Psychiatry 1966; 15: 183-189.

137. Karacan I, Moore CA. Genetics and human sleep. Psychiatr Ann 1979; 9: 11-23.

138. Kato K, Hirai K, Nishiyama K et al. Neurochemical properties of ramelteon (TAK-375), a selective MT1/MT2 receptor agonist. Neuropharma-

cology 2005; 48: 301-310.

139. Katz RS, Kravitz HM. Fibromyalgia, depression, and alcoholism: a family history study. J Rheumatol 1996; 23: 149-154.

140. Kazis LE, Meenan RF, Anderson JJ. Pain in the rheumatic diseases: investigations of a key health status component. Arthritis Rheum 1983; 26: 1017-1022.

141. Keller S, Frishman WH. Neuropsychiatric effects of cardiovascular drug therapy. Cardiol Rev 2003;11:73-93.

142. Kent JM. SNaRIs, NaSSAs, and NaRIs: New agents for the treatment of depression. Lancet 2000; 335: 911-918.

143. Kim, HC, Young, T, Mathews, CG et al. Sleep-disordered breathing and neuropsychological deficits. Am J Respir Crit Care Med 1997; 156: 1813-1819.

144. Klink ME, Quan SF, Kaltenborn WT et al. Risk factors associated with complaints of insomnia in a general adult population: Influence of previous complaints of insomnia. Arch Intern Med 1992; 152: 1634-1637.

145. Knutsson A, Akerstedt T, Jonsson BG et al. Increased risk of ischaemic heart disease in shift workers. Lancet 1986; 2: 89-92.

146. Knutsson A, Hallquist J, Reuterwall C et al. Shiftwork and myocardial infarction: A case-control study. Occup Environ Med 1999; 56: 46-50.

147. Kollar EJ, Namerow N, Pasnau RO et al. Neurological findings during prolonged sleep deprivation. Neurology 1968; 18: 836-840.

148. Koller M. Health risks related to shift work. Int Arch Occup Environ Health 1983; 53: 59-75.

149. Koopman C, Nouriani B, Erickson V et al. Sleep disturbances in women with metastatic breast cancer. Breast J 2002; 6: 362-370.

150. Krasowski MD, Finn SE, Ye Q et al: Trichloroethanol modulation of recombinant GABA-A, glycine, and GABA pI receptors. J Pharmacol Exp Ther 1998; 284: 934-942.

151. Kripke DF, Garfinkel L, Wingard DL et al. Mortality associated with sleep duration and insomnia. Arch Gen Psychiatry 2002; 59: 131-136.

152. Kruyer WB, Hickman JR Jr. Medication-induced performance decrements: Cardiovascular medications. J Occup Med 1990; 32: 342-349.

153. Kupfer DJ, Reynolds CF III, Ulrich RF et al. Comparison of automated REM and slow-wave sleep analysis in young and middle-aged depressed subjects. Biol Psychiatry 1986; 21: 189-200.

154. Kupfer DJ, Reynolds CF III. Management of insomnia. N Engl J Med 1997; 336: 341-346.

155. Kupfer DJ, Spiker DG, Coble P et al. Amitriptyline and EEG sleep in depressed patients: I. Drug effect. Sleep 1978; 1: 149-159.

156. Kurtze N, Gundersen KT, Svebak S. Quality of life, functional disability and lifestyle among subgroups of fibromyalgia patients: the significance of anxiety and depression. Br J Med Psychol 1999; 72: 471-484.

157. Lavie P. To nap, perchance to sleep: Ultradian aspects of napping. In Dinges DF, Broughton RJ eds. Sleep and Alertness: Chronobiological, Behavioral, and Medical Aspects of Napping. New York: Raven Press; 1989: 99-120.

158. Leger D, Guilleminault C, Bader G et al. Medical and socio-professional impact of insomnia. Sleep 2002; 25: 625-629.

159. Lentz MJ, Landis CA, Rothermel J et al. Effects of selective slow wave sleep disruption on musculoskeletal pain and fatigue in middle aged women. J Rheumatol 1999; 26: 1586-1592.

160. Lexi-Comp, Inc. Diazepam: Drug information. UpToDate Online 2006: 1-8. 8 August 2006 <http://www.utdol.com>.

161. Lexi-Comp, Inc. Eszopiclone: Drug information. UpToDate Online 2006: 1-4. 8 August 2006 <http://www.utdol.com>.

162. Lexi-Comp, Inc. Zaleplon: Drug information. UpToDate Online 2006: 1-4. 8 August 2006 <http://www.utdol.com>.

163. Lexi-Comp, Inc. Zolpidem: Drug information. UpToDate Online 2006: 1-5. 8 August 2006 <http://www.utdol.com>.

164. Lieberman HR, Tharion WJ, Shukitt-Hale B et al. Effects of caffeine, sleep loss, and stress on cognitive performance and mood during U.S. Navy SEAL training. Sea-Air-Land. Psychopharmacology (Berl) 2002; 164: 250-261.

165. Light AI, Sun JH, McCool C et al. The effects of acute sleep deprivation on level of resident training. Curr Surg 1989; 46: 29-30.

166. Liu Y, Tanaka H, The Fukuoka Heart Study Group. Overtime work, insufficient sleep, and risk of nonfatal acute myocardial infarction in Japanese men. Occup Environ Med 2002; 59: 447-451.

167. Lobo LL, Tufik S. Effects of alcohol on sleep parameters of sleep-deprived healthy volunteers. Sleep 1997; 20: 52-59.

168. Magni G, Caldieron C, Rigatti-Luchini S et al. Chronic musculoskeletal pain and depressive symptoms in the general population. An analysis of the 1st National Health and Nutrition Examination survey data. Pain 1990; 43: 299-307.

169. Mahowald MW, Chokroverty S, Kader G et al. Sleep disorders. Continuum. A Program of the American Academy of Neurology; 1997

170. Mahowald ML, Mahowald MW. Nighttime sleep and daytime functioning (sleepiness and fatigue) in less well-defined chronic rheumatic diseases with particular reference to the "alpha-delta NREM

sleep anomaly.". Sleep Med 2000; 1: 195–207.

171. McBeth J, Macfarlane GJ, Benjamin S et al. Features of somatization predict the onset of chronic widespread pain: results of a large population-based study. Arthritis Rheum 2001; 44: 940-946.

172. McBeth J, Silman AJ. The role of psychiatric disorders in fibromyalgia. Curr Rheumatol Rep 2001; 3: 157-164.

173. McCracken LM, Iverson GL. Disrupted sleep patterns and daily functioning in patients with chronic pain. Pain Res Manage 2002; 7: 75-79.

174. McFarlane AC, Brooks PM. An analysis of the relationship between psychological morbidity and disease activity in rheumatoid arthritis. J Rheumatol 1988; 15: 926-931.

175. Meier-Ewert HK, Ridker PM, Rifai N et al. Effect of sleep loss on C-reactive protein, an inflammatory marker of cardiovascular risk. J Am Coll Cardiol 2004; 43: 678-683.

176. Mellinger GD, Balter MB, Uhlenhuth EH. Insomnia and its treatment: Prevalence and correlates. Arch Gen Psychiatry 1985; 42 :225-232.

177. Mendelson WB, James SP, Garnett D et al. A psychophysiological study of insomnia. Psychiatry Res 1986; 19: 267-284.

178. Mendelson WB, Roth T, Cassella J et al. The treatment of chronic insomnia: Drug indications, chronic use and abuse liability: Summary of a 2001 New Clinical Drug Evaluation Unit (NCDEU) meeting symposium. Sleep Med Rev 2003; 8: 7-17.

179. Mendelson WB, Thompson C, Franko T. Adverse reactions to sedative/hypnotics: Three years' experience. Sleep 1996; 19: 702-706.

180. Mendelson WB. Human Sleep: Research and Clinical Care. New York: Plenum Press; 1987.

181. Mendelson WB. Hypnotic medications: mechanisms of action and pharmacologic effects. In: Kryger MH, Roth T, Dement WC eds. Principles and Practice of Sleep Medicine, Fourth Edition. Philadelphia: Elsevier Saunders; 2005: 444-451.

182. Menefee LA, Cohen M, Anderson WR et al. Sleep disturbance and nonmalignant chronic pain: A comprehensive review of the literature. Pain Med 2000; 1: 156-172.

183. Meuser T, Pietruck C, Radbruch L et al. Symptoms during cancer pain treatment following WHO-guidelines: A longitudinal follow-up study of symptom prevalence, severity and etiology. Pain 2001; 93: 247-257.

184. Miller JC, Horvath SM. Sleep and altitudes. Aviat Space Environ Med 1977; 48: 615-620.

185. Mitler MM, Dinges DF, Dement WC. Sleep medicine, public policy, and public Health. In: Kryger MH, Roth T, Dement WC eds. Principles and Practice of Sleep Medicine, Second Edition. Philadelphia: WB Saunders; 1994: 453-462.

186. Mitler MM, Gujavarly KS, Browman CP. Maintenance of wakefulness test: A polysomnographic technique for evaluating treatment in patients. Electroencephalogr Clin Neurophysiol 1982; 53: 658-661.

187. Mitler MM, Miller JC. Methods of testing for sleeplessness. Behav Med 1996; 21: 171-183.

188. Mohler H, Okada T. Benzodiazepine receptor: Demonstration in the central nervous system. Science 1977; 198: 849-851.

189. Moldofsky H, Lue FA, Mously C et al. The effect of zolpidem in patients with fibromyalgia: a dose ranging, double-blind, placebo controlled, modified crossover study. J Rheumatol 1996; 23: 529–533.

190. Moldofsky H, Scarisbrick P, England R et al. Musculoskeletal symptoms and non-REM sleep disturbance in patients with "fibrositis syndrome" and healthy subjects. Psychosom Med 1975; 37: 341-351.

191. Moldofsky H, Scarisbrick P. Induction of neurasthenic musculoskeletal pain syndrome by selective sleep stage deprivation. Psychosom Med 1976; 38: 35-44.

192. Moldofsky H. Sleep and pain: Clinical review. Sleep Med Rev 2001; 5: 387-398.

193. Molony RR, MacPeek DM, Schiffman PL et al. Sleep, sleep apnea, and fibromyalgia syndrome. J Rheumatol 1986; 13: 797-800.

194. Monk TH, Buysse DJ, Reynolds CF III et al. Circadian determinants of the postlunch dip in performance. Chronobiol Int 1996; 13: 123-133.

195. Monti JM, Monti D. Sleep disturbance in generalized anxiety disorder and its treatment. Sleep Med Rev 2000; 4: 263-276.

196. Montplaisir J, Allen RP, Walters AS et al. Restless legs syndrome and periodic limb movements during sleep. In: Kryger MH, Roth T, Dement WC eds. Principles and Practice of Sleep Medicine, Fourth Edition. Philadelphia: Elsevier Saunders; 2005: 839-852.

197. Montplaisir J, Boucher S, Poirier G et al. Clinical, polysomnographic and genetic characteristics of restless legs syndrome: A study of 133 patients diagnosed with new standard criteria. Mov Disord 1997; 12: 61-65.

198. Morgan K, Clarke D. Longitudinal trends in late-life insomnia: Implications for prescribing. Age Ageing 1997; 26: 179-184.

199. Morin CM, Gibson D, Wade J. Self-reported sleep and mood disturbance in chronic pain patients. Clin J Pain 1998; 14: 311-314.

200. Morin CM, Gramling SE. Sleep patterns and aging: Comparison of older adults with and without insomnia complaints. Psychol Aging 1989; 4: 290-294.

201. Mullington JM, Chan JL, Van Dongen HP et al. Sleep loss reduces diurnal rhythm amplitude of

leptin in healthy men. J Neuroendocrinol 2003; 15: 851-854.

202. Murphy P, Badia P, Myers B et al. Nonsteroidal anti-inflammatory drugs affect normal sleep patterns in humans. Physiol Behav 1994; 55: 1063-1066.

203. National Sleep Foundation. Sleep in America Poll 2002. Washington, DC, National Sleep Foundation, 2002.

204. Nausieda PA, Weiner WJ, Kaplan LR et al. Sleep disruption in the course of chronic levodopa therapy: an early feature of levodopa psychosis. Clin Neuropharmacol 1982; 5: 183–194.

205. Nebes RD, Pollock BG, Houck PR et al. Persistence of cognitive impairment in geriatric patients following antidepressant treatment: A randomized, double-blind clinical trial with nortriptyline and paroxetine. J Psychiatr Res 2003; 37: 99-108.

206. Newman AB, Enright PL, Manolio TA et al. Sleep disturbance, psychosocial correlates, and cardiovascular disease in 5201 older adults: The Cardiovascular Health Study. J Am Geriatr Soc 1997; 45: 1-7.

207. Newman AB, Spiekerman CF, Enright P et al. Daytime sleepiness predicts mortality and cardiovascular disease in older adults. The Cardiovascular Health Study Research Group. J Am Geriatr Soc 2000; 48: 115-123.

208. Nicholson AN, Smith PA, Stone BM et al. Altitude insomnia: Studies during an expedition to the Himalayas. Sleep 1988; 11: 354-361.

209. Nicholson AN, Stone BM. Antihistamines: Impaired performance and the tendency to sleep. Eur J Clin Pharmacol 1986; 30: 27-32.

210. Nicholson B. Responsible prescribing of opioids for the management of chronic pain. Drugs 2003; 63: 17-32.

211. Nielson WR, Merskey H. Psychosocial aspects of fibromyalgia. Curr Pain Headache Rep 2001; 5: 330-337.

212. Nilsson LG, Backman L, Karlsson T. Priming and cued recall in elderly, alcohol intoxicated and sleep deprived subjects: A case of functionally similar memory deficits. Psychol Med 1989; 19: 423-433.

213. Obermeyer WH, Benca RM. Effects of drugs on sleep. Neurol Clin 1996; 14: 827-840.

214. Ohayon M, Partinen M. Insomnia and global sleep dissatisfaction in Finland. J Sleep Res 2002; 11: 339-346.

215. Ohayon MM, Carskadon MA, Guilleminault C et al. Meta-analysis of quantitative sleep parameters from childhood to old age in healthy individuals: developing normative sleep values across the human lifespan. Sleep 2004; 27: 1255-1273.

216. Ohayon MM, Caulet M, Guilleminault C. How a general population perceives its sleep and how this relates to the complaint of insomnia. Sleep 1997; 20: 715-723.

217. Ohayon MM, Roth T. What are the contributing factors for insomnia in the general population? J Psychosom Res 2001; 51: 745-755.

218. Ohayon MM, Zulley J. Correlates of global sleep dissatisfaction in the German population. Sleep 2001; 24: 780-787.

219. Ohayon MM. Epidemiology of insomnia: What we know and what we still need to learn. Sleep Med Rev 2002; 6: 97-111.

220. Ohayon MM. Prevalence of DSM-IV diagnostic criteria of insomnia: distinguishing insomnia related to mental disorders from sleep disorders. J Psychiatr Res 1997; 31: 333–346.

221. Okifuji A, Turk DC, Sherman JJ. Evaluation of the relationship between depression and fibromyalgia syndrome: why aren't all patients depressed? J Rheumatol 2000; 27: 212-219.

222. Onen SH, Alloui A, Gross A et al. The effects of total sleep deprivation selective sleep interruption and sleep recovery on pain tolerance thresholds in healthy subjects. J Sleep Res 2001; 10: 35-42.

223. Pacher P, Kohegyi E, Kecskemeti V et al. Current trends in the development of new antidepressants. Curr Med Chem 2001; 8: 89-100.

224. Papineau KL, Roehrs TA, Petrucelli N et al. Electrophysiological assessment (the multiple sleep latency test) of the biphasic effects of ethanol in humans. Alcohol Clin Exp Res 1998; 22: 231-235.

225. Parmeggiani PL. Temperature regulation during sleep: A study in homeostasis. In Orem J, Barnes CD eds: Physiology in Sleep. New York: Academic Press; 1980: 98-143.

226. Patat A, Rosenzweig P, Enslen M et al. Effects of a new slow release formulation of caffeine on EEG, psychomotor and cognitive functions in sleep-deprived subjects. Hum Psychopharmacol 2000; 15: 153-170.

227. Peigneux P, Laureys S, Fuchs S et al. Are spatial memories strengthened in the human hippocampus during slow wave sleep? Neuron 2004; 44: 535-545.

228. Perlis ML, Giles DE, Bootzin RR et al. Alpha sleep and information processing, perception of sleep, pain and arousability in fibromyalgia. Int J Neurosci 1997; 89: 265-280.

229. Phillips BA, Cooper KR, Burke TV. The effect of sleep loss on breathing in chronic obstructive pulmonary disease. Chest 1987; 91: 29-32.

230. Pollak CP, Perlick D, Linsner JP et al. Sleep problems in the community elderly as predictors of death and nursing home placement. J Community Health 1990; 15: 123-135.

231.Practice parameters for the use of polysomnography in the evaluation of insomnia. Standards of Practice Committee of the American Sleep Disorders Association. Sleep 1995; 18: 55-57.

232.Preskorn SH. Comparison of the tolerability of bupropion, fluoxetine, imipramine, nefazodone, paroxetine, sertraline, and venlafaxine. J Clin Psychiatry 1995; 56(Suppl 6): 12-21.

233.Pressman MR. Stages and architecture of normal sleep. UpToDate Online 2006; 14.2: 1-6. 13 July 2006 <http://www.utdol.com>.

234.Prinz P. Sleep patterns in the healthy aged: Relationship with intellectual function. J Gerontol 1977; 32: 179-186.

235.Prinz PN, Peskind ER, Vitaliano PP et al. Changes in the sleep and waking EEGs of nondemented and demented elderly subjects. J Am Geriatr Soc 1982; 30: 86-93.

236.Prinzmetal M, Alles GA. The central nervous system stimulant effects of dextro-amphetamine sulphate. Am J Med Sci 1940; 200: 665-673.

237.Punjabi NM, Bandeen-Roche K, Young T. Predictors of objective sleep tendency in the general population. Sleep 2003; 26: 678-683.

238.Quera-Salva MA, Orluc A, Goldenberg F et al. Insomnia and use of hypnotics: Study of a French population. Sleep 1991; 14: 386-391.

239.Qureshi A, Lee-Chiong T Jr. Medications and their effects on sleep. Med Clin North Am 2004; 88: 751-766,

240.Qureshi AI, Giles WH, Croft JB et al. Habitual sleep patterns and risk for stroke and coronary heart disease: A 10-year follow-up from NHANES I. Neurology 1997; 48: 904-911.

241.Radanov BP, Sturzenegger M, Di Stefano G. Longterm outcome after whiplash injury. A 2-year follow-up considering features of injury mechanism and somatic, radiologic and psychosocial findings. Medicine (Baltimore) 1995; 74: 281-297.

242.Radomski MW, Hart LE, Goodman JM et al. Aerobic fitness and hormonal responses to prolonged sleep deprivation and sustained mental work. Aviat Space Environ Med 1992; 63: 101-106.

243.Rains JC, Penzien DB. Chronic headache and sleep disturbance. Curr Pain Headache Rep 2002; 6: 498-504.

244.Rechtschaffen A. Current perspectives on the function of sleep. Perspect Biol Med 1998; 41: 359-390.

245.Rechtschaffen A. Polygraphic aspects of insomnia: The abnormalities of sleep in man. In: Proceedings of the XVth European Meeting on Electroencephalography. Gastaut H, Lugaresi L, Berti G, Coccagna G eds. Bologna; 1976: 109.

246.Reid KJ, Chang AM, Zee PC. Circadian rhythm sleep disorders. Med Clin North Am 2004; 88: 631-651.

247.Reynolds CF III, Coble PA, Kupfer DJ et al. Application of the multiple sleep latency test in disorders of excessive sleepiness. Electroencephalogr Clin Neurophysiol 1982; 53: 443-452.

248.Reynolds CF III, Kupfer DJ. Sleep research in affective illness: State of the art circa 1987. Sleep 1987; 10: 199-215.

249.Ribeiro S, Gervasoni D, Soares ES et al. Longlasting novelty-induced neuronal reverberation during slow-wave sleep in multiple forebrain areas. PLoS Biol 2004; 2: E24.

250.Richardson GS, Carskadon MA, Flagg W et al. Excessive daytime sleepiness in man: Multiple sleep latency measurement in narcoleptic and control subjects. Electroencephalogr Clin Neurophysiol 1978; 45: 621-627.

251.Richardson GS, Malin HV. Circadian rhythm sleep disorders: Pathophysiology and treatment. J Clin Neurophysiol 1996; 13: 17-31.

252.Rickles K, Schweizer E. Clinical overview of serotonin reuptake inhibitors. J Clin Psychiatry 1990; 51: 9–12.

253.Riley III JL, Benson MB, Gremillion HA et al. Sleep disturbances in orofacial pain patients: Pain-related or emotional distress? J Craniomandib Pract 2001; 19: 106-113.

254.Rockwood K, Davis HS, Merry HR et al. Sleep disturbances and mortality: Results from the Canadian Study of Health and Aging. J Am Geriatr Soc 2001; 49: 639-641.

255.Roehrs T, Merlotti L, Halpin D et al. Effects of theophylline on nocturnal sleep and daytime sleepiness/alertness. Chest 1995; 108: 382-387.

256.Roehrs T, Tietz E, Zorick F et al. Daytime sleepiness and antihistamines. Sleep 1984; 7: 137-141.

257.Rogers GS, Van de Castle RL, Evans WS et al. Vaginal pulse amplitude response patterns during erotic conditions and sleep. Arch Sex Behav 1985; 14: 327-342.

258.Roizenblatt S, Moldofsky H, Benedito-Silva AA et al. Alpha sleep characteristics in fibromyalgia. Arthritis Rheum 2001; 44: 222-230.

259.Roizenblatt S, Tufik S, Goldenberg J et al. Juvenile fibromyalgia: Clinical and polysomnographic aspects. J Rheumatol 1977; 24: 579-585.

260.Ross JJ. Neurological findings after prolonged sleep deprivation. Arch Neurol 1965; 12: 399-403.

261.Roth T, Roehrs T. Determinants of residual effects of hypnotics. Accid Anal Prev 1985; 17: 291-296.

262.Roth T, Zorick F, Wittig R et al. Pharmacological and medical considerations in hypnotic use. Sleep 1982; 5: S46-S52.

263.Roth T, Zorick F, Wittig R et al. The effects of doxepin HCl on sleep and depression. J Clin Psychiatry 1982; 43: 366-368.

264.Rozerem [package insert]. Lincolnshire, IL; Takeda Pharmaceuticals America, Inc; 2006.

265.Rumble R, Morgan K. Hypnotics, sleep, and mortality in elderly people. J Am Geriatr Soc 1992; 40: 787-791.

266.Salin-Pascual RJ, De La Fuente JR, Galicia-Polo L et al. Effects of transdermal nicotine on mood and sleep in nonsmoking major depressed patients. Psychopharmacology (Berl) 1995; 121: 476-479.

267.Sateia MJ, Doghramji K, Hauri PJ et al. Evaluation of chronic insomnia. An American Academy of Sleep Medicine review. Sleep 2000; 23: 243-308.

268.Sateia MJ, Nowell PD. Insomnia. Lancet 2004; 364: 1959-1973.

269.Sateia MJ, Pigeon WR. Identification and management of insomnia. Med Clin North Am 2004; 88: 567-596.

270.Sawynok J. Pharmacological rationale for the clinical use of caffeine. Drugs 1995; 49: 37-50.

271.Schiavi RC, Schreiner-Engel P. Nocturnal penile tumescence in healthy aging men. J Gerontol 1988; 43: M146-M150.

272.Schiffman PL, Trontell MC, Mazar ME et al. Sleep deprivation decreases ventilatory response to CO2 but not load compensation. Chest 1983; 84: 695-698.

273.Schug S, Garrett W, Gillespie G. Opioid and nonopioid analgesics. Best Pract Res Clin Anaesthesiol 2003; 17: 91-110.

274.Schwartz SW, Cornoni-Huntley J, Cole SR et al. Are sleep complaints an independent risk factor for myocardial infarction? Ann Epidemiol 1998; 8: 384-392.

275.Schweitzer PK. Drugs that disturb sleep and wakefulness. In: Kryger MH, Roth T, Dement WC eds. Principles and Practice of Sleep Medicine, Fourth Edition. Philadelphia: Elsevier Saunders; 2005: 499-518.

276.Scudds RA, McCain GA, Rollman GB et al. Improvements in pain responsiveness in patients with fibrositis after successful treatment with amitriptyline. J Rheumatol 1989; 16: 98-103.

277.Seidel WF, Dement WC. Sleepiness in insomnia: evaluation and treatment. Sleep 1982; 5 Suppl 2: S182.

278.Seifritz E, Hemmeter U, Trachsel L et al. Effects of flumazenil on recovery sleep and hormonal secretion after sleep deprivation in male controls. Psychopharmacology 1995; 120: 449-456.

279.Sewitch DE. The perceptual uncertainty of having slept: The inability to discriminate electroencephalographic sleep from wakefulness. Psychophysiology 1984; 21: 243-259.

280.Sharpley AL, Cowen PJ. Effect of pharmacologic treatments on the sleep of depressed patients. Biol Psychiatry 1995; 37: 85-98.

281.Shaver JL, Lentz M, Landis CA et al. Sleep, psychological distress, and stress arousal in women with fibromyalgia, Res Nurs Health 1997; 20: 247-257.

282.Shaw PJ, Cirelli C, Greenspan RJ et al. Correlates of sleep and waking in Drosophila melanogaster. Science 2000; 287: 1834-1837.

283.Shearer WT, Reuben JM, Mullington JM et al. Soluble TNF-alpha receptor 1 and IL-6 plasma levels in humans subjected to the sleep deprivation model of spaceflight. J Allergy Clin Immunol 2001; 107: 165-170.

284.Shipley JE, Kupfer DJ, Griffin SJ et al. Comparison of effects of desipramine and amitriptyline on EEG sleep of depressed patients. Psychopharmacology (Berl) 1985; 85: 14-22.

285.Silber MH. Clinical practice. Chronic insomnia. N Engl J Med 2005; 353: 803-810.

286.Sjogren P. Psychomotor and cognitive functioning in cancer patients. Acta Anaesthesiol Scand 1997; 41: 159-161.

287.Smith MT, Perlis ML, Smith MS et al. Sleep quality and presleep arousal in chronic pain. J Behav Med 2000; 23: 1-13.

288.Somers VK, Dyken ME, Mark AL et al. Sympathetic nerve activity during sleep in normal subjects. N Engl J Med 1993; 328: 303-307.

289.Spiegel K, Sheridan JF, Van Cauter E. Effect of sleep deprivation on response to immunization. JAMA 2002; 288: 1471-1472.

290.Spiegel K, Tasali E, Penev P et al. Brief communication: Sleep curtailment in healthy young men is associated with decreased leptin levels, elevated ghrelin levels, and increased hunger and appetite. Ann Intern Med 2004; 141: 846-850.

291.Squires RF, Braestrup C. Benzodiazepine receptors in rat brain. Nature 1977; 266: 732-734.

292.Staedt J, Windt H, Hajaki G et al. Cluster arousal analysis in chronic pain-disturbed sleep. J Sleep Res 1993; 2: 134-137.

293.Stepanski E, Lamphere J, Badia P et al. Sleep fragmentation and daytime sleepiness. Sleep 1984; 7: 18-26.

294.Steyvers FJJM, Gaillard AWK. The effects of sleep deprivation and incentives on human performance. Psychol Res 1993; 55: 64-70.

295.Summala, H, Mikkola, T. Fatal accidents among car and truck drivers: effects of fatigue, age, and alcohol consumption. Hum Factors 1994; 36:315-326.

296.Tenkanen L, Sjoblom T, Harma M. Joint effect of shift work and adverse life-style factors on the risk of coronary heart disease. Scand J Work Environ Health 1998; 24: 351-357.

297.Thase ME. Treatment issues related to sleep and depression. J Clin Psychiatry 2000; 61(Suppl 11): 46-50.

298.The Gallup Organization: Sleep in America. Princeton, NJ, Gallup Organization, 1995.

299.The Gallup Organization: The Gallup study of sleeping habits. Princeton, NJ, Gallup Organization, 1979.

300.Touchon J, Besset A, Billiard M et al. Fibrositis syndrome: Polysomnographic and psychological aspects. In Koella WP, Obál F, Schulz H et al eds. SLEEP '86. New York: Gustav Fischer Verlag; 1988: 445-447.

301.Trenkwalder C, Walters AS, Hening W. Periodic limb movements and restless legs syndrome. Neurol Clin 1996; 14: 629-650.

302.Van Dongen HPA, Maislin G, Mullington JM et al. The cumulative cost of additional wakefulness: Dose-response effects on neurobehavioral functions and sleep physiology from chronic sleep restriction and total sleep deprivation. Sleep 2003; 26: 117-126.

303.Van Dongen HPA, Rogers NL, Dinges DF. Understanding sleep debt: Theoretical and empirical issues. Sleep Biol Rhythms 2003; 1: 4-12.

304.van Laar MW, Volkerts ER, Vertaten MN et al. Differential effects of amitriptyline, nefazodone and paroxetine on performance and brain indices of visual selective attention and working memory. Psychopharmacology 2000; 162: 351-363.

305.Vaswani M, Linda FK, Ramesh S. Role of selective serotonin reuptake inhibitors in psychiatric disorders: A comprehensive review. Prog Neuropsychopharmacol Biol Psychiatry 2003; 27: 85-102.

306.Volz H-P, Sturm Y. Antidepressant drugs and psychomotor performance. Neuropsychobiology 1995; 31: 146-155.

307.Wagner DR. Disorders of the circadian sleep-wake cycle. Neurol Clin 1996; 14: 651-670.

308.Walder B, Tramer M, Blois R. The effects of two single doses of tramadol on sleep: A randomized, cross-over trial in healthy volunteers. Eur J Anaesthesiol 2001; 18: 36-42.

309.Walters AS. Toward a better definition of the restless legs syndrome. The International Restless Legs Syndrome Study Group. Mov Disord 1995; 10: 634-642.

310.Ware JC, Brown FW, Moorad PJ et al. Effects on sleep: A double-blind study comparing trimipramine to imipramine in depressed insomniac patients. Sleep 1989; 12: 537-549.

311.Ware JC, Russell IJ, Campos E. Alpha intrusions into the sleep of depression and fibromyalgia syndrome (fibrositis) patients (abstract). Sleep Res 1986; 15: 210.

312.Wehr TA, Moul DE, Barbato G et al. Conservation of photoperiod-responsive mechanisms in humans. Am J Physiol 1993; 265: R846-R857.

313.Weil JV. Respiratory physiology: sleep at high altitudes. In: Kryger MH, Roth T, Dement WC eds. Principles and Practice of Sleep Medicine, Fourth Edition. Philadelphia: Elsevier Saunders; 2005: 245-255.

314.Weiser S, Cedrashi C. Psychosocial issues in the prevention of chronic low back pain - a literature review. Ballieres Best Pract Res Clin Rheumatol 1992; 6: 657-684.

315.Weissman MM, Greenwald S, Nino-Murcia G et al. The morbidity of insomnia uncomplicated by psychiatric disorders. Gen Hosp Psychiatry 1997; 19: 245-250.

316.Weitzman ED, Zimmerman JC, Czeisler CA et al. Cortisol secretion is inhibited during sleep in normal man. J Clin Endocrinol Metab 1983; 56: 352-358.

317.Wetter DW, Young TB, Bidwell TR et al. Smoking as a risk factor for sleep-disordered breathing. Arch Intern Med 1994; 154: 2219-2224.

318.White, DP Douglas NJ, Pickett CK et al. Sleep deprivation and control of ventilation. Am Rev Respir Dis 1983; 128: 984-986.

319.Whiting PJ, McKernan RM, Wager-Srdar SA. Structure and pharmacology of vertebrate GABA-A receptor subtypes. Int Rev Neurobiol 1995; 38: 95-138.

320.Widerstrom-Noga EG, Felipe-Cuervo E, Yezierski RP. Chronic pain after spinal injury: Interference with sleep and daily activities. Arch Phys Med Rehabil 2001; 82: 1571-1577.

321.Williams HL, Gieseking CF, Lubin A. Some effects of sleep loss on memory. Percept Mot Skills 1966; 23: 1287-1293.

322.Williams HL, Lubin A. Speeded addition and sleep loss. J Exp Psychol 1967; 73: 313-317.

323.Winokur A, Gary KA, Rodner S et al. Depression, sleep physiology, and antidepressant drugs. Depress Anxiety 2001; 14: 19-28.

324.Wisor JP, Nishino S, Sora I et al. Dopaminergic role in stimulant-induced wakefulness. J Neurosci 2001; 21: 1787-1794.

325.Wittig RM, Zorick FJ, Blumer D et al. Disturbed sleep in patients complaining of chronic pain. J Nerv Ment Dis 1982; 70: 429-431.

326.Wolfe F, Smythe HA, Yunus MB et al. The American College of Rheumatology 1990 criteria for the classification of fibromyalgia : Report of the Multicenter Criteria Committee. Arthritis Rheum 1990; 33: 160-172.

327.Yoss RE, Daly DD. Treatment of narcolepsy with Ritalin. Neurology 1959; 9: 171-173.

328.Yules RB, Lippman ME, Freedman DX. Alcohol administration prior to sleep: The effect of EEG sleep stages. Arch Gen Psychiatry 1967; 16: 94-97.

329.Yunus MB. Psychological aspects of fibromyalgia syndrome: a component of the dysfunctional spectrum syndrome. Ballieres Best Pract Res Clin Rheumatol 1994; 8: 811-837.

330.Zulley J. Distribution of REM sleep in entrained 24 hour and free-running sleep-wake cycles. Sleep 1980; 2: 377-389.

331.Zwyghuizen-Doorenbos A, Roehrs T, Lamphere J et al. Increased daytime sleepiness enhances ethanol's sedative effects. Neuropsychopharmacology 1988; 1: 279-286.

References Chapter 12

1. Aaron LA, Bradley LA, Alarcon GS et al. Perceived physical and emotional trauma as precipitating events in fibromyalgia. Associations with heal care seeking and disability status but not pain severity. Arthritis Rheum 1997; 40: 453-460.

2. Aaron LA, Bradley LA, Alarcon GS et al. Psychiatric diagnoses in patients with fibromyalgia are related to health care-seeking behavior rather than to illness. Arthritis Rheum 1996; 39: 436-445.

3. Affleck G, Tennen H, Keefe FJ et al. Everyday life with osteoarthritis or rheumatoid arthritis: independent effects of disease and gender on daily pain, mood, and coping. Pain 1999; 83: 601-609.

4. Ahles TA, Yunus MB, Gaulier B et al. The use of contemporary MMPI norms in the study of chronic pain patients. Pain 1986; 24: 159-163.

5. Ahles TA, Yunus MB, Riley SD et al. Psychological factors associated with primary fibromyalgia syndrome. Arthritis Rheum 1984; 27: 1101-1106.

6. Alexander RW, Bradley LA, Alarcón GS et al. Sexual and physical abuse in women with fibromyalgia: association with outpatient health care utilization and pain medication usage. Arthritis Care Res 1998; 11: 102-115.

7. Alfici S, Sigal M, Landau M. Primary fibromyalgia syndrome-a variant of depressive disorder? Psychother Psychosom 1989; 51: 156-161.

8. American Psychiatric Association. Diagnostic and Statistical Manual of Mental Disorders, Fourth Edition, Text Revision. Washington, DC: American Psychiatric Association; 2000.

9. And AKK, Schanberg L. Juvenile fibromyalgia syndrome. Curr Rheumatol Rep 2001; 3; 165-171.

10. Antony MM, Brown TA, Barlow DH. Current perspectives on panic and panic disorder. Curr Dir Psychol Sci 1992; 1: 79-82.

11. Bandura A. Social learning theory. New York: Prentice-Hall; 1977.

12. Bandura A. Self-efficacy: Toward a unifying theory of behavioral change. Psychol Rev 1977; 84: 191-215.

13. Bantick SJ, Wise RG, Ploghaus A et al. Imaging how attention modulates pain in humans using functional MRI. Brain 2002; 125: 310-319.

14. Beck AT, Rush AJ, Shaw BF et al.. Cognitive Therapy of Depression. In: New York: Guilford Press; 1979.

15. Bennett RM, Burckhardt CS, Clark SR et al. Group treatment of fibromyalgia: a 6 month outpatient program. J Rheumatol 1996; 23: 521-528.

16. Bennett RM. Fibromyalgia and the disability dilemma. A new era in understanding a complex, multidimensional pain syndrome. Arthritis Rheum 1996; 39: 1627-1643.

17. Bennett, RM. Fibromyalgia. In: Wall PD, Melzack R eds. Textbook of Pain. Fourth ed. Edinburgh: Churchill Livingston; 1999; 579-601.

18. Berscheid E. Interpersonal attraction. In: Lindzey G, Aronson E eds. The Handbook of Social Psychology. New York: Random House; 1985.

19. Beydoun A, Morrow TJ, Shen JF et al. Variability of laser-evoked potentials: attention, arousal and lateralized differences. Electroencephalogr Clin Neurophysiol 1993; 88: 173-181.

20. Bigos SJ, Battie MC, Spengler DM et al.. A longitudinal, prospective study of industrial back injury reporting. Clin Orthop 1992; 279: 21-34.

21. Blake DJ, Maisiak R, Graciela S et al. Sexual quality of life of patients with arthritis compared to arthritis free controls. J Rheumatol 1987; 14: 570-576.

22. Block AR, Kremer AF, Gaylor M. The spouse as a discriminative cue for pain behavior. Pain 1980; 9: 245-252.

23. Boisset-Pioro MH, Esdaile JM, Fitzcharles MA. Sexual and physical abuse in women with fibromyalgia syndrome. Arthritis Rheum 1995; 38: 235-241.

24. Boothby JL, Thorn BE, Stroud MW et al. Coping with pain. In: Gatchel RJ, Turk DC eds. Psychosocial Factors in Pain. New York: Guilford Press; 1999: 343-359.

25. Bouton ME, Mineka S, Barlow DH. A modern learning theory perspective on the etiology of panic disorder. Psychol Rev 2001; 108: 4-32.

26. Bradley LA. Adherence with treatment regimens among adult rheumatoid arthritis patients: current status and future directions. Arthritis Care Res 1989; 2: 33-39.

27. Brooks JC, Nurmikko TJ, Bimson WE et al. fMRI of thermal pain: effects of stimulus laterality and attention. Neuroimage 2002; 15: 293-301.

28. Brown JD. Accuracy and bias in delf-knowledge. In: Snyder CR, Forsyth DF eds. Handbook of Social and Clinical Psychology: The Health Perspective. New York: Pergamon Press; 1991.

29. Buckelew SP, Conway R, Parker J et al. Biofeed-

back/relaxation training and exercise interventions for fibromyalgia: a prospective trial. Arthritis Care Res 1998; II: 196-209.

30. Buckelew SP, Parker JC, Keefe FJ et al. Self-efficacy and pain behavior among subjects with fibromyalgia. Pain 1994; 59: 377-385.

31. Burckhardt CS, Bjelle A. Perceived control: a comparison of women with fibromyalgia, rheumatoid arthritis, and systemic lupus erythematosus using a Swedish version of the Rheumatology Attitudes Index. Scand J Rheumatol 1996; 25: 300-306.

32. Burckhardt CS, Clark SR, O'Reilly CA et al. Pain-coping strategies of women with fibromyalgia: a relationship to pain, fatigue and quality of life. J Musculoskel Med 1997; 5: 5-21.

33. Burke LE, Ockene IS eds. Compliance in healthcare and research. New York: Futura; 2001.

34. Bushnell MC, Duncan GH, Hofbauer RK et al. Pain perception: is there a role for primary somatosensory cortex? Proc Natl Acad Sci U S A 1999; 96: 7705-7709.

35. Callahan LF, Smith WJ, Pincus T. Self-report questionnaires in five rheumatic diseases: comparison of health status constructs and associations with formal educational level. Arthritis Care Res 1989; 2: 122-131.

36. Campbell DT. On the conflicts between biological and social evolution and between psychology and moral tradition. Am Psychol 1975; 30: 1103-1126.

37. Carey G. Genes, fears, phobias, and phobic disorders. J Couns Dev 1990; 68: 628-632.

38. Case RB, Moss AJ, Case N et al. Living alone after myocardial infarction. Impact on prognosis. JAMA 1992; 267: 515-519.

39. Cassisi JE, Sypert GW, Lagana L et al. Pain, disability, and psychological functioning in chronic low back pain subgroups: Myofascial versus herniated disc syndrome. Neurosurgery 1993; 33: 379-385.

40. Chabal C, Erjavec MK, Jacobson L. Prescription opiate abuse in chronic pain patients: Clinical criteria, incidence and predictors. Clin J Pain 1997; 13: 150-155.

41. Chambers CT, Craig KD, Bennett SM. The impact of maternal behavior on children's pain experiences: an experimental analysis. J Pediatr Psychol 2002; 27: 293-301.

42. Chambless DL, Baker MJ, Baucom DH et al. Update on empirically validated therapies, II. Clinical Psychologist 1998; 51: 3-16.

43. Ciccone DS, Elliott DK, Chandler HK et al. Sexual and physical abuse in women with fibromyalgia syndrome: a test of the trauma hypothesis. Clin J Pain 2005; 21: 378-386.

44. Clinical Standards Advisory Group. Report of a Clinical Standards Advisory Group committee on back pain. London: HMSO; 1994.

45. Cohen H, Neumann L, Haiman Y et al. Prevalence of post-traumatic stress disorder in fibromyalgia patients: overlapping syndromes or post-traumatic fibromyalgia syndrome? Semin Arthritis Rheum 2002; 32: 38-50.

46. Cohen S. Psychosocial models of the role of social support in the etiology of physical disease. Health Psychol 1988; 7: 269-297.

47. Colon EA, Callies AL, Popkin MK et al. Depressed mood and other variables related to bone marrow transplantation survival in acute leukemia. Psychosomatics 1991; 32: 420-425.

48. Craig KD, Patrick CJ. Facial expression during induced pain. J Pers Soc Psychol 1985; 48: 1080-1091.

49. Craig KD, Prkachin KM. Nonverbal measures of pain. In: Melzack R ed. Pain measurement and assessment. New York: Raven Press; 1983.

50. Craig KD. Consequences of caring: pain in the human context. Can Psychol 1987; 28: 311-321.

51. Craig KD. Emotions and psychobiology. In: McMahon SB, Koltzenburg M eds. Wall and Melzack's Textbook of Pain, Fifth Edition. Edinburgh: Elsevier Churchill Livingstone; 2006: 231-239.

52. Craig KD. Social modeling influences: pain in context. In: Sternbach R A ed. The Psychology of Pain. New York: Raven Press; 1986.

53. Crisson JE, Keefe FJ. The relationship of locus of control to pain coping strategies and psychological distress in chronic pain patients. Pain 1988; 35: 147-154.

54. Crocker J, Wolfe CT. Contingencies of self-worth. Psychol Rev 2001; 108: 593-623.

55. D'Zurilla TJ, Goldfried MR. Problem solving and behavior modification. J Abnorm Psychol 1971; 78: 107-126.

56. Daltroy LH. Doctor-patient communication in rheumatological disorders. Baillières Clin Rheumatol 1993; 7: 221-239.

57. Davey GCL. Preparedness and phobias: specific evolved associations or a generalized expectancy bias? Behav Brain Sci 1995; 18: 289-297.

58. Deale A, Chalder T, Marks I et al. Cognitive behavior therapy for chronic fatigue syndrome: a randomized controlled trial. Am J Psychiatry 1997; 154: 408-414.

59. DeGood DE, Tait RC. 2001 Assessment of pain beliefs and coping. In: Turk DC, Melzack R eds. Handbook of pain assessment. New York: Guilford Press; 2001: 320-345.

60. DeNeve KM, Cooper H. The happy personality: A meta-analysis of 137 personality traits and sub-

jective well-being. Psychol Bull 1998; 124: 197-229.

61. Dermer M, Cohen SJ, Jacobsen E et al. Evaluative judgments of aspects of life as a function of vicarious exposure to hedonic extremes. J Pers Soc Psychol 1979; 37: 247-260.

62. DeVellis RF, Callahan LF. A brief measure of helplessness in rheumatic disease: The helplessness subscale of the rheumatology attitudes index. J Rheumatol 1993; 20: 866–869.

63. Deyo RA. Compliance with therapeutic regimens in arthritis: issues, current status, and a future agenda. Semin Arthritis Rheum 1982; 12: 233-244.

64. Doeglas D, Suurmeijer T, Krol B et al. Social support, social disability, and psychological well-being in rheumatoid arthritis. Arthritis Care Res 1994; 7: 10–15.

65. Duckworth KL, Bargh JA, Garcia M et al. The automatic evaluation of novel stimuli. Psychol Sci 2002; 13: 513-519.

66. Eckert ED, Heston LL, Bouchard TJ Jr. MZ twins reared apart: preliminary findings of psychiatric disturbances and traits. Prog Clin Biol Res 1981; 69 Pt B: 179-188.

67. Eisenberg DM, Davis RB, Ettner SL et al. Trends in alternative medicine use in the United States, 1990-1997. JAMA 1998; 280: 1569-1575.

68. Ellison CG, George LK. Religious involvement, social ties, and social support in a Southeastern community. J Sci Study Relig 1994; 33: 46-61.

69. Epstein SA, Kay G, Clauw D et al. Psychiatric disorders in patients with fibromyalgia. A multicenter investigation. Psychosomatics. 1999; 40: 57-63.

70. Ercolani M, Trombini G, Chattat R et al. Fibromyalgic syndrome: depression and abnormal illness behavior. Multicenter investigation. Psychother Psychosom 1994; 61: 178-186.

71. Evans PJD. Narcotic addiction in patients with chronic pain. Anaesthesia 1981; 36: 597–602.

72. Faymonville ME, Laureys S, Degueldre C et al. Neural mechanisms of antinociceptive effects of hypnosis. Anesthesiology 2000; 92: 1257-1267.

73. Ferguson ED. Adler's motivational theory: An historical perspective on belonging and the fundamental human striving. Individ Psychol 1989; 45: 354-361.

74. Fernandez E, Milburn TW. Sensory and affective predictors of overall pain and emotions associated with affective pain. Clin J Pain 1994; 10: 3–9.

75. Ferraccioli G, Ghirelli L, Scita F et al. EMG-biofeedback training in fibromyalgia syndrome. J Rheumatol 1987; 14: 820-825.

76. Fields HL. Pain modulation: expectation, opioid analgesia and virtual pain. Prog Brain Res 2000; 122: 163-172.

77. Fishbain DA. Approaches to treatment decisions for psychiatric comorbidity in the management of the chronic pain patient. Med Clin North Am 1999; 83: 737-760.

78. Fishbain DA, Cutler R, Rosomoff HL et al. Chronic pain-associated depression: Antecedent or consequence of chronic pain? A review. Clin J Pain 1997; 13: 116-137.

79. Fishbain DA, Goldberg M, Meagher BR et al. Male and female chronic pain patients categorized by DSM-III psychiatric diagnostic criteria. Pain 1986; 26: 181-197.

80. Fishbain DA, Steele-Rosomoff R, Rosomoff HL. Drug abuse, dependence, and addiction in chronic pain patients. Clin J Pain 1992; 8: 77–85.

81. Flor H, Breitenstein C, Birbaumer N et al. A psychophysiological analysis of spouse solicitousness toward pain behaviors, spouse interaction, and pain perception. Behav Ther 1995; 26: 255-272.

82. Folkman S, Lazarus RS, Dunkel-Schetter C et al. The dynamics of a stressful encounter: cognitive appraisal, coping and encounter outcomes. J Pers Soc Psychol 1986; 50: 992-1003.

83. Fordyce WE. Behavioral methods for chronic pain and illness. St Louis; Mosby: 1976.

84. Fordyce WE. Operant or contingency therapies. In: Loeser JD, Butler SD, Chapman CR et al eds. The Management of Pain, Third Edition. Philadelphia: Lippincott, Williams and Wilkins; 2000.

85. Frank JD. Therapeutic components shared by all psychotherapies. In: Harvey JH, Parks MM eds. The Master Lecture Series: Volume I. Psychotherapy research and behavior change. Washington, D.C.: American Psychological Association; 1982.

86. Frankenstein UN, Richter W, McIntyre MC et al. Distraction modulates anterior cingulate gyrus activations during the cold pressor test. Neuroimage 2001; 14: 827-836.

87. Fredrickson BL. Positive emotions. In: Snyder CR, Lopez SJ eds. Handbook of Positive Psychology. New York: Oxford; 2002.

88. Gallup G. Religion in America: 1990. In: Princeton: Princeton Religious Research Center; 1990.

89. Garnham A, Oakhill JV. Accounting for belief bias in a mental model framework: comment on Klauer, Musch, and Naumer (2000). Psychol Rev 2005; 112: 509-518.

90. Gaston-Johansson F, Gustafsson F, Felldin R et al. A comparative study of feelings, attitudes and behaviors of patients with fibromyalgia and rheumatoid arthritis. Soc Sci Med 1990; 31: 941-957.

91. Geisser ME, Haig AJ, Theisen ME. Activity avoidance and function in persons with chronic back pain. J Occup Rehabil 2000; 10: 215-227.

92. Geisser ME, Roth RS. Knowledge of and agreement with pain diagnosis: relation to pain beliefs,

pain severity, disability and psychological distress. J Occup Rehabil 1998; 8: 73-88.

93. Giescke T, Williams DA, Harris RE et al. Subgrouping of fibromyalgia patients on the basis of pressure-pain thresholds and psychological factors. Arthritis Rheum 2003, 48: 2916-2922.

94. Gil KM, Ross SL, Keefe FJ. Behavioral treatment of chronic pain: four pain management protocols. In: France RD, Krishnan KRR eds. Chronic Pain. New York: American Psychiatric Press; 1988.

95. Gil KM, Williams DA, Keefe FJ et al.. The relationship of negative thoughts to pain and psychological distress. Behav Ther 1990; 21: 349-362.

96. Goldberg RT. Childhood abuse, depression, and chronic pain. Clin J Pain 1994; 10: 277-281.

97. Goldenberg DL, Kaplan KH, Nadeau MG. A controlled study of stress-reduction, cognitive-behavioral treatment program in fibromyalgia. J Musculoskel Pain 1994; 2: 53-65.

98. Goldenberg DL. Psychological symptoms and psychiatric diagnosis in patients with fibromyalgia. J Rheumatol 1989; 16(Suppl. 19): 127-130.

99. Goldenberg DL, Mossey CJ, Schmid CH. A model to assess severity and impact of fibromyalgia. J Rheumatol 1995; 22: 2313-2318.

100.Goldfried MR, Davidson G. Clinical Behavioural Therapy. New York: Holt, Rinehart & Winston; 1976.

101. Goodenow C, Reisine ST, Gradey KE. Quality of social support and associated social and psychological functioning in women with rheumatoid arthritis. Health Psychol 1990 ;9: 266–284.

102.Goodman JE, McGrath PJ. Modeling mothers' influences on children's pain during a cold pressor task. Pain 2002; 104: 559-565.

103.Gottlieb NH, Green LW. Lifestyle events, social network, lifestyle, and health: An analysis of the 1979 National Survey of Personal Health Practices and Consequences. Health Educ Q 1984; 11: 91-105.

104.Granges G, Zilko P, Littlejohn GO. Fibromyalgia syndrome: assessment of the severity of the condition 2 years after diagnosis. J Rheumatol 1997; 36: 1318-1323.

105.Greenfield S, Fitzcharles MA, Esdaile JM. Reactive fibromyalgia syndrome. Arthritis Rheum 1992; 35: 678-681.

106.Gruder CL. Choice of comparison persons in evaluating oneself. In: Suls JM, Miller RL eds. Social Comparison Processes. New York: Hemisphere; 1977.

107.Guest GH, Drummond PD. Effect of compensation on emotional state and disability in chronic back pain. Pain 1992; 48: 125-130.

108.Gustafsson M, Gaston-Johansson F. Pain intensity and health locus of control: a comparison of patients with fibromyalgia syndrome and rheumatoid arthritis. Patient Educ Couns 1996; 29: 179–188.

109.Hadhazy VA, Ezzo J, Creamer P et al. Mind-body therapies for the treatment of fibromyalgia. A systematic review. J Rheumatol 2000; 27: 2911-2918.

110. Hagglund KJ, Haley WE, Reveille JD et al. Predicting individual differences in pain and functional impairment among patients with rheumatoid arthritis. Arthritis Rheum 1989; 32: 851–858.

111. Hassett AL, Cone JD, Patella SJ et al. The role of catastrophizing in the pain and depression of women with fibromyalgia syndrome. Arthritis Rheum 2000, 43: 2493-2500.

112. Hawley DJ, Wolfe F, Cathey MA. Pain, functional disability, and psychological status: a 12-month study of severity in fibromyalgia. J Rheumatol 1988; 15: 1551-1556.

113. Hawley DJ, Wolfe F. Pain, disability, and pain/disability relationships in seven rheumatic disorders: a study of 1,522 patients. J Rheumatol 1991; 10: 1552-1557.

114. Haythornthwaite JA, Clark MR, Pappagallo M et al. Pain coping strategies play a role in the persistence of pain in post-herpetic neuralgia. Pain 2003; 106: 453-460.

115. Henriksson CM. Living with continuous muscular pain – patient perspectives. Part I: Encounters and consequences. Scand J Caring Sci 1995; 9: 67-76.

116. Hensing G, Spak F. Psychiatric disorders as a factor in sick-leave due to other diagnoses: A general population-based study. Br J Psychiatry 1998; 172: 250–256.

117. Highfield MEF. Providing spiritual care to patients with cancer. Clin J Oncol Nurs 2000: 4; 115-120.

118. Hill J, Bird H, Thorpe R. Effects of rheumatoid arthritis on sexual activity and relationships. Rheumatology 2003; 42: 280-286.

119. Hofbauer RK, Fiset P, Plourde G et al. Dose-dependent effects of propofol on the central processing of thermal pain. Anesthesiology 2004; 100: 386-394.

120.Hoffmann NG, Olofsson O, Salen B et al. Prevalence of abuse and dependency in chronic pain patients. Int J Addict 1995; 30: 919–927.

121. Hoshiyama M, Kakigi R. After-effect of transcutaneous electrical nerve stimulation (TENS) on pain-related evoked potentials and magnetic fields in normal subjects. Clin Neurophysiol 2000; 111: 717-724.

122.House JS, Landis KR, Umberson D. Social relationships and health. Science 1988; 241:540-545.

123.Hudson JI, Goldenberg DL, Pope HG Jr et al. Comorbidity of fibromyalgia with medical and psychiatric disorders. Am J Med 1992; 92: 363-367.

124. Hudson JI, Pope HG Jr. Does childhood sexual abuse cause fibromyalgia? Arthritis Rheum 1995; 38: 161-163.

125. Hudson JI, Pope HG Jr. The relationship between fibromyalgia and major depressive disorder. Rheum Dis Clin N Am 1996; 22: 285-303.

126. Ickes W, Snyder M, Garcia S. Personality influences on the choice of situations. In: Hogan R, Johnson J, Briggs S eds. Handbook of Personality Psychology. San Diego: Academic Press; 1997.

127. Idler EL, Kasl SV. Religion, disability, depression, and the timing of death. AJS 1992; 97: 1052-1079.

128. Jackson T, Iezzi A, Lafreniere K. The impact of psychosocial features of employment status on emotional distress in chronic pain and healthy comparison samples. J Behav Med 1997; 20: 241-256.

129. Jacobs WJ, Nadel L. Stress-induced recovery of fears and phobias. Psychol Rev 1985; 92: 512-531.

130. Janis I. The patient as decision-maker. In: Gentry WD ed. Handbook of Behavioral Medicine. New York: Guilford Press; 1983: 326-368.

131. Jensen MP, Turner JA, Romano JM et al. Coping with chronic pain: a critical review of the literature. Pain 1991; 47: 249-283.

132. Jones M, Rivett D. Clinical reasoning for manual therapists. Oxford: Butterworth Heinemann; 2004.

133. Kabat-Zinn J, Lipworth L, Burney R. The clinical use of mindfulness meditation for the self-regulation of chronic pain. J Behav Med 1985; 8: 163-190.

134. Kabat-Zinn J, Massion AO, Kristeller J et al. Effectiveness of a meditation-based stress reduction program in the treatment of anxiety disorders. Am J Psychiatry 1992; 149: 936-943.

135. Kaplan KH, Goldenberg DL, Galvin-Nadeau M. The impact of a meditation-based stress reduction program on fibromyalgia. Gen Hosp Psychiatry 1993; 15: 284-289.

136. Katon W, Egan K, Millder D. Chronic pain: Lifetime psychiatric diagnoses and family history. Am J Psychiatry 1985; 142: 1156-1160.

137. Kazis LE, Meenan RF, Anderson JJ. Pain in the rheumatic diseases: investigations of a key health status component. Arthritis Rheum 1983; 26: 1017-1022.

138. Keefe F, Brown G, Wallston K et al. Coping with rheumatoid arthritis pain: catastrophizing as a maladaptive strategy. Pain 1989; 37: 51-56.

139. Keefe FJ, Block AR. Development of an observation method for assessing pain behavior in chronic low back pain patients. Behav Ther 1983; 13: 363-375.

140. Keefe FJ, Dolan E. Pain behavior and pain coping strategies in low back pain and myofascial pain dysfunction syndrome patients. Pain 1986; 24: 49-56.

141. Keefe FJ, Williams DA. Assessment of pain behaviors. In: Turk DC, Melzack R eds. Handbook of Pain Assessment. New York: Guilford Press; 1992; 277–292.

142. Keel PJ, Bodoky C, Gerhard U et al. Comparison of integrated group therapy and group relaxation training for fibromyalgia. Clin J Pain 1998; 14: 232-238.

143. Kennedy M, Felson DT. A prospective long-term study of fibromyalgia syndrome. Arthritis Rheum 1996; 39: 682-685.

144. Kerns RD, Haythornthwaite J, Southwick S et al. The role of marital interaction in chronic pain and depressive symptom severity. J Psychosom Res 1990; 34: 401–408.

145. Kerns RD, Turk DC. Depression and chronic pain: The mediating role of the spouse. J Marriage Fam 1984; 46: 845–852.

146. Kiecolt-Glaser JK, Newton TL. Marriage and health: his and hers. Psychol Bull 2001; 127: 472-503.

147. King SA. The clinical application of DSM-IV for patients with pain. International Association for the Study of Pain, 8th World Congress on Pain, Vancouver, Canada. 1996; 304: abstr 288.

148. King DE, Bushwick B. Beliefs and attitudes of hospital inpatients about faith healing and prayer. J Fam Pract 1994; 39: 349-352.

149. Klaber Moffett J. Pain: perception and attitudes. In: Gifford L (ed) Topical issues in pain 2. Biopsychosocial assessment and management. Relationships and pain. Falmouth: CNS Press; 2000: 141-151.

150. Klayman J, Ha YW. Confirmation, disconfirmation, and information in hypothesis testing. Psychol Rev 1987; 94: 211-228.

151. Koenig HG, Cohen HJ, Blazer DG et al. Religious coping and depression among elderly, hospitalized medically ill men. Am J Psychiatry 1992; 149: 1693-1700.

152. Kraaimaat FW, van Dam-Baggen RMJ, Bijlsma JWJ. Association of social support and the spouse's reaction with psychological distress in male and female patients with rheumatoid arthritis. J Rheumatol 1995; 22: 644–648.

153. Kraimaat FW, Bakker AH, Janssen E et al. Intrusiveness of rheumatoid arthritis on sexuality in male and female patients living with a spouse. Arthritis Care Res 1996; 9: 120-125.

154. Kurtz ME, Wyatt G, Kurtz JC. Psychological and sexual well-being, philosophical/spiritual views and health habits of long-term cancer survivors. Health Care for Women International 1995; 16: 253-262.

155. Kurtze N, Gundersen KT, Svebak S. Quality of life, functional disability and lifestyle among subgroups of fibromyalgia patients: the significance

of anxiety and depression. Br J Med Psychol 1999; 72: 471-484.

156. Large RG. DSM-III diagnoses in chronic pain: Confusion or clarity?. J Nerv Ment Dis 1986; 174: 295-302.

157. Larsen RJ, Diener E, Cropanzano RS. Cognitive operations associated with individual differences in affect intensity. J Pers Soc Psychol 1987; 53: 767-774.

158. Lautenbacher S, Rollman GB. Possible deficiencies of pain modulation in fibromyalgia. Clin J Pain 1997; 13: 189-196.

159. Lazarus RS. Progress on a cognitive-motivational-relational theory of emotion. Am Psychol 1991; 46: 819-834.

160. Leary MR, Haupt AL, Strausser KS et al. Calibrating the sociometer: the relationship between interpersonal appraisals and state self-esteem. J Pers Soc Psychol 1998; 74: 1290-1299.

161. Leary MR, Schreindorfer LS, Haupt AL. The role of low self-esteem in emotional and behavioral problems: Wy is low self-estem dysfunctional? J Soc Clin Psychol 1995; 14: 297-314.

162. Leary MR. The social and psychological importance of self-esteem. In: Kowalski RM, Leary MR eds. The Social Psychology of Emotional and Behavioral Problems. Washington, DC: American Psychological Association; 1999.

163. Leavitt F, Katz RS. Is the MMPI invalid for assessing psychological disturbance in pain related organic conditions? Journal of Rheumatology 1989; 16: 521-526.

164. Lee J, Giles K, Drummond PD. Psychological disturbances and an exaggerated response to pain in patients with whiplash injury. J Psychosom Res 1993; 37: 105-110.

165. Lepper MR, Anderson CA, Ross L. Perseverance of social theories: The role of explanation in the persistence of discredited information. J Pers Soc Psychol 1980; 39: 1037-1049.

166. LeResche L. Facial expression in pain: a study of candid photographs. J Nonverbal Behav 1982; 7: 56-76.

167. Lewinsohn PM. The behavioral study and treatment of depression. In: Hersen M, Eisler RM, Miller PM eds. Progress in Behavior Modification. New York: Academic Press; 1975.

168. Ley P. Psychological studies of doctor-patient communication. In: Rachman S ed. Contributions to Medical Psychology. Oxford: Pergamon Press; 1977: 9-42.

169. Lindstrom I, Ohlund C, Eek C et al. The effect of graded activity on patients with subacute low back pain: a randomized prospective clinical study with an operant-conditioning behavioral approach. Phys Ther 1992; 72: 279-290.

170. Lipchik GL, Milles K, Covington EC. The effects of multidisciplinary pain management treatment on locus of control and pain beliefs in chronic non-terminal pain. Clin J Pain 1993; 9: 49-57.

171. Longe SE, Wise R, Bantick S et al. Counter-stimulatory effects on pain perception and processing are significantly altered by attention: an fMRI study. Neuroreport 2001; 12: 2021-2025.

172. Lord CG, Ross L, Lepper M. Biased assimilation and attitude polarization: The effects of prior theories on subsequently considered eveidence. J Pers Soc Psychol 1979; 37: 2098-2109.

173. Lousberg R, Schmidt AJM, Groenmann NH. The relationship between spouse solicitousness and pain behavior: searching for more experimental evidence. Pain 1992; 51: 75-79.

174. Lykken DT, Tellegen A. Happiness is a stochastic phenomenon. Psychol Sci 1996; 7: 186-189.

175. Lyubomirsky S, King L, Diener E. The benefits of frequent positive affect: does happiness lead to success? Psychol Bull 2005; 131: 803-855.

176. MacFarlane GJ, Thomas E, Papageorgiou AC et al. The natural history of chronic pain in the community: a better prognosis than in the clinic? J Rheumatol 1996; 23: 1617-1620.

177. Magni G, Caldieron C, Regatti-Luchini S. Chronic musculoskeletal pain and depressive symptoms in the general population: An analysis of the First National Health and Nutrition Examination Survey data. Pain 1990; 43: 299-307.

178. Manne SL, Zautra AJ. Spouse criticism and support: Their association with coping and psychological adjustment among women with rheumatoid arthritis. J Pers Soc Psychol 1989;56:608-617.

179. Marshall M, Helmes E, Deathe AB. A comparison of psychosocial functioning and personality in amputee and chronic pain populations. Clin J Pain 1992; 8: 351-357.

180. Martin MY, Bradley LA, Alexander RW et al. Coping strategies predict disability in patients with primary fibromyalgia. Pain 1996; 68: 45-53.

181. Maslow AH. Motivation and Personality, Second Edition. New York: Harper & Row; 1970.

182. Matthews DA, Marlowe SM, MacNutt FS. Effects of intercessory prayer on patients with rheumatoid arthritis. South Med J 2000; 93: 1177-1186.

183. McBeth J, MacFarlane GJ, Benjamin J et al. The association between tender points, psychological distress, and adverse childhood experiences: a community-based study. Arthritis Rheum 1999; 42: 1397-1404.

184. McBeth J, Silman AJ. The role of psychiatric disorders in fibromyalgia. Curr Rheumatol Rep 2001; 3: 157-164.

185. McCarberg B, Wolf J, Oliver K et al. The rela-

tionship between health locus of control and well-being in fibromyalgia patients. J Pain 2002; 3: 14.

186. McDaniel LK, Anderson KO, Bradley LA et al. Development of an observation method for assessing pain behavior in rheumatoid arthritis patients. Pain 1986; 24: 165-184.

187. McDermid AJ, Rollman GB, McCain GA. Generalized hypervigilance in fibromyalgia: evidence of perceptual amplification. Pain 1996; 66: 133-144.

188. Medina JL, Diamond S. Drug dependency in patients with chronic headache. Headache 1997; 17: 12–14.

189. Melzack R. The McGill Pain Questionnaire: major properties and scoring methods. Pain 1975; 1: 277-299.

190. Merskey H. Pain and psychological medicine. In: Wall PD, Melzack R eds. Textbook of Pain. Fourth ed. Edinburgh: Churchill Livingston; 1999: 929-949.

191. Mineka S, Zinbarg R. A contemporary learning theory perspective on the etiology of anxiety disorders: it's not what you thought it was. Am Psychol 2006; 61: 10-26.

192. Mineka S, Zinbarg R. Conditioning and ethological models of anxiety disorders: stress-in-dynamic-context anxiety models. Nebr Symp Motiv 1996; 43 : 135-210.

193. Moore JE, McFall ME, Kivlahan DR et al. Risk of misinterpretation of MMPI Schizophrenia scale elevations in chronic pain patients. Pain 1986; 32: 207-213.

194. Morin CM, Culbert JP, Schwartz SM. Nonpharmacological interventions for insomnia: a meta-analysis of treatment efficacy. Am J Psychiatry 1994; 151: 1172-1180.

195. Murray JE. Marital protection and marital selection: evidence from a historical-prospective sample of American men. Demography 2000; 37: 511-521.

196. Murray SL, Rose P, Bellavia GM et al. When rejection stings: how self-esteem constrains relationship-enhancement processes. J Pers Soc Psychol 2002; 83:556-573.

197. Myers DG, Diener E. The pursuit of happiness. Sci Am 1996; 5: 54-56.

198. Myers DG, Diener E. Who is happy? Psychol Sci 1995; 6: 10-19.

199. Myers DG. Psychology, Seventh Edition. New York: Worth Publishers; 2004.

200. Myers DG. Social Psychology. New York; McGraw Hill: 2002.

201. Myers DG. The American Paradox: Spiritual Hunger in an Age of Plenty. New Haven: Yale University Press: 2000.

202. Myers DG. The Pursuit of Happiness. New York: Avon; 1993.

203. Nelson N. A meta-anlysis of the life-event/health paradigm: The influence of social support. Philadelphia: Temple University Ph.D. dissertation; 1988.

204. Nicassio PM, Radojevic V, Weisman MH et al. A comparison of behavioral and educational interventions for fibromyalgia. J Rheumatol 1997; 24: 2000-2007.

205. Nicassio PM, Radojevic V. Models of family functioning and their contribution to patient outcomes in chronic pain. Motiv Emot 1993; 17: 295-316.

206. Nielson WR, Merskey H. Psychosocial aspects of fibromyalgia. Curr Pain Headache Rep 2001; 5: 330-337.

207. Nielson WR, Walker C, McCain GA. Cognitive behavioral treatment of fibromyalgia syndrome: preliminary findings. J Rheumatol 1992; 19: 98-103.

208. NIH. Integration of behavioral and relaxation approaches into the treatment of chronic pain and insomnia. NIH Technology Assessment Panel on Integration of Behavioral and Relaxation Approaches into the Treatment of Chronic Pain and Insomnia. JAMA 1996; 276: 313-318.

209. Oakhill J, Garnham A. On theories of belief bias in syllogistic reasoning. Cognition 1993; 46: 87-92.

210. Ohman A. Face the beast and fear the face: animal and social fears as prototypes for evolutionary analyses of emotion. Psychophysiology 1986; 23: 123-145.

211. Okifuji A, Turk DC, Sherman JJ. Evaluation of the relationship between depression and fibromyalgia syndrome: why aren't all patients depressed? J Rheumatol 2000; 27: 212-219.

212. Parducci A. Happiness, Pleasure, and Judgment: The Contextual Theory and Its Applications. Hillsdale: Erlbaum; 1995.

213. Pargament KI, Olsen H, Reilly B et al. God help me (II): The relationship for religious orientations to religious coping with negative life events. J Sci Study Relig 1992; 31: 504-513.

214. Parker JC, Smarr KL, Buescher KL et al. Pain control and rational thinking: Implications for rheumatoid arthritis. Arthritis Rheum 1989; 32: 984–990.

215. Pastor MA, Salas E, Lopez S et al. Patients' beliefs about their lack of pain control in primary fibromyalgia syndrome. Br J Rheumatol 1993; 32: 484–489.

216. Patrick CJ, Craig KD, Prkachin KM. Observer judgments of acute pain: facial action determinants. J Pers Soc Psychol 1986; 50: 1291-1298.

217. Pattison EM, Lapins NA, Doerr HA. Faith healing: A study of personality and function. J Nerv Ment Dis 1973;157:397-409.

218.Payne TC, Leavitt F, Garron DC et al. Fibrositis and psychologic disturbance. Arthritis Rheum 1982 ; 25 : 213-217.

219.Pennebaker JW, Barger SD, Tiebout J. Disclosure of traumas and health among Holocaust survivors. Psychosom Med 1989; 51: 577-589.

220.Pennebaker JW, O'Heeron RC. Confiding in others and illness rate among spouses of suicide and accidental-death victims. J Abnorm Psychol 1984; 93: 473-476.

221.Penninx BWJH, van Tilburg T, Deeg DJH et al. Direct and buffer effects of social support and personal coping resources in individuals with arthritis. Soc Sci Med 1997; 44: 393–402.

222.Petrovic P, Kalso E, Petersson KM et al. Placebo and opioid analgesia - imaging a shared neuronal network. Science 2002; 295: 1737-1740.

223.Pincus T, Callahan LF, Bradley LA et al. Elevated MMPI scores for hypochondriasis, depression, and hysteria in patients with rheumatoid arthritis reflect disease rather than psychological status. Arthritis Rheum 1986; 29: 1456-1466.

224.Plaghki L, Delisle D, Godfraind JM. Heterotopic nociceptive conditioning stimuli and mental task modulate differently the perception and physiological correlates of short CO_2 laser stimuli. Pain 1994; 57:181-192.

225.Polatin PB, Kinney RK, Gatchel RJ et al. Psychiatric illness and chronic low-back pain. Spine 1993; 18: 66–71.

226.Poloma MM, Pendleton BF. The effects of prayer and prayer experiences on measures of general well-being. J Psychol Theol 1991; 19: 71-83.

227.Portenoy RK, Foley K. Chronic use of opioid analgesics in non-malignant pain: Report of 38 cases. Pain 1986; 25: 171–186.

228.Posner J, Russell JA, Peterson BS. The circumplex model of affect: an integrative approach to affective neuroscience, cognitive development, and psychopathology. Dev Psychopathol 2005; 17: 715-734.

229.Rafii A, Haller DL, Poklis A. Incidence of recreational drug use among chronic pain clinic patients. Presented at American Pain Society Ninth Annual Meeting, St. Louis, MO. 1990; A33: abstr.

230.Rainville P, Duncan GH, Price DD et al. Pain affect encoded in human anterior cingulate but not somatosensory cortex. Science 1997; 277: 968-971.

231.Regan CA, Lorig K, Thorensen CE. Arthritis appraisal and ways of coping: Scale development. Arthritis Care Res 1988; 1: 139–150.

232.Reich J, Rosenblatt RM, Tupen J. DSM-III: A new nomenclature for classifying patients with chronic pain. Pain 1983; 16: 201–206.

233.Reinert A, Treede R, Bromm B. The pain inhibiting pain effect: an electrophysiological study in humans. Brain Res 2000; 862: 103-110.

234.Remick RA, Blasberg B, Campos PE et al. Psychiatric disorder associated with atypical facial pain. Can J Psychiatry 1983; 28: 178–181.

235.Revenson TA, Schiaffino KM, Majerovitz SD et al. Social support as a double-edged sword: The relation of positive and problematic support to depression among rheumatoid arthritis patients. Soc Sci Med 1991; 33: 807–813.

236.Richards DG. The phenomenology and psychological correlates of verbal prayer. J Psychol Theol 1991; 19: 354-363.

237.Rickard K. The occurrence of maladaptive health-related behaviors and teacher-related conduct problems in children of chronic low back pain patients. J Behav Med 1988; 11: 107-116.

238.Risdon A, Eccleston C, Crombez G et al. How can we learn to live with pain? A Q-methodological analysis of the diverse understandings of acceptance of chronic pain. Soc Sci Med 2003; 56: 375-386.

239.Romano JM, Turner JA, Friedman LS et al. Sequential analysis of chronic pain behaviors and spouse responses. J Consult Clin Psychol 1992; 60: 777-782.

240.Romano JM, Turner JA. Chronic pain and depression: Does the evidence support a relationship. Psychol Bull 1985; 97: 18–34.

241.Rosenthal RN. Comorbidity of psychiatric and substance use disorders. Primary Psychiatry 1995; Jul/Aug: 42–45.

242.Russell JA, Lewicka M, Niit T. A cross-cultural study of a circumplex model of affect. J Pers Soc Psychol 1989; 57: 848-856.

243.Schachter S, Singer JE. Cognitive, social, and physiological determinants of emotional state. Psychol Rev 1962; 69: 379-399.

244.Schiaffino KM, Revenson TA, Gibofsky A. Assessing the impact of self-efficacy beliefs on adaptation to rheumatoid arthritis. Arthritis Care Res 1991; 4: 150-157.

245.Schkade DA, Kahneman D. Does living in California make people happy? A focusing illusion in judgments of life satisfaction. Psychol Sci 1998; 9: 340-346.

246.Schoeneman TJ. Individualism. In: Ramachandran VS ed. Encyclopedia of Human Behavior. San Diego: Academic Press; 1994.

247.Seligman MEP. Helplessness: On Depression, development and death. San Francisco: Freeman; 1975.

248.Seligman MEP. Learned Optimism. New York: Knopf; 1991.

249.Sewitch MJ, Dobkin PL, Bernatsky S et al. Medication non-adherence in women with fibromyalgia.

Rheumatology (Oxford) 2004; 43: 648-654.

250. Shaver PR, Morgan HJ, Wu S. Is love a basic emotion? Pers Relatsh 1996; 3: 81-96.

251. Simmonds MJ. The effect of pain and illness on movement: assessment methods and their meanings. In: Giamberardino MA ed. Pain 2002-an updated review: refresher course syllabus. Seattle: IASP Press; 2002: 179-187.

252. Singh BB, Berman BM, Hadhazy VA et al. A pilot study of cognitive behavioral therapy in fibromyalgia. Altern Ther Health Med 1998; 4: 67-70.

253. Skov RB, Sherman SJ. Information-gathering processes: Diagnosticity, hypothesis-confirmatory strategies, and perceived hypothesis confirmation. J Exp Soc Psychol 1986; 22: 93-121.

254. Smarr KL, Parker JC, Wright GE et al. The importance of enhancing self-efficacy in rheumatoid arthritis. Arthritis Care Res 1997; 10: 18–26.

255. Smith TW, Christensen AJ, Peck JR et al. Cognitive distortion, helplessness, and depressed mood in rheumatoid arthritis: A four-year longitudinal analysis. Health Psychol 1994; 13: 213–217.

256. Smith TW, Peck JR, Ward JR. Helplessness and depression in rheumatoid arthritis. Health Psychol 1990; 9: 377–389.

257. Smythe HA. Problems with the MMPI. Journal of Rheumatology 1984; 11: 417-418.

258. Stapel DA, Koomen W, Ruys KI. The effects of diffuse and distinct affect. J Pers Soc Psychol 2002; 83: 60-74.

259. Steele-Rosomoff R, Fishbain DA, Goldberg M et al. Chronic pain patients who lie in this psychiatric examination about current drug/alcohol use. Pain 1990; 5(suppl): S299.

260. Strupp HH. The outcome problem in psychotherapy: Contemporary perspectives. In: Harvey JH, Parks MM eds. The Master Lecture Series: Volume I. Psychotherapy Research and Behavior Change. Washington DC: American Psychological Association; 1982.

261. Suhr JA. Neuropsychological impairment in fibromyalgia: relation to depression, fatigue, and pain. J Psychosom Res 2003; 55: 321-329.

262. Sullivan MJ, Thorn B, Haythornthwaite JA et al. Theoretical perspectives on the relation between catastrophizing and pain. Clin J Pain 2001; 17: 52-64.

263. Suls JM, Tesch F. Students' preferences for information bout their test performance: A social comparison study. J Exp Soc Psychol 1978; 8: 189-197.

264. Taylor ML, Trotter DR, Csuka ME. The prevalence of sexual abuse in women with fibromyalgia. Arthritis Rheum 1995; 38: 229-234.

265. Thieme K, Turk DC, Flor H. Comorbid depression and anxiety in fibromyalgia syndrome: relationship to somatic and psychosocial variables. Psychosom Med 2004; 66: 837-844.

266. Toomey TC, Seville JL, Mann JD et al. Relationship of sexual and physical abuse to pain description, coping, psychological distress, and health-care utilization in a chronic pain sample. Clin J Pain 1995; 11: 307-315.

267. Tracey I, Ploghaus A, Gati JS et al. Imaging attentional modulation of pain in the periaqueductal gray in humans. J Neurosci 2002; 22: 2748-2752.

268. Triandis HC. Culture and Social Behavior. New York: McGraw-Hill; 1994.

269. Trier KK, Sufpe A. Prayer, religiosity, and healing in the heartland, USA: A research note. Rev Relig Res 1991; 32: 351-358.

270. Turk DC, Flor H. The cognitive-behavioural approach to pain management. In: McMahon SB, Koltzenburg M eds. Wall and Melzack's Textbook of Pain, Fifth Edition. Edinburgh: Elsevier Churchill Livingstone; 2006: 339-348.

271. Turk DC, Kerns RD, Rosenberg R. Effects of marital interaction on chronic pain and disability: examining the down side of social support. Rehabil Psychol 1992; 37: 259-274.

272. Turk DC, Okifuji A, Sherman JJ. Psychological factors in chronic pain: implications for physical therapists. In: Towney JW, Taylor JT eds. Low back pain, Third Edition. Baltimore: Williams and Wilkins; 2000.

273. Turk DC, Okifuji A, Sinclair JD et al. Differential responses by psychosocial subgroups of fibromyalgia syndrome patients to an interdisciplinary treatment. Arthritis Care Res 1998; 11: 397-404.

274. Turk DC, Okifuji A, Sinclair JD et al. Interdisciplinary treatment for fibromyalgia syndrome: clinical and statistical significance. Arthritis Care Res 1998; 11: 186-195.

275. Turk DC, Okifuji A, Starz TW et al. Effects of type of symptom onset on psychological distress and disability in fibromyalgia syndrome patients. Pain 1996; 68: 423-430.

276. Turnbull JM. Anxiety and physical illness in the elderly. J Clin Psychiatry 1989; 50(suppl): 40–45.

277. Vaillant GE. Aging Well: Surprising Guideposts to a Happier Life from the Landmark Harvard Study of Adult Development. Boston: Little, Brown; 2002.

278. Vaughan KB, Lanzetta JT. The effect of modification of expressive displays on vicarious emotional arousal. J Exp Soc Psychol 1981; 17: 16-30.

279. Vaughan KB, Lanzetta JT. Vicarious instigation and conditioning of facial expressive and autonomic responses to a model's expressive display

of pain. J Pers Soc Psychol 1980; 38: 909-923.

280. Villemure C, Bushnell MC. Cognitive modulation of pain: how do attention and emotion influence pain processing? Pain 2002; 95:195-199.

281. Vlaeyen JW, Teeken-Gruben NJ, Goossens ME et al. Cognitive-educational treatment of fibromyalgia: a randomized clinical trial. I. Clinical effects. J Rheumatol 1996; 23: 1237-1245.

282. Waddell G. The back pain revolution. Edinburgh: Churchill Livingstone; 1998.

283. Wade JB, Price DD, Hamer RM et al. An emotional component analysis of chronic pain. Pain 1990; 40: 303-310.

284. Walker EA, Keegan D, Gardner G et al. Psychosocial factors in fibromyalgia compared with rheumatoid arthritis: I. Psychiatric diagnoses and functional disability. Psychosom Med 1997; 59: 565-571.

285. Watson D, Suls J, Haig J. Global self-esteem in relation to structural models of personality and affectivity. J Pers Soc Psychol 2002; 83: 185-197.

286. Watson D, Wiese D, Vaidya J et al. The two general activation systems of affect: Structured findings, evolutionary considerations, and psychobiological evidence. J Pers Soc Psychol 1999; 76: 820-838.

287. Watson D. Mood and Temperament. New York: Guilford; 2000.

288. Watson PC. On the failure to eliminate hypotheses in a conceptual task. Q J Exp Psychol 1960; 12: 129-140.

289. Weinberger M, Tierney WM, Booher P et al. Social support, stress, and functional status in patients with osteoarthritis. Soc Sci Med 1990; 30: 503–508.

290. Weiner B. An attributional theory of achievement motivation and emotion. Psychol Rev 1985; 92: 548-573.

291. White KP, Nielson WR, Harth M et al. Chronic widespread musculoskeletal pain with or without fibromyalgia: psychological distress in a representative community adult sample. J Rheumatol 2002; 29: 588-594.

292. White KP, Nielson WR. Cognitive behavioral treatment of fibromyalgia syndrome: a followup assessment. J Rheumatol 1995; 22: 717-721.

293. Wigers SH. Fibromyalgia outcome: the predictive values of symptom duration, physical activity, disability pension, and critical life events – a 4.5 year prospective study. J Psychosom Res 1996; 41: 235-243.

294. Williams DA, Cary MA, Groner KH et al. Improving physical functional status in patients with fibromyalgia: a brief cognitive behavioral intervention. J Rheumatol 2002; 29: 1280-1286.

295. Williams DA. Psychological and behavioral therapies in fibromyalgia and related syndromes. Best Pract Res Clin Rheumatol 2003; 17: 649-665.

296. Williams RB, Barefoot JC, Califf RM et al. Prognostic importance of social and economic resources among medically treated patients with angiographically documented coronary artery disease. JAMA 1992; 267 :520-524. Erratum in: JAMA 1992; 268: 2652.

297. Wise MG, Taylor SE. Anxiety and mood disorders in medically ill patients. J Clin Psychiatry 1990; 51: 27–32.

298. Wolfe F, Anderson J, Harkness D et al. A prospective, longitudinal, multicenter study of service utilization and costs in fibromyalgia. Arthrtis Rheum 1997; 40: 1560-1570.

299. Wolfe F, Anderson J, Harkness D et al. Health status and disease severity in fibromyalgia: results of a six-center longitudinal study. Arthritis Rheum 1997; 40: 1571-1579.

300. Wolfe F, Cathey MA, Kleinheksel SM et al. Psychological status in primary fibrositis and fibrositis associated with rheumatoid arthritis. J Rheumatol 1984; 11: 500-506.

301. Worrel LM, Krahn LE, Sletten CD et al. Treating fibromyalgia with a brief interdisciplinary program: initial outcomes and predictors of response. Mayo Clin Proc 2001; 76: 384-390.

302. Yates JW, Chalmer BJ, St James P et al. Religion in persons with advanced cancer. Med Pediatr Oncol 1981; 9: 121-128.

303. Yoshino S, Uchida S. Sexual problems of women with rheumatoid arthritis. Arch Phys Med Rehabil 1981; 62: 122-123.

304. Zborowski M. People in pain. San Francisco: Jossey-Bass; 1969.

References Chapter 13

1. Andersen BL. Sexual functioning morbidity among cancer survivors. Current status and future research directions. Cancer 1985; 55: 1835-1842.

2. Andersen KV, Bovim G. Impotence and nerve entrapment in long distance amateur cyclists. Acta Neurol Scand 1997; 95: 233-240.

3. Araujo AB, Mohr BA, McKinlay JB. Changes in sexual function in middle-aged and older men: longitudinal data from the Massachusetts Male Aging Study. J Am Geriatr Soc 2004; 52: 1502-1509.

4. Avis NE, Zhao X, Johannes CB et al. Correlates of sexual function among multi-ethnic middle-aged women: results from the Study of Women's Health Across the Nation (SWAN). Menopause 2005; 12: 385-398.

5. Bancroft J, Loftus J, Long JS. Distress about sex: a national survey of women in heterosexual relationships. Arch Sex Behav 2003; 32: 193-211.

6. Basson R. Sexual Desire and Arousal Disorders in Women. N Engl J Med 2006; 354: 1497-1506.

7. Baumeister RF. Passion, intimacy, and time: passionate love as a function of change in intimacy. Pers Soc Psychol Rev 1999; 3: 49-67.

8. Baumhakel M, Bohm M. Erectile dysfunction correlates with left ventricular function and precedes cardiovascular events in cardiovascular high-risk patients. Int J Clin Pract 2007; 61: 361-366.

9. Berman JR, Berman LA, Werbin TJ et al. Clinical evaluation of female sexual function: effects of age and estrogen status on subjective and physiologic sexual responses. Int J Impot Res 1999; 11: S31-38.

10. Bhadauria S, Moser DK, Clements PJ et al. Genital tract abnormalities and female sexual function impairment in systemic sclerosis. Am J Obstet Gynecol 1995; 172(2 Pt 1): 580-587.

11. Blake DJ, Maisiak R, Graciela S et al. Sexual quality of life of patients with arthritis compared to arthritis free controls. J Rheumatol 1987; 14: 570–576.

12. Blumstein P, Schwartz P. American Couples. New York: William Morrow; 1983.

13. Bruce RA, Fisher LD, Cooper, MN et al. Separation of effects of cardiovascular disease and age on ventricular function with maximal exercise. Am J Cardiol 1974; 34: 757-763.

14. Carter JN, Tyson JE, Tolis G, et al. Prolactin-screening tumors and hypogonadism in 22 men. N Engl J Med 1978; 299: 847-852.

15. Chiurlia E, D'Amico R, Ratti C et al. Subclinical coronary artery atherosclerosis in patients with erectile dysfunction. J Am Coll Cardiol 2005; 46: 1503-1506.

16. Collins NL, Miller LC. Self-disclosure and liking: a meta-analytic review. Psychol Bull 1994; 116: 457-475.

17. Curry SL, Levine SB, Corty E et al. The impact of systemic lupus erythematosus on women's sexual functioning. J Rheumatol 1994; 21: 2254-2260.

18. Davis SR, Davison SL, Donath S et al. Circulating androgen levels in self-reported sexual function in women. JAMA 2005; 294: 91-96.

19. Dennerstein L, Lehert P. Modeling mid-aged women's sexual functioning: a prospective, population-based study. J Sex Marital Ther 2005; 30: 173-183.

20. Dennerstein L, Smith AM, Morse CA et al. Sexuality and the menopause. J Psychosom Obstet Gynaecol 1994; 15: 59-66.

21. Diamond M. and Karlen A. The sexual response cycle. In Lief H ed. Sexual Problems in Medical Practice. Chicago: American Medical Association Press; 1981: 37-51.

22. Ellenberg M. Impotence in diabetes: The neurologic factor. Ann Intern Med 1971; 75: 213-219.

23. Ende J, Rockwell S, Glasgow M. The sexual history in general medicine practice. Arch Intern Med 1984; 144: 558-561.

24. Feldman HA, Goldstein I, Hatzichristou DG et al. Impotence and its medical and psychosocial correlates: Results of the Massachusetts Male Aging Study. J Urol 1994; 151: 54-61.

25. Flor H, Turk DC, Scholz OB. Impact of chronic pain on the spouse: marital, emotional and physical consequences. J Psychosom Res 1987; 31: 63-71.

26. Folomeev M, Alekberova Z. Impotence in systemic lupus erythematosus. J Rheumatol 1990; 17: 117–118.

27. Frank E, Anderson C, Rubenstein D. Frequency of sexual dysfunction in "normal" couples. N Engl J Med 1978; 299: 111-115.

28. Fung MM, Bettencourt R, Barrett-Connor E. Heart disease risk factors predict erectile dysfunction 25 years later: the Rancho Bernardo Study. J Am Coll Cardiol 2004; 43: 1405-1411.

29. Ganz PA, Kwan L, Stanton AL et al. Quality of life at the end of primary treatment of breast cancer: first results from the moving beyond cancer randomized trial. J Natl Cancer Inst 2004; 96: 376-387.

30. George LK, Weiler SJ. Sexuality in middle and later life. Arch Gen Psychiatry 1981; 38; 919-923.

31. Godschalk MF, Sison A, Mulligan T. Management of erectile dysfunction by the geriatrician. J Am Geriatr Soc 1997; 45: 1240-1246.

32. Grover SA, Lowensteyn I, Kaouache M et al. The prevalence of erectile dysfunction in the primary care setting: importance of risk factors for diabetes and vascular disease. Arch Intern Med 2006; 166: 213-219.

33. Haboubi NH, Lincoln N. Views of health professionals on discussing sexual issues with patients. Disabil Rehabil 2003; 25: 291-296.

34. Harman SM, Tsitouras PD. Reproductive hormones in aging men. I. Measurement of sex steroids, basal luteinizing hormone, and Leydig cell response to chorionic gonadotropin. J Clin Endocrinol Metab 1980; 51: 35-40.

35. Hartmann U, Philippsohn S, Heiser K et al. Low sexual desire in midlife and older women: personality factors, psychosocial development, present sexuality. Menopause 2004; 11: 726-740.

36. Hellerstein HK, Friedman EH. Sexual activity and the postcoronary patient. Arch Intern Med 1970; 125: 987-999.

37. Hill J, Bird H, Thorpe R. Effects of rheumatoid arthritis on sexual activity and relationships. Rheumatology (Oxford) 2003; 42: 280-286.

38. Holmberg L, Anderson H. HABITS (hormonal

replacement therapy after breast cancer—is it safe?), a randomised comparison: trial stopped. Lancet 2004; 363: 453-455.

39. Howlett C, Swain M, Fitzmaurice N et al. Sexuality: The neglected component in palliative care. Int J Palliat Nurs 1997; 3: 218-221.

40. Kaplan HS. Psychiatric evaluation and therapy: What's new? In: World Book of Impotence. Lue TF Ed. London: Smith Gordon; 1992: 59.

41. Kaplan, HS. The New Sex Therapy. New York, NY: Brunner/Mazel; 1974.

42. Karacan I, Aslan C, Hirshkowitz M. Erectile mechanisms in man. Science 1983; 220: 1080-1082.

43. Karacan I, Goodenough DR, Shapiro A et al. Erection cycle during sleep in relation to dream anxiety. Arch Gen Psychiatry 1966; 15: 183-189.

44. Katz, A. The sounds of silence: Sexuality information for cancer patients. J Clin Oncol 2005; 23: 238-241.

45. Kedia KR. Vascular disorders and male erectile dysfunction. Current status in diagnosis and male erectile dysfunction. Current status in diagnosis and management by revascularization of the corpora cavernosa. Urol Clin North Am 1981; 8: 153-168.

46. Kolodny RC. Sexual dysfunction in diabetic females. Diabetes 1971; 20: 557-559.

47. Kool MB, Woertman L, Prins MA et al. Low relationship satisfaction and high partner involvement predict sexual problems of women with fibromyalgia. J Sex Marital Ther 2006; 32: 409-423.

48. Kraimaat FW, Bakker AH, Janssen E et al. Intrusiveness of rheumatoid arthritis on sexuality in male and female patients living with a spouse. Arthritis Care Res 1996; 9: 120–125.

49. Kwan M, Greenleaf WJ, Mann J et al. The nature of androgen action on male sexuality: A combined laboratory-self-report study on hypogonadal men. J Clin Endocrinol Metab 1983; 57: 557-562.

50. Laumann EO, Nicolosi A, Glasser DB et al. Sexual problems among women and men aged 40-80 y: prevalence and correlates identified in the Global Study of Sexual Attitudes and Behaviors. Int J Impot Res 2005; 17: 39-57.

51. Laumann EO, Paik A, Rosen RC. Sexual dysfunction in the United States: prevalence and predictors. JAMA 1999; 281: 537-544.

52. Levine SB, Rosenthal M. Marital sexual dysfunction: Female dysfunctions. Ann Intern Med 1977; 86: 588-597.

53. Levine SB. Marital sexual dysfunction: Erectile dysfunction. Ann Intern Med 1976; 85: 340-350.

54. Longcope C, Johnston CC Jr. Androgen and es-

trogen dynamics: stability over a two year interval in peri-menopausal women. J Steroid Biochem 1990; 35:91-95.

55. Mannino DM, Klevens RM, Flanders WD. Cigarette smoking: an independent risk factor for impotence? Am J Epidemiol 1994; 140: 1003-1008.

56. Maravilla KR, Heiman JR, Garland PA et al. Dynamic MR imaging of the sexual arousal response in women. J Sex Marital Ther 2003; 29(Suppl 1): 71-76.

57. Marceau L, Kleinman K, Goldstein I et al. Does bicycling contribute to the risk of erectile dysfunction? Results from the Massachusetts Male Aging Study (MMAS). Int J Impot Res 2001; 13: 298-302.

58. Maruta T, Osborne D, Swanson DW et al. Chronic pain patients and spouses: marital and sexual adjustment. Mayo Clin Proc 1981; 56: 307-310.

59. Marwick C. Survey says patients expect little physician help on sex. JAMA 1999; 281: 2173-2174.

60. Masters WH, Johnson VE, Kolodny RC. Human Sexuality. New York, NY: Longman; 1995.

61. Masters WH, Johnson VE, Kolodny RC. Sex and Human Loving. Boston: Little, Brown and Company; 1986.

62. Masters WH, Johnson VE. Human Sexual Response. Boston: Little, Brown and Company; 1966.

63. Mehta J, Krop HO. The effect of myocardial infarction on sexual functioning. Sex Disabil 1979; 2: 115-121.

64. Mills TM, Wiedmeier VT, Stopper VS. Androgen maintenance of erectile function in the rat penis. Biol Reprod 1992; 46: 342-348.

65. Min JK, Williams KA, Okwuosa TM et al. Prediction of coronary heart disease by erectile dysfunction in men referred for nuclear stress testing. Arch Intern Med 2006; 166: 201-206.

66. Morse WI, Morse JM. Erectile impotence precipitated by organic factors and perpetuated by performance anxiety. Can Med Assoc J 1982; 127: 599-601.

67. Mushayandebvu T, Castracane VD, Gimpel T et al. Evidence for diminished midcycle ovarian androgen production in older reproductive aged women. Fertil Steril 1996; 65: 721-723.

68. Myers LS, Dixen J, Morrissette D et al. Effects of estrogen, androgen, and progestin on sexual psychophysiology and behavior in postmenopausal women. J Clin Endocrinol Metab 1990; 70: 1124-1131.

69. NFO Research, Inc. AARP/Modern Maturity Sexuality Study. AARP 1999. 22 May 2008 <http://www.aarp.org/research/reference/publicopinions/Articles/aresearch-import-726.html>

70. Oliven J. Clinical Sexuality: A Manual for the Physician and the Professions. Philadelphia: JB Lippincott Company; 1974.

71. Osborne D. Psychosocial aspects of male sexual dysfunction: Diagnosis and management. Urol Clin North Am 1981; 8: 135-132.

72. Ostensen M, Almberg K, Koksvik HS. Sex, reproduction, and gynecological disease in young adults with a history of juvenile chronic arthritis. J Rheumatol. 2000; 27: 1783-1787.

73. Ostensen M. New insights into sexual functioning and fertility in rheumatic diseases. Best Pract Res Clin Rheumatol 2004; 18: 219-232.

74. Packham JC, Hall MA. Long-term follow-up of 246 adults with juvenile idiopathic arthritis: social function, relationships and sexual activity. Rheumatology (Oxford). 2002; 41: 1440-1443.

75. Palmer BF. Sexual dysfunction in men and women with chronic kidney disease and end-stage kidney disease. Adv Ren Replace Ther 2003; 10: 48-60.

76. Pauly I, Goldstein S. Prevalence of significant sexual problems in medical practice. Med Aspects Hum Sex 1979; 13; 48.

77. Pfeiffer E, Verwoerdt A, Wang HS. Sexual behavior in aged men and women. I. Observations on 254 community volunteers. Arch Gen Psychiatry 1968; 19: 753-758.

78. Pinderhughes CA, Grace ED, Reyna LJ et al. Interrelationships between sexual functioning and medical conditions. Med Aspects Hum Sex 1972; 6: 52.

79. Prins MA, Woertman L, Kool MB et al. Sexual functioning of women with fibromyalgia. Clin Exp Rheumatol 2006; 24: 555-561.

80. Purifoy FE, Koopmans LH, Mayes DM. Age differences in serum androgen levels in normal adult males. Hum Biol 1981; 53: 499-511.

81. Renshaw DC. Profile of 2376 patients treated at Loyola Sex Clinic between 1972 and 1987. Sex Marital Ther 1988; 3: 111-117.

82. Reynolds CF, Frank E III, Thase ME et al. Assessment of sexual function in depressed, impotent, and healthy men: Factor analysis of a Brief Sexual Function Questionnaire for men. Psychiatry Res 1988; 24: 231-250.

83. Rogers GS, Van de Castle RL, Evans WS et al. Vaginal pulse amplitude response patterns during erotic conditions and sleep. Arch Sex Behav 1985; 14: 327-342.

84. Sadoughi W, Leshner M, Fine HL. Sexual adjustment in a chronically ill and physically disabled population: a pilot study. Arch Phys Med Rehabil 1971; 52: 311-317.

85. Saigal CS, Wessells H, Pace J et al. Predictors and prevalence of erectile dysfunction in a racially diverse population. Arch Intern Med 2006; 166: 207-212.

86. Sant SM, O'Connell D. Cauda equina syndrome in ankylosing spondylitis: a case report and review of the literature. Clin Rheumatol 1995; 14: 224-226.

87. Schiavi RC, Schreiner-Engel P. Nocturnal penile tumescence in healthy aging men. J Gerontol 1988; 43: M146-M150.

88. Schover LR, Jensen SB. Sexuality and Chronic Illness. New York, NY: The Guilford Press; 1988.

89. Schover LR. Sexuality and fertility in urologic cancer patients. Cancer 1987; 60(3 Suppl): 553-558.

90. Schover LR. The impact of breast cancer on sexuality, body image, and intimate relationships. CA Cancer J Clin 1991; 41: 112-120.

91. Schwarzer U, Sommer F, Klotz T et al. Cycling and penile oxygen pressure: the type of saddle matters. Eur Urol 2002; 41: 139-143.

92. Seagraves RT, Balon R. Sexual Pharmacology Fast Facts. New York: W. W. Norton & Company; 2003.

93. Semmens JP, Wagner G. Estrogen deprivation and vaginal function in postmenopausal women. JAMA 1982; 248:445-448.

94. Skopouli FN, Papanikolaou S, Malamou-Mitsi Vet al. Obstetric and gynaecological profile in patients with primary Sjögren's syndrome. Ann Rheum Dis 1994; 53: 569-573.

95. Stenberg A, Heimer G, Ulmster U et al. Prevalence of genitourinary and other climacteric symptoms in 61-year-old women. Maturitas 1996; 24: 31-36.

96. Sullivan ME, Keoghane SR, Miller MA. Vascular risk factors and erectile dysfunction. BJU Int 2001; 87: 838-845.

97. Thompson IM, Tangen CM, Goodman PJ et al. Erectile dysfunction and subsequent cardiovascular disease. JAMA 2005; 294: 2996-3002.

98. Tikiz C, Muezzinoglu T, Pirildar T et al. Sexual dysfunction in female subjects with fibromyalgia. J Urol 2005; 174: 620-623.

99. Torrens MJ. Neurologic and neurosurgical disorders associated with impotence. In: Krane RJ, Siroky MB, Goldstein I Eds. Male Sexual Dysfunction. Boston: Little, Brown & Company; 1983: 55-62.

100. Unlu E, Ulas UH, Gurcay E et al. Genital sympathetic skin responses in fibromyalgia syndrome. Rheumatol Int 2006; 26: 1025-1030.

101. van Lunsen RHW, Laan E. Genital vascular responsiveness in sexual feelings in midlife women: psychophysiologic, brain, and genital imaging studies. Menopause 2004; 11: 741-748.

102. Verwoerdt A, Pfeiffer E, Wang HS. Sexual behavior in senescence. II. Patterns of sexual activity and interest. Geriatrics 1969; 24: 137-154.

103. Walsh PC, Mostwin JL. Radical prostatectomy and cystoprosatectomy with preservation of potency: Results using a nerve sparing technique.

Br J Urol 56: 1984; 694-697.

104. Winters SJ, Sherins RJ, Troen P. The gonadotropin-suppressive activity of androgen is increased in elderly men. Metabolism 1984; 33: 1052-1059.

105. Yoshino S, Uchida S. Sexual problems of women with rheumatoid arthritis. Arch Phys Med Rehabil 1981; 62: 122–123.

106. Zorzon M, Zivadinov R, Bosco A et al. Sexual dysfunction and multiple sclerosis: a case-control study. I. Frequency and comparison groups. Mult Scler 1999; 5: 418-427.

Glossary

Accommodation – a process by which the interventions allows the task to be carried out to completion in the face of intervention.

Acetylcholine – a neurotransmitter.

Actigraphy – recording limb movements while awake and asleep.

Agonist – a drug or molecule that stimulates a receptor to generate a response.

Allodynia – perception of a stimulus considered non-painful by normal individuals as being painful.

Alpha wave – predominant brain electrical activity while awake as measured by electroencephalogram (EEG).

Alpha-1 adrenergic – the effect of stimulating a specific adrenalin receptor.

Amino acids – a group of molecules that are the basic building blocks of proteins some of which can modulate nerve cell responses.

Amygdala – an area of the brain involved in the integration and processing of pain signals.

Analgesics – medications that modify pain message processing to increase pain thresholds and reduce the perceived severity of pain.

Androgens – a group of hormonal compounds responsible for the development and maintenance of male sexual characteristics and other metabolic effects such as maintenance of bone density.

Anemia – a reduction in the number of red blood cells below normal.

Anorexia – diminished appetite or aversion to food.

Antagonist – a drug or molecule that inhibits a receptor from generating a response.

Anticholinergic – inhibiting acetylcholine effects.

Antihistamine – inhibiting histamine effects.

Aplastic anemia – a severe reduction in the production of all blood cells.

Arrhythmia – abnormality of the rhythm of the heartbeat.

Aseptic meningitis – inflammation of the lining of the brain or spinal cord not due to an infection.

Asthenia – weakness or debility.

Benzodiazepine – a category of sedative and/or sleep inducing medication.

Bias – the tendency to interpret or analyze information beyond what the facts or logic would support.

Bradycardia – slow heart rate.

Bursa – a closed sac lined with the same tissue that lines a joint (synovium) containing a small amount of fluid found in areas to reduce friction and wear where tendons or ligaments pass adjacent to other ligaments, tendons, or bones.

Bursae – plural of bursa.

Bursitis – inflammation of a bursa.

Cardiac conduction block – interference of the normal conduction of electrical impulses in the heart.

Cardiac ischemia – reduction of the blood flow to the heart causing impairment in the function of the tissues of the heart and, if severe enough, causes tissue damage or death.

Cardiovascular – having to do with the heart and blood vessels.

Central nervous system sensitization – see central sensitization.

Central sensitization – spinal cord pain pathways and dorsal horn of the spinal cord develop increased sensitivity to pain with reduced pain thresholds, increased intensity, prolonged persistence after discontinuance, broader local distribution, and referred distribution of the pain stimulus.

Chemoreceptor trigger zone – an area in the brain through which chemicals can trigger nausea and vomiting.

Chronic – of long duration and slow progress.

Circadian – biological variations or rhythms following a 24 hour cycle comprising the body's internal clock.

Cognitive impairment – difficulty or inability to acquire, retain, or process information beyond what is normally expected for the given environment.

Congestive heart failure – the condition that develops when heart muscle is sufficiently damaged and weakened such that it cannot pump blood adequately.

Coronary thromboembolic disease – blood clots blocking blood flow to the arteries supplying the heart.

COX – cyclooxygenase.

COX-1 – a specific form of cyclooxygenase.

COX-2 – another specific form of cyclooxygenase.

Cyclooxygenase – an enzyme family controlling the production of prostaglandins.

Degenerative disc disease – disc, joint, and periarticular structure symptoms and signs related to related to the degeneration and breakdown of the of the discs in the spine.

Delta wave – brain electrical activity during deeper phases of sleep as measured by electroencephalogram (EEG) increasing in prevalence as the depth of Non-Rapid Eye Movement sleep increases.

Dermatomal nerve root – area of skin sensation served by the nerves of a specific spinal cord nerve root level.

Descending modulation – neurons that transmit signals from various areas of the brain to the dorsal horn to regulate and modify by inhibition or facilitation the incoming pain message before it is conducted upward to the brain.

Diabetes mellitus – diabetes.

Diarthroidial joint – the most common type of joint in humans in which two bones capped by hyaline cartilage meet and are nourished and lubricated by a tissue known as synovial tissue to provide for free joint motion.

Diffuse noxious inhibitory control – a central nervous system pathway originating in the brain that normally suppresses the severity of a painful stimulus through the application of a painful or non-painful stimulus locally or to another site.

Dorsal horn – a region of the spinal cord where incoming pain signals are processed and modulated before being conducted upward to the brain.

Dynorphins – endogenous internally produced neurotransmitters simulating the effect of opioids on the Delta opioid receptor.

Dyspepsia – indigestion or upset stomach.

Emotional lability – emotional instability.

Endorphins – endogenous internally produced neurotransmitters simulating the effect of opioids on the Mu opioid receptor.

Enkephalins – endogenous internally produced neurotransmitters simulating the effect of opioids on the Mu and Kappa opioid receptors.

Ergonomics – the physical interaction of individuals with their surrounding environment and the analysis of such.

Estrogen – a group of hormonal compounds responsible for the development and maintenance of female sexual characteristics, ovulation, and other metabolic effects such as maintenance of bone density.

Fascia – a sheet of fibrous tissue.

Fasciae – plural of fascia.

Fasciitis – inflammation in a fascia area.

Female urethral syndrome – see irritable bladder.

Fibromyalgia-like diseases – diseases that have features of fibromyalgia but are not diagnosed as fibromyalgia.

Gait disturbance – abnormality of walking.

Gamma-aminobutyric acid – a neurotransmitter involved in the integration and processing of pain signals, inducing sleep, and other brain and spinal cord functions.

Gastric erosion – a shallow breakdown of the stomach lining usually accompanied by inflammation.

Gastrointestinal – having to do with the stomach and intestine.

Genetic – biologically inherited characteristic from a parent.

Glucocorticoid – a steroid-like compound that exerts various metabolic effects and anti-inflammatory effects.

Hematological – having to do with blood and blood forming tissues.

Hepatic – having to do with the liver.

Hepatitis – inflammation of the liver.

Histamine – a chemical produced by various cells that among its effects promotes inflammation and pain.

HIV infection – infection with the human immunodeficiency virus.

Hyaline cartilage – the cartilage material contact surface in a freely moving diarthroidial joint.

Hyperalgesia – increased sensitivity to a painful stimulus compared to normal individuals.

Hypermobility – loose or double-jointedness with joints moving beyond normal, expected ranges.

Hypermobility syndromes – syndromes characterized by joint laxity.

Hypertension – high blood pressure.

Hypochondriasis – the fear of having or the belief that one has a serious disease based on the exaggeration or misinterpretation of physical or mental sensations.

Hypotension – low blood pressure.

Hypothalamus – an area of the brain involved in the integration and processing of pain signals.

Inflammation – the cellular and tissue changes that occur in response to an injury or tissue stimulation caused by a mechanical-physical, chemical, thermal, or biological source.

Interconnecting neurons – neurons within the dorsal horn that interconnect and modulate various incoming and outgoing pain signals in the dorsal horn.

Ion channel – a cell membrane pore or opening that allows the flow of electrically charged atoms in and out of the cell.

Irritable bladder – a disorder characterized by bladder pain of variable severity with symptoms of urinary urgency and frequency, lasting over a protracted period of time. Also known as painful bladder syndrome or interstitial cystitis.

Irritable bowel syndrome – a gastrointestinal syndrome characterized by chronic abdominal pain and altered bowel habits absent any organic cause.

Leukotrienes – are products of a metabolic pathway that comprise a group of molecules that mediate inflammation as well as having effects on the function of other tissues.

Libido – sexual desire.

Lyme disease – a tick-borne illness caused by the one of several spirochetes of the Borrelia family which can affect the skin, nervous system, joints, or heart and/or other organs of the body.

Melatonin – a sleep promoting hormone.

Modification – a process by which the elements of a task are reduced such that the task cannot be fully carried out despite ideal accommodation.

Morbidity – disease states related to a given condition or the ratio of the presence of disease states related to a condition for a given population.

Mortality – the death rate as defined by the ratio of the number of deaths for a given population.

Multiple sleep latency test – a test that repeatedly measures the time it takes to fall asleep during the day given the opportunity to do so.

Myocardial infarction – the death of heart tissue due to obstructed blood flow in the arteries to the heart commonly referred to as a heart attack.

Myofascial trigger points – tender nodules in muscle. These are not the same as fibromyalgia tender points.

Negative predictive value – see text.

Nerve root – the nerves of a specific spinal cord nerve root level.

Neuroendocrine – relating to hormones and their interactions.

Neurological – having to do with the nerves, spinal cord, brain, and nervous system.

Neuromuscular re-education – the retraining of the brain and nerve pathways involved in muscle function and the muscles themselves to alter muscular tone and the balance of muscular pull and relaxation to improve joint posture, alignment, loading, and ergonomics.

Neuron – nerve cell.

Neuropathy – disease of nerves impairing nerve function.

Neurotransmitter – molecule that stimulates a nerve cell.

Neurotransmitters – molecules stimulating nerve cell responses.

Neutral position – the position of a joint or group of joints and joint related structures that optimizes the posture, alignment and biomechanics to minimize joint and joint structure loading and other forces.

Neutropenia – a reduction in the number a certain type of white blood cells, called neutrophils, below normal.

N-methyl-D-aspartate – a neurotransmitter involved in the integration and processing of pain signals and other brain and spinal cord functions.

Nociception – the sensing of painful sensation.

Norepinephrine – a neurotransmitter involved in the integration and processing of pain signals, modulating mood, and other brain and spinal cord functions.

Noxious – injurious.

NREM – non-rapid eye movement sleep.

Opioids – opium-like compounds that produce effects on the body similar to morphine.

Orthostatic hypotension – low blood pressure when standing upright.

Orthotics – specially designed physical devices used to align and/or support joints and joint related structures.

Osteoarthritis – joint and periarticular structure symptoms and signs related to the degeneration and breakdown of the cartilage in the joint.

Pain amplification – increased intensity, prolonged persistence after discontinuance, and broader distribution of a painful stimulus compared to normal individuals.

Pain magnification – see pain amplification.

Pain processing – the process by which the severity and quality of pain is modified by the nervous system.

Paralytic ileus – paralysis of the contractions of the gastrointestinal tract.

Parenteral – introduction of treatment by means other than the intestinal canal usually meaning intravenously (through the veins) or into vascular tissues such subcutaneously (through the tissues under the skin) or intramuscularly (into the muscle).

Patellofemoral – the portion of the knee joint involving the kneecap.

Pathogenesis – the mechanism by which a disease develops.

Pathologic – structural and functional tissue changes that arise from a disease.

Peptic ulcer – breakdown of the lining of the stomach or duodenum usually accompanied by inflammation.

Performance characteristics – when applied to classification criteria, the conditions and populations to which they are applicable.

Periaqueductal grey matter – an area of the brain involved in the integration and processing of pain signals.

Periarticular structures – structures related to the joint and joint function including bursae, tendon insertions, tendon sheaths, and fasciae.

Peripheral sensitization – sensitization directly at the pain site from the pain stimulus.

Placebo – an intervention or treatment with no known effect on the condition being treated.

Placebo effect – an outcome that occurs as a result of an intervention or treatment that has no known effect on the condition being treated.

Platelet – blood cell involved with clotting.

Polypain – acronym for polyregional pain and increased nociception.

Polysomnography – study of electrical brain wave activity and eye movements during sleep and possibly other physiologic variables.

Positive predictive value – see text.

Posttraumatic stress disorder – see text.

Primary afferent neurons (sensory) – nerve cells that convert thermal, chemical, or mechanical pain stimuli into electrical signals that are conducted to the dorsal horn of the spinal cord.

Primary generalized osteoarthritis – widespread generalized osteoarthritis at multiple sites unrelated to another primary cause.

Probability – the use of data and statistics to predict what has not yet occurred or is not yet factually known.

Projecting neurons – neurons in the dorsal horn of the spinal cord that directly conduct pain message through the spinal cord via the spinothalamic tract to the brain.

Prostaglandins – are products of a metabolic pathway that comprise a group of molecules that mediate inflammation as well as having effects on the function of other tissues.

Quadriceps muscle – the large muscle at the front of the thigh that straightens the knee joint.

Reactive hyperemia – excess and persistent redness from pressure on the skin.

Receptor – a structure on the surface of a cell that specifically recognizes a particular molecule.

Recidivism – the tendency to relapse into a former, undesirable condition.

Referred pain – pain felt away from the site of the original pain stimulus.

REM sleep – rapid eye movement sleep.

Renal – having to do with the kidney.

Renin-angiotensin-aldosterone system – a chemical system involved in the maintenance of blood pressure.

Respiratory – having to do with the breathing system and lungs.

Restless legs syndrome – a syndrome characterized by spontaneous, continuous leg movements associated with uncomfortable or painful sensations at rest and relieved by movement.

Reuptake – the uptake of a neurotransmitter by a nerve cell following its initial release by the nerve cell.

Rheumatoid arthritis – a symmetrical arthritis involving multiple joints of the extremities of unknown cause that may lead to joint deformity and destruction.

Rostroventral medulla – an area of the brain involved in the integration and processing of pain signals.

Rotoscoliosis – a curve in the spine with twist or rotational component.

Scoliosis – a curve in the spine.

Sensitivity (statistical) – see text.

Serotonin – a neurotransmitter involved in the integration and processing of pain

signals, modulating mood, and other brain and spinal cord functions.

Sjogren's syndrome – a chronic inflammatory disorder characterized by impaired tear and saliva production.

Somnambulism – sleep walking.

Specificity (statistical) – see text.

Spinothalamic tract – spinal cord pain pathway conducting pain message from the dorsal horn of the spinal cord to the brain.

Statistics – the collection, organizing, summarizing, and analysis of factual data to explain existing patterns and relationships.

Sublingual – under the tongue.

Substance P – a neurotransmitter involved in the integration and processing of pain signals.

SWS – slow wave sleep.

Synovial fluid – fluid found within structures lined by synovial tissue.

Synovial lining – lining of synovial tissue.

Synovial tissue – also known as synovium; tissue found in freely moving diarthroidial joints that nourish and lubricate the hyaline cartilage and joint and also found in other structures lined with synovium such as bursae and tendon sheaths.

Systemic lupus erythematosus – a chronic inflammatory disease of unknown cause which can affect the skin, joints, kidneys, lungs, nervous system, lining membranes of the lungs, heart, and gut, and/or other organs of the body accompanied by immune system abnormalities.

Tachycardia – rapid heart rate.

Temporal summation – in response to a repeated painful stimulus, the pain intensity to any one stimulation is greater than the response to the preceding stimulus.

Tendinitis – inflammation of a tendon.

Tendon – a fibrous tissue or band connecting a muscle to bone or other tissue.

Tendon sheath – an enveloping covering of a tendon lined with the same tissue that lines a joint (synovium).

Tenosynovitis – inflammation of a tendon sheath.

Testosterone – the hormone responsible for male characteristics, other metabolic effects in men, and libido (sex drive) in men and women.

Thalamus – an area of the brain involved in the integration and processing of pain signals.

Thrombocytopenia – a reduction in the number of platelets, the cells involved in making blood clots, below normal.

Thromboembolic – having to do with the development of blood clots in blood vessels and the dislodgement of blood clots in blood vessels to form blockages in blood flow.

Thromboxanes – products of the prostaglandin metabolic pathway.

Tinnitus – noises or sounds in the ear arising from the hearing system itself.

Transdermal – through the skin.

Ulcer – a breakdown of tissue usually accompanied by inflammation.

Valium – brand name for diazepam, a benzodiazepine sedative/hypnotic.

Wind-up – see temporal summation.

Index

Other Resources

Information

American College of Rheumatology (www.rheumatology.org)
National Library of Medicine
(www.nlm.nih.gov/medlineplus/healthtopics.html)
National Institute of Arthritis, Musculoskeletal, and Skin Diseases
(www.niams.nih.gov/, search for "fibromyalgia")
National Fibromyalgia Research Association (www.nfra.net)
National Fibromyalgia Association (www.fmaware.org)
The Arthritis Foundation (www.arthritis.org)

Fibromyalgia Polypain Arthritis Center

www.fmpolypain.com

Products to Manage Fibromyalgia and Chronic Musculoskeletal Pain

www.fibromyalgiapainstore.com

Book

The Missing Pieces of the Fibromyalgia Puzzle
(www.missingpiecesfibromyalgia.com)

About the Author

Jeff Sarkozi, M.D., F.R.C.P.C., F.A.C.R. is an internationally trained and board certified rheumatologist and internal medicine specialist with more than 25 years of experience in clinical practice and research. Dr. Sarkozi has specialized in the diagnosis and management of patients with unexplained chronic widespread musculoskeletal pain and fibromyalgia for over two decades and has seen thousands of patients with chronic widespread musculoskeletal pain and fibromyalgia. Dr. Sarkozi has researched, developed, and patented numerous unique orthotic devices and created original, innovative treatment programs to relieve symptoms and improve function in patients with fibromyalgia, chronic widespread musculoskeletal pain, and other arthritic conditions. He currently directs the Fibromyalgia Polypain Arthritis Center in Orange County, California.

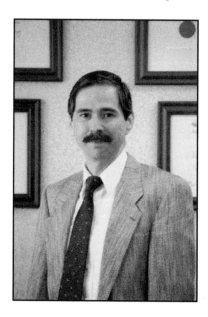